Lecture Notes in Computer Science   8090

Commenced Publication in 1973
Founding and Former Series Editors:
Gerhard Goos, Juris Hartmanis, and Jan van Leeuwen

Hongen Liao   Cristian A. Linte
Ken Masamune   Terry M. Peters
Guoyan Zheng (Eds.)

Augmented Reality Environments for Medical Imaging and Computer-Assisted Interventions

6th International Workshop, MIAR 2013 and
8th International Workshop, AE-CAI 2013
Held in Conjunction with MICCAI 2013
Nagoya, Japan, September 22, 2013
Proceedings

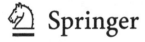 Springer

Volume Editors

Hongen Liao
Tsinghua University, Department of Biomedical Engineering, Beijing, China
E-mail: liao@tsinghua.edu.cn

Cristian A. Linte
Mayo Clinic, Biomedical Imaging Resource, Rochester, MN, USA
E-mail: linte.cristian@mayo.edu

Ken Masamune
The University of Tokyo, Department of Mechano-Informatics, Tokyo, Japan
E-mail: masa@i.u-tokyo.ac.jp

Terry M. Peters
Robarts Research Institute, Imaging Research Laboratories, London, ON, Canada
E-mail: tpeters@robarts.ca

Guoyan Zheng
University of Bern, Institute for Surgical Technology and Bioinformatics
Bern, Switzerland
Email: guoyan.zheng@istb.iunibe.ch

ISSN 0302-9743   e-ISSN 1611-3349
ISBN 978-3-642-40842-7   e-ISBN 978-3-642-40843-4
DOI 10.1007/978-3-642-40843-4
Springer Heidelberg New York Dordrecht London

Library of Congress Control Number: 2013947172

CR Subject Classification (1998): J.3, I.4, I.6, I.5, I.2.10, I.3.5, F.1

LNCS Sublibrary: SL 6 – Image Processing, Computer Vision, Pattern Recognition, and Graphics

Typesetting: Camera-ready by author, data conversion by Scientific Publishing Services, Chennai, India

Printed on acid-free paper

Springer is part of Springer Science+Business Media (www.springer.com)

Preface

This year, the 6th edition of the *Medical Imaging and Augmented Reality (MIAR)* meeting joined forces with the 8th edition of the *Augmented Reality for Computer-Assisted Interventions (AE-CAI)* workshop. As organizers of this joint meeting, we are pleased to present the proceedings of this exciting workshop held in conjunction with MICCAI 2013 on September 22nd, 2013 in Nagoya, Japan.

Over the past several years, the satellite workshops and tutorials at MICCAI have experienced increased popularity. MIAR/AE-CAI 2013 is a joint venture between the prestigious *MIAR* workshop series held bi-annually since 2002, and the *AE-CAI* workshop series affiliated with MICCAI and featured on an almost annual basis since 2003. This year's joint workshop received over 40 submissions and reached over 50 registrants, not including the members of the organizing and program committees, making MIAR/AE-CAI one of the best received and best attended workshops at MICCAI 2013.

The event was jointly organized by scientists from The University of Tokyo (Tokyo, Japan), Mayo Clinic (Rochester, MN, USA), and Robarts Research Institute (London, ON, Canada), who have had a long standing tradition in the development and application of augmented & virtual environments for medical imaging and image-guided interventions. In addition, a Program Committee (PC) consisting of more than 70 international experts served as reviewers for the submitted papers.

Rapid technical advances in medical imaging, including its growing applications to drug delivery, gene therapy, and invasive/interventional procedures, as well as a symbiotic development of protein science, imaging modalities, and nano-technological devices, have attracted significant interests in recent years. This has been fueled by the clinical and basic science research endeavors to obtain more detailed physiological and pathological information about the human body, to facilitate the study of localized genesis and progression of diseases. Current research has also been motivated by the increased movement of medical imaging from being a primarily diagnostic modality toward its role as a therapeutic and interventional aid, driven by the need to streamline the diagnostic and therapeutic processes via minimally invasive visualization and therapy.

The objective of the MIAR/AE-CAI workshop was to attract scientific contributions that offer solutions to the technical problems in the area of augmented and virtual environments for computer-assisted interventions, and to provide a venue for dissemination of papers describing both complete systems and clinical applications. The community also encourages a broad interpretation of the field – from macroscopic to molecular imaging, passing the information on to scientists and engineers to develop breakthrough therapeutics, diagnostics, and medical devices, which can then be seamlessly delivered back to patients. The workshop attracted researchers in computer science, biomedical engineering, computer vision, robotics, and medical imaging. This meeting featured a single track of oral and poster presentations showcasing original research engaged in the development of virtual and augmented environments for medical image visualization and image-guided interventions.

In addition to the proffered papers and posters, we were pleased to welcome as keynote speakers Dr. Pierre Jannin (Université de Rennes I, France), speaking on the modeling of surgical processes for intelligent computer-assisted interventions, and Dr. Maki Sugimoto (Kobe University, Japan), describing state-of-the-art developments in patient-based augmented reality and bio-texture manufacturing for minimally invasive and robotic surgery.

MIAR/AE-CAI 2013 attracted 44 paper submissions from 10 countries. The submissions were distributed for review to the PC and each paper was evaluated by at least three experts, who provided detailed critiques and constructive comments to the authors and workshop editorial board. Based on the reviews, 29 papers were selected for oral & poster presentation and publication in these proceedings. The authors revised their submissions according to the reviewers' suggestions, and resubmitted their manuscripts, along with their response to reviewers, for a final review by the volume editors (to ensure that all reviewers' comments were properly addressed) prior to publication in this collection.

On behalf of the MIAR/AE-CAI 2013 Organizing Committee, we would like to extend our sincere thanks to all PC members for providing detailed and timely reviews of the submitted manuscripts. We also thank all authors, presenters and attendees at MIAR/AE-CAI 2013 for their scientific contribution, enthusiasm and support. We hope that you will all enjoy reading this volume and we look forward to your continuing support and participation in future MIAR meetings, as well as our next AE-CAI event to be hosted at MICCAI 2014 in Boston, USA.

July 2013

Hongen Liao
Cristian A. Linte
Ken Masamune
Terry M. Peters
GuoyanZheng

Organization

Proceedings of the MICCAI 2013 Joint Workshop on Medical Imaging and Augmented Reality & Augmented Environments for Computer-Assisted Interventions: MIAR/AE-CAI 2013

MIAR/AE-CAI 2013 Workshop Committees

Organizing Committee

Hongen Liao, PhD	Tsinghua University, Beijing, China & The University of Tokyo, Tokyo, Japan
Cristian A. Linte, PhD	Mayo Clinic, Rochester, MN, USA
Ken Masamune, PhD	The University of Tokyo, Tokyo, Japan
Terry M. Peters, PhD	Robarts Research Institute, London, ON, Canada
Guoyan Zheng, PhD	University of Bern, Switzerland

Program Committee

Purang Abolmaesumi	University of British Columbia, Canada
Leon Axel	NYU Medical Center, USA
Marie-Odile Berger	IRISA, Rennes, France
Wolfgang Birkfellner	Medical University of Vienna, Austria
Adrien Bartoli	ISIT, Université d'Auvergne, France
Eddie Edwards	Imperial College London, UK
Gary Egan	University of Melbourne, Australia
Gabor Fichtinger	Queen's University, Canada
James Gee	University of Pennsylvania, USA
Lixu Gu	Shanghai Jiaotong University, China
Makoto Hashizume	Kyushu University, Japan
David Hawkes	University College London, UK
Pierre Jannin	Inserm, Université de Rennes, France
Tianzi Jiang	NLPR, Institute of Automation, CAS, China
Leo Joskowicz	The Hebrew University of Jerusalem, Israel
Ron Kikinis	Harvard Medical School, USA
Tianming Liu	University of Georgia, USA
Anthony Maeder	CSIRO, Australia
Nassir Navab	Technische Universität, Munich, Germany
Stephen J. Riederer	Mayo Clinic, USA
Dinggang Shen	UNC at Chapel Hill, USA
Pengcheng Shi	Rochester Institute of Technology, USA
Theo Van Walsum	Erasmus MC, The Netherlands

Guangzhi Wang   Tsinghua University, China
Jaw-Lin Wang   National Taiwan University, Taiwan
Stephen T.C. Wong   The Methodist Hospital - Weill Cornell Medical
                         College, USA
Yasushi Yamauchi   Toyo University, Japan
Guang-Zhong Yang   Imperial College London, UK

Review Committee

Takehiro Ando   The University of Tokyo, Japan
Christos Bergeles   Imperial College London, UK
Tobias Blum   Technical University Munich, Germany
Yiyu Cai   Nanyang Technological University, Singapore
Chung-Ming Chen   National Taiwan University, Taiwan
Cheng Chen   University of Bern, Switzerland
Elvis Chen   Robarts Research Institute, Canada
Xinjian Chen   Soochow University, China
Simon Drouin   Laval University in Quebec City, Canada
Yong Fan   Institute of Automation,
                         Chinese Academy of Sciences, China
Kenko Fujii   Imperial College London, UK
Stamatia Giannarou   Imperial College London, UK
Ali Gooya   University of Pennsylvania, USA
David Holmes III   Mayo Clinic, USA
Jaesung Hong   Daegu Gyeongbuk Institute of Science and
                         Technology, Korea
Bernhard Kainz   Graz University of Technology, Austria
Ali Khamene   Siemens Corp. Research, USA
Jan Klein   Fraunhofer MEVIS, Germany
Rudy Lapeer   University of East Anglia, UK
Su-Lin Lee   Imperial College London, UK
Ming Li   National Institutes of Health, USA
Jimmy Liu   Agency for Science, Technology and Research,
                         Singapore
Benny Lo   Imperial College London, UK
Xiongbiao Luo   Nagoya University, Japan
Gian-Luca Mariottini   University Texas at Arlington, USA
Robert Merrifield   Imperial College London, UK
Coert Metz   Erasmus MC, Netherlands
John Moore   Roberts Research Institute, Canada
Ryoichi Nakamura   Chiba University, Japan
Kilian Pohl   IBM Research, USA
Philip Pratt   Imperial College London, UK
Maryam Rettmann   Mayo Clinic, USA
Jannick Rolland   University of Rochester, USA
Steffen Schumann   University of Bern, Switzerland

Amber Simpson	Vanderbilt University, USA
Danail Stoyanov	University College London, UK
Tamas Ungi	Queen's University, Canada
Kirby Vosburgh	BWH/Harvard, USA
Junchen Wang	The University of Tokyo, Japan
Kelvin K. Wong	Methodist Hospital - Weill Cornell Medical College, USA
Stefan Wesarg	Fraunhofer IGD, Germany
Jue Wu	Upenn, USA
Zhong Xue	Weill Cornell Medical College, USA
Pew-Thian Yap	UNC-Chapel Hill, USA
Jong Chul Ye	Korea Advanced Institute of Science & Technology, Korea
Daoqiang Zhang	Nanjing University of Aeronautics and Astronautics, China
Bo Zheng	The University of Tokyo, Japan

Hosting Institutions

The University of Tokyo, Tokyo, Japan
Mayo Clinic, Rochester, MN, USA
Robarts Research Institute, London, ON, Canada
University of Bern, Bern, Switzerland

Sponsors

NDI - Northern Digital Inc.

Table of Contents

Simultaneous Tensor and Fiber Registration (STFR) for Diffusion Tensor Images of the Brain

Zhong Xue[*] and Stephen T.C. Wong

The Methodist Hospital Research Institute, Weill Cornell Medical College, Cornell University, Houston, Texas, United States
zxue@tmhs.org

Abstract. Accurate registration of diffusion tensor imaging (DTI) data of the brain among different subjects facilitates automatic normalization of structural and neural connectivity information and helps quantify white matter fiber tract differences between normal and disease. Traditional DTI registration methods use either tensor information or orientation invariant features extracted from the tensors. Because tensors need to be re-oriented after warping, fibers extracted from the deformed DTI often suffer from discontinuity, indicating lack of fiber information preservation after registration. To remedy this problem and to improve the accuracy of DTI registration, in this paper, we introduce a simultaneous tensor and fiber registration (STFR) algorithm by matching both tensor and fiber tracts at each voxel and considering re-orientation with deformation simultaneously. Because there are multiple fiber tracts passing through each voxel, which may have different orientations such as fiber crossing, incorporating fiber information can preserve fiber information better than only using the tensor information. Additionally, fiber tracts also reflect the spatial neighborhood of each voxel. After implementing STFR, we compared the registration performance with the current state-of-the art tensor-based registration algorithm (called DTITK) using both simulated images and real images. The results showed that the proposed STFR algorithm evidently outperforms DTITK in terms of registration accuracy. Finally, using statistical parametric mapping (SPM) package, we illustrate that after normalizing the fractional anisotropy (FA) maps of both traditional developing (TD) and Autism spectrum disorder (ASD) subjects to a randomly selected template space, regions with significantly different FA highlighted by STFR are with less noise or false positive regions as compared with DTITK. STFR methodology can also be extended to high-angular-resolution diffusion imaging and Q-ball vector analysis.

1 Introduction

Diffusion tensor imaging (DTI) has been widely and effectively used to study the neural connectivity in the brain [1, 2]. Deformable registration and automatic labeling of DTI images of different subject act as important roles in such applications. It is also a fundamental step in other DTI image analysis such as generating the group averaged atlas of the brain or in comparing different groups after normalization.

---

[*] Corresponding author.

C.A. Linte et al. (Eds.): MIAR/AE-CAI 2013, LNCS 8090, pp. 1–8, 2013.

In DTI, a trivariate Gaussian distribution is used to model the anisotropic water diffusion at each voxel and is characterized by a diffusion tensor. Tractography can be performed to the tensor field to extract fiber tracts that reflect white matter or axon orientations. Thus, how to align the tensor field of one subject onto another globally and locally while preserving the fiber tracts information after warping is the major goal for DTI registration. In the literature, orientation invariant features were extracted to drive such a deformation. For example, Yang *et al.* combined geometrical and fiber orientation features to define the image similarity [3]. However, the extracted scalar features from tensors and fibers only represent partial information of the tensor, and the orientation information is neglected. To fully take the advantage of the tensor information algorithms directly rely on the tensor were proposed [4-6]. Typical similarity measures include mutual information, multichannel DTI feature similarity or tensor similarity, and different transformation mechanisms were introduced in DTI registration studies, including elastic deformation, diffeomorphism, B-Spline, and piece-wise affine transformations. Comparative studies suggested that high dimensional approaches utilizing full tensor features instead of tensor-derived indices can further improve the alignment of white matter (WM) tracts.

One important factor needed to be considered is tensor re-orientation. Different from scalar image registration, the tensor at each voxel needs to be re-oriented to match the two images [7]. In [8], a finite strain algorithm and a preservation of principal direction algorithm were proposed to determine the tensor re-orientation, and re-orientation can be performed in each iteration. Recent advances such as the piece-wise affine transformation and the diffeomorphic non-linear registration algorithms adopted and integrated analytical gradients of the registration objective functions by considering the re-orientation of tensor during the registration. However, as mention above, only tensor information was utilized in these methods. Because tractography on newly warped images does not generate fiber bundles as accurate as those from the original DTI due to the registration errors, it is highly desirable that both tensor and fiber information need to be incorporated in the registration process. Although recent works showed that combining the tensor and fiber information is promising [9], they extracted the orientation-invariant features and did not consider the orientation of tensors and fibers during the procedure of the registration.

In this paper, we propose a new DTI registration method that combines the tensor and fiber information simultaneously in the registration procedure, called simultaneous tensor and fiber registration (STFR). The image similarity measures are defined as the similarity of the voxel-wise tensors and that of the orientation of the fiber tracts, and the deformation and re-orientation is simultaneously updated by minimizing the cost function consisting of the new similarity subjected to the smoothness constraints of the deformation field. In this way, not only tensors but also local fiber tracts are aligned. Both simulated and real human brain DTI data sets were used to evaluate the registration performance in the experiments. By using simulated images with known deformations, the registration errors of the proposed STFR algorithm and DTITK were calculated and compared [5]. The results showed the new algorithm yielded more accurate registration, with an average decrease of 12% of registration errors. Visual inspection also showed that the registered images of real human brain data sets are more similar to the template. Finally, we illustrated that by applying STFR to DTI images from ASD and TD groups, two-sample t-tests using SPM software showed regions with significantly different FA are with less noise or false positive regions. The methodology of STFR can also be extended to high-angular-resolution diffusion imaging and Q-ball vector analysis.

2   Methods

2.1   Algorithm Formulation

Image registration aims to find a deformation field fthat maps a subject image Sonto the template image$T$ by minimizing the objective function:

$$E(\mathbf{f}) = E_{SIM}(T, S, \mathbf{f}) + \lambda E_{CON}(\mathbf{f}), \tag{1}$$

where $E_{SIM}(T, S, \mathbf{f})$ stands for the distance measure between the two DTI images (T and S) using deformation field $\mathbf{f}$, and $E_{CON}(\mathbf{f})$ represents the smoothness constraint of $\mathbf{f}$. λ is the weight of the smoothness constraint. To incorporate both tensor and fiber orientation and consider re-orientation simultaneously, the objective function of STFR is defined as,

$$E(\mathbf{f}) = \frac{1}{|\Omega|}\sum_{\mathbf{x}\in\Omega}\left\{S_D\left(R(\mathbf{f}(\mathbf{x}))D_T(\mathbf{x})R^T(\mathbf{f}(\mathbf{x})), D_S(\mathbf{f}(\mathbf{x}) + \mathbf{x})\right)\right.$$
$$\left. + \xi S_F\left(R(\mathbf{f}(\mathbf{x}))F_T(\mathbf{x}), F_S(\mathbf{f}(\mathbf{x}) + \mathbf{x})\right)\right\} + \lambda E_{CON}(\mathbf{f}), \tag{2}$$

where $\mathbf{x}$ is a voxel in the template image domain Ω, $|\Omega|$ is the number of voxels. $D_T(\mathbf{x})$ denotes the tensor at voxel $\mathbf{x}$ in the template image, and $D_S(\mathbf{f}(\mathbf{x}) + \mathbf{x})$ represents the tensor at the corresponding location in the subject image. $F_T(\mathbf{x})$ stands for the fiber tract orientations at voxel $\mathbf{x}$ in the template image, and $F_S(\mathbf{f}(\mathbf{x}) + \mathbf{x})$ represents the fiber tract orientations at the corresponding location in the subject image. $R(\mathbf{f}(\mathbf{x}))$ is the respective rotation matrix, calculated from the deformation field at voxel $\mathbf{x}$. It can be seen from Eq. (2) that both the tensor and the fiber tracts in the template image needs to be deformed (by using $\mathbf{f}$) and re-oriented (by using R) in order to be compared with the corresponding tensor and fiber tracts in the subject image. ξindicates the tradeoff between tensor distance and fiber distance, and λ is the weight for the smoothness constraints of $\mathbf{f}$.

The first term in Eq.(2) calculates the distance between two tensors. Tensor similarity measures can be defined by different metrics such as full tensor distance, tensor scalar product and so on. In [10], different tensor similarity measures have been compared and the best registration performance was obtained by the Euclidean distance measure using full tensor. Utilizing this tensor metric, the tensor similarity in the Eq. (2) is defined as:

$$S_D(,) = \sqrt{tr\left(\left(R(\mathbf{f}(\mathbf{x}))D_T(\mathbf{x})R^T(\mathbf{f}(\mathbf{x})) - D_S(\mathbf{f}(\mathbf{x}) + \mathbf{x})\right)^2\right)}. \tag{3}$$

The second term in Eq. (2) calculates the similarity between the fiber tracts passing voxel $\mathbf{x}$ in image T and those passing the corresponding voxel $\mathbf{f}(\mathbf{x}) + \mathbf{x}$ in image S. We used the tractography algorithm in DTI-Studio to extract the fiber tracts on each image. Because the tractography was performed on sub-voxel resolution, there are multiple tracts passing through each voxel with different numbers. To define the distance between M fibers at a template voxel and N fibers at the corresponding subject voxel, we adopted a pair-wise cosine distance metric to compute the distances. Considering the deformation and re-orientation, the distance of fiber tracts of Eq. (2) is defined as:

$$S_F(,) = \frac{1}{M}\sum_{m=1}^{M} min_{n=1}^{N} \left\{1 - < R_F(\mathbf{f}(\mathbf{x}))F_{T,m}(\mathbf{x}), F_{S,n}(\mathbf{f}(\mathbf{x}) + \mathbf{x}) >\right\}. \tag{4}$$

The third term $E_{CON}(\mathbf{f})$ of Eq. (2) is the smoothness constraint of the deformation field, and it is defined as $||\nabla \mathbf{f}||^2$. In this way, by minimizing $E(\mathbf{f})$ we obtain the deformation field that matches not only the tensor but also the fiber tracts between the template image and the subject image (after deformation and re-orient the tensors and fiber tracts). Topology of the deformation field was also regularized using [11] to ensure realistic elastic transformation.

2.2   Algorithm Implementation

After getting the tractography results using DTI-Studio, orientations of the fiber tracts passing through each voxel are collected. Global affine registration was first performed before applying the proposed algorithm. Images are then down-sampled so the registration is performed in pyramid fashion. At the lowest resolution, the initial deformation was set to zero, and the deformation at the lower resolution was up-sampled to higher resolution as initialization. At each resolution, the following two steps were performed iteratively:

Step 1: Calculate the voxel-wise orientation matrix R from the current deformation field $\mathbf{f}$. We first calculate the Jacobian matrix, $J_f(\mathbf{x})$, and the orientation matrix is calculated as follows[12]:

$$\begin{cases} U(\mathbf{x}) = I + J_f(\mathbf{x}), \\ R(\mathbf{x}) = (U(\mathbf{x})U^T(\mathbf{x}))^{-\frac{1}{2}}U(\mathbf{x}). \end{cases} \tag{5}$$

Step 2: Update $\mathbf{f}$. Using cubic B-Spline to model the deformation and applying the finite differential method, the partial derivatives of the objective function with respect to the deformation field can be calculated as $\partial E/\partial \mathbf{f}$, and $\mathbf{f}$ is updated by:

$$\mathbf{f} \leftarrow \mathbf{f} - \varepsilon\, \partial E/\partial \mathbf{f}. \tag{6}$$

The iteration will stop until the change of objective function is smaller than a prescribed value or the maximal number of iterations is reached. Because fiber orientation in the lower resolutions does not affect much the final registration results and collecting all the fiber tracts passing through a low-resolution voxel may involve more fibers with multiple orientations, the fiber orientation is only used in the highest resolution.

3   Experiments

3.1   Comparing Registration Accuracy Using Simulated DTI Data

To evaluate the performance of the registration, we used simulated images with known underlying deformation fields to compare the registration accuracy. The proposed STFR algorithm and the DTITK algorithm were compared using these simulated images. The statistical model-based deformation simulation algorithm [13] was adopted to simulate deformation fields and to generate a series of simulated DTI images. First, we used the free-form deformation (FFD) algorithm[10] to register 150 MRI T1-weighted images onto the T1 image of our template and generated the global affine transformations and deformation fields. Then, a wavelet-based statistical model was trained using these fields to capture their variability [13]. This wavelet-based statistical model was then used to simulate 10 deformation fields by randomly sampling the statistical model space. Using the DTI image of the template, we generated the simulated DTI images by applying the simulated deformation fields [12]. The tensors of the template DTI image had been undergone both warping and re-orientation operations in order to generate the warped DTI images.

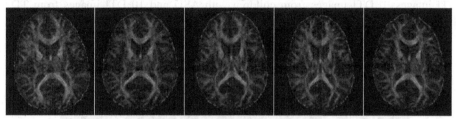

Fig. 1. Examples of simulated DTI images (left: template image; others: simulated images)

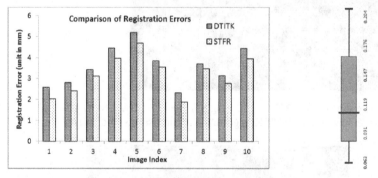

Fig. 2. Comparison of registration errors of STFR and DTITK using 10 simulated DTI images. The box plot shows he improvement of registration error of STFR as compared with DTITK (ranging from 6.3% to 20.4%).

We evaluated the performance of STFR and DTITK using these simulated images. Fig. 1 shows examples of the simulated images. After applying STFR and DTITK to register the simulated images with the template, we calculated registration accuracy using:

$$e = \frac{1}{|\Omega|}\sum_{\mathbf{x}\in\Omega}|(\mathbf{f}_s(\mathbf{x}) - \mathbf{f}(\mathbf{x})|, \tag{7}$$

where $\mathbf{f}_s$ represents the simulated deformation field, and $\mathbf{f}$ is the resultant deformation field, both defined on the space of the template image Ω. Fig. 2 plots the average registration errors of the 10 simulated images using STFR and DTITK, respectively. It can be seen that the proposed STFR yielded less errors as compared to DTITK. We also showed the box plot for the improvement of the registration errors of

STFR compared with DTITK. The improvement ranges from 6.3% to 20.4%, with a median value of 11% and a mean value of 12%.

3.2   Applying STFR to Real DTI Images

To quantitatively evaluation the registration performance we registered 15 normal adult data (resolution: $0.9375mm \times 0.9375mm \times 2mm$) onto the template. The computational speed was about 25 minutes for a machine with Intel Core i7 CPU with 8G memory running Linux x86 system. Fig. 3 shows two sample results. It can be seen that the images generated by STFR are much more similar with the template image.

To illustrate the performance of STFR, we applied it to register another set of real DTI images:10 DTI images from children with ASD and 10 DTI images from TD

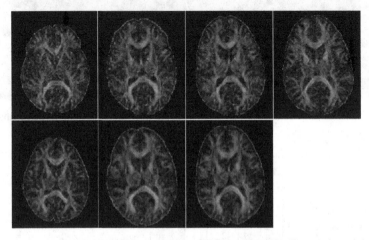

Fig. 3. Example results of real DTI images using STFR and DTITK. From left to right: subject image; registration results using DTITK; registration results using STFR; and the template.

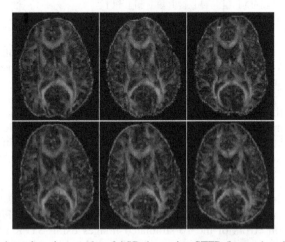

Fig. 4. Example registration results of ASD data using STFR (bottom) and DTITK (top)

children. Each data set contains 1 B0 image and 32 diffusion weighting image sequences along different directions. The image resolution is $2mm \times 2mm \times 2.7mm$, with size 128×128×70. We used the same template as the above experiment. Fig. 4 shows some registration results of ASD children using DTITK and STFR, respectively (we didn't show original DTI data because of the page limit). Compared to the previous registration results, because the image resolution herein is lower, the registration performance is not as good as that in Section 3.1, but from Fig. 4, we can clearly see that STFR yielded better registration. For some images DTITK results were not satisfactory.

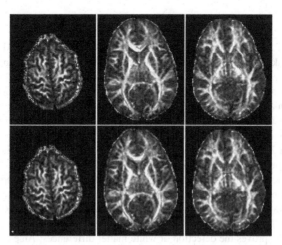

Fig. 5. SPM two-sample t-test results for normalized FA maps of ASD and TD data using STFR (bottom) and DTITK (top), respectively

In addition to compare the results visually, we normalized the FA maps of these subjects and performed two-sample t-tests on them using the SPM software package to highlight the regions with significant different FA values. All the normalized FA maps are first smoothed using the same parameters (Full width at half maximum (FWHM)=4mm) and p-value threshold was set to 0.05 with FDR correction. Some regions with significantly different FA are highlighted on the FA map of the template image in Fig. 5. Detailed analysis of the anatomical differences about the two groups is beyond the scope of this paper, but from the difference maps we can notice that because of larger registration errors, DTITK did not align the cortical areas of the brain well, resulting in some false positive regions marked by the SPM software. These results further indicate that STFR is a potential tool for aligning brain DTI images. We plan to make the software toolkit publicly available on *http://www.nitrc.org projects/mias*.

Although validated the algorithm using simulated and real DTI data. We have not yet applied statistical power analysis for evaluating the performance of the algorithm. In the future, further validation with sufficient statistical power is necessary in the future study, and we would like to explore brain connectivity studies on ASD after registering the DTI images.

4   Conclusion

In conclusion, we proposed a simultaneous tensor and fiber registration algorithm for DTI images. Full tensor information and fiber orientation information were utilized by simultaneously considering their re-orientations during the registration. The registration performance was evaluated through simulated and real DTI images and compared with DTITK. The results confirmed the advantage of the proposed algorithm for better preserving fiber orientation. Our future work is to extend the registration algorithm for use in a neural connectivity network study of Autism.

References

1. Eluvathingal, T.J., Chugani, H.T., Behen, M.E., Juhasz, C., Muzik, O., Maqbool, M., Chugani, D.C., Makki, M.: Abnormal brain connectivity in children after early severe socioemotional deprivation: A DTI study. Pediatrics 117, 2093–2100 (2006)
2. Keller, T.A., Kana, R.K., Just, M.A.: A developmental study of the structural integrity of white matter in autism. Neuroreport 18, 23–27 (2007)
3. Yang, J., Shen, D., Davatzikos, C., Verma, R.: Diffusion tensor image registration using tensor geometry and orientation features. In: Metaxas, D., Axel, L., Fichtinger, G., Székely, G. (eds.) MICCAI 2008, Part II. LNCS, vol. 5242, pp. 905–913. Springer, Heidelberg (2008)
4. Wang, Y., Gupta, A., Liu, Z., Zhang, H., Escolar, M.L., Gilmore, J.H., Gouttard, S., Fillard, P., Maltbie, E., Gerig, G., Styner, M.: DTI registration in atlas based fiber analysis of infantile Krabbe disease. Neuroimage 55, 1577–1586 (2011)
5. Zhang, H., Avants, B.B., Yushkevich, P.A., Woo, J.H., Wang, S., McCluskey, L.F., Elman, L.B., Melhem, E.R., Gee, J.C.: High-dimensional spatial normalization of diffusion tensor images improves the detection of white matter differences: An example study using amyotrophic lateral sclerosis. IEEE Trans. Med. Imaging 26, 1585–1597 (2007)
6. Ziyan, U., Sabuncu, M.R., O'Donnell, L.J., Westin, C.-F.: Nonlinear registration of diffusion MR images based on fiber bundles. In: Ayache, N., Ourselin, S., Maeder, A. (eds.) MICCAI 2007, Part I. LNCS, vol. 4791, pp. 351–358. Springer, Heidelberg (2007)
7. Xue, Z., Li, H., Guo, L., Wong, S.T.: A local fast marching-based diffusion tensor image registration algorithm by simultaneously considering spatial deformation and tensor orientation. Neuroimage 52, 119–130 (2010)
8. Yeo, B.T., Vercauteren, T., Fillard, P., Peyrat, J.M., Pennec, X., Golland, P., Ayache, N., Clatz, O.: DT-REFinD: diffusion tensor registration with exact finite-strain differential. IEEE Trans. Med. Imaging 28, 1914–1928 (2009)
9. Wang, Q., Yap, P.-T., Wu, G., Shen, D.: Diffusion tensor image registration with combined tract and tensor features. In: Fichtinger, G., Martel, A., Peters, T. (eds.) MICCAI 2011, Part II. LNCS, vol. 6892, pp. 200–208. Springer, Heidelberg (2011)
10. Alexander, D.C., Gee, J.C., Bajcsy, R.: Similarity measures for matching diffusion tensor images. In: British Machine Vision Conference, pp. 93-102 (1999)
11. Karacali, B., Davatzikos, C.: Estimating topology preserving and smooth displacement fields. IEEE Trans. Med. Imaging 23, 868–880 (2004)
12. Alexander, D.C., Pierpaoli, C., Basser, P.J., Gee, J.C.: Spatial transformations of diffusion tensor magnetic resonance images. IEEE Trans. Med. Imaging 20, 1131–1139 (2001)
13. Xue, Z., Shen, D., Davatzikos, C.: Statistical representation of high-dimensional deformation fields with application to statistically constrained 3D warping. Med. Image Anal. 10, 740–751 (2006)

Real-Time Marker-Free Patient Registration and Image-Based Navigation Using Stereovision for Dental Surgery

Junchen Wang[1], Hideyuki Suenaga[2], Liangjing Yang[1], Hongen Liao[1,3],
Etsuko Kobayashi[1], Tsuyoshi Takato[2], and Ichiro Sakuma[1]

[1] Graduate School of Engineering, The University of Tokyo, Tokyo, Japan
[2] Department of Oral-Maxillofacial Surgery, Dentistry and Orthodontics,
The University of Tokyo Hospital, Tokyo, Japan
[3] School of Medicine, Tsinghua University, Beijing, China

Abstract. Surgical navigation techniques have been evolving rapidly in the field of oral and maxillofacial surgery (OMS). However, challenges still exist in the current state of the art of computer-assisted OMS especially from the viewpoint of dental surgery. The challenges include the invasive patient registration procedure, the difficulty of reference marker attachment, navigation error caused by patient movement, bulky optical markers and maintenance of line of sight for commercial optical tracking devices, inaccuracy and susceptibility of electromagnetic (EM) sensors to magnetic interference for EM tracking devices. In this paper, a new solution is proposed to overcome the mentioned challenges. A stereo camera is designed as a tracking device for both instrument tracking and patient tracking, which is customized optimally for the limited surgical space of dental surgery. A small dot pattern is mounted to the surgical tool for instrument tracking, which can be seen by the camera at all times during the operation. The patient registration is achieved by patient tracking and 3D contour matching with the preoperative patient model, requiring no fiducial marker and reference marker. In addition, the registration is updated in real-time. Experiments were performed to evaluate our method and an average overall error of 0.71 mm was achieved.

Keywords: marker-free registration, image-based navigation, image tracking, stereovision, dental surgery.

1   Introduction

Computer-assisted oral and maxillofacial surgery (OMS) has been rapidly evolving in the last decade [1]. The categories of the computer-assisted OMS technology can be roughly divided into surgical simulation and surgical navigation in terms of whether it is performed in the surgical planning phase or the surgical phase. In preoperative simulation, 3D models of the surgical site are created from preoperative medical images as the counterparts in the virtual space. Surgeons can perform various inspections, measurements and labeling on the models and make detailed surgical planning

C.A. Linte et al. (Eds.): MIAR/AE-CAI 2013, LNCS 8090, pp. 9–18, 2013.
© Springer-Verlag Berlin Heidelberg 2013

with the help of a computer. In addition, virtual surgical procedures could also be carried out to simulate the real ones by means of special software and haptic devices [2-4]. In intra-operative navigation, a tracking device is used to track the surgical instrument whose position and orientation are mapped into the corresponding model space via a registration procedure. By this way, the relative spatial relationship between the instrument and the surgical site is related and visualized, hence being able to transfer the premade surgical plan accurately.

In one branch of OMS, dental surgery is carried out within the limited space (i.e. the mouth) and the surgical navigation for dental surgery is subjected to patient movement especially when the surgical site is located on the mandible. Some commercially available navigation systems and prototypes for dental surgery have been reported and evaluated [5-11]. However, several disadvantages still exist in these navigation systems. Firstly, all of the systems employ either optical trackers or electromagnetic (EM) trackers to locate surgical instruments intra-operatively. Currently used optical markers are bulky compared with the small operative field, which makes it inappropriate to be attached on either the patient or the instrument. An EM tracker has relatively lower accuracy and is susceptible to metallic materials, which may cause the tracking to be unstable in an operating room environment. Secondly, a reference marker is required to be attached to the patient to deal with patient movement. The use of a reference marker is either invasive (screwed into the bone) or error-prone (attached on the skin or using specific casts). Lastly, the image registration procedures are cumbersome and invasive. For better registration accuracy, fiducial markers are usually used. Similar to the attachment of the reference marker, the attachment of fiducial markers either is invasive to patients or requires a cumbersome patient-specific casts which is error-prone.

In this paper, a new solution is proposed to overcome the mentioned disadvantages. A stereo camera is designed as a tracking device for both instrument tracking and patient tracking, which is optimized and configured for the limited surgical space of dental surgery. A small dot pattern with the size 30 ×30 mm is mounted to the surgical tool for instrument tracking, which can be seen by the camera at all times during the operation. The patient registration is achieved by patient tracking followed by real-time 3D contour matching with the preoperative patient model, which requires no fiducial marker or reference marker.

2   Stereo Camera Tracking System

2.1   Stereo Camera

The stereo camera consists of two CMOS cameras with USB3.0 interface separated at a distance of approximate 120mm, as shown in Fig. 1(a). The maximum frame rate is 60 frames per second (fps) with image resolution 1280×1024 pixels. The stereo camera is calibrated using a 7×7 dot array pattern plate with the size 100×100 mm. The left and right images are undistorted and rectified so that only horizontal parallax exits between them. The intra-operative configuration of the stereo camera is illustrated in Fig. 1(b). The camera is looking down at the operative field (including the upper and lower teeth) at a distance of approximate 460 mm. The overlap view of the two cameras sufficiently covers the entire range of motion for the surgical instruments. This configuration has two advantages: one is that the measurement geometry is customized optimally for the limited operative field so as to achieve better accuracy; the other is that it is easy to maintain the line of sight between the camera and the instrument during the operation.

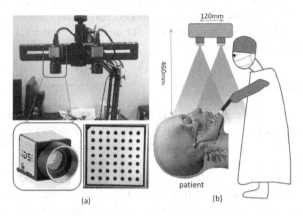

(a)   (b)

Fig. 1. (a) Stereo camera and calibration plate (b) Intra-operative configuration

2.2   Instrument Tracking

A small tool marker is designed to be attached on the surgical tool for the instrument tracking task. As shown in Fig. 2(a), the tool marker is composed of a resin mounting base fabricated by a 3D printer and a 3×3 dot array pattern for stereo tracking. The surgical tool has a cylindrical profile whose axis is perpendicular to the plane of the pattern. Fig. 2(b) shows the assembly of the two parts. The tip offset of the tool in the tool marker frame is determined by the geometry of the design (or, pivot calibration). The dot array patterns are recognized in both left and right images after which dot centroids are extracted with sub-pixel accuracy. Three-dimensional coordinates of the dot centroids are then calculated by triangulation. The pose of the tool marker frame is therefore calculated by matching the local coordinates in the marker frame to the calculated coordinates in the stereo camera frame. The pose of the tool tip frame is further obtained by a post concatenation of the fixed transformation matrix from the tool marker frame to the tool tip frame.

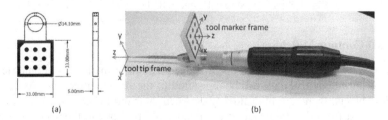

(a)   (b)

Fig. 2. (a) Tool marker (b) Surgical instrument with the tool marker

3   Real-Time Marker-Free Patient Registration

Patient registration or image registration is a key procedure to associate the surgical object with its virtual counterpart. The resulting transformation matrix is used to map the pose of the surgical tool tracked by the stereo camera to the pose in the preoperative image frame, by which computer graphics (CG) techniques could be applied to navigate the surgical procedure. The proposed patient registration is achieved by patient tracking followed by matching the 3D contour of the tracked object to its preoperative image in real-time.

3.1   Patient Tracking

The patient tracking here refers to the 3D contour tracking of the teeth. Fig. 3 shows the stereo images of a surgical scene (simulated) of dental surgery on lower teeth. The operative field indicated by the red rectangles is exposed to the stereo camera using a dental clamp. Owing to the high contrast between the teeth and the background oral cavity, the 3D contour of the teeth (front teeth) could be easily extracted by the following algorithm. The region of interest (ROI) indicated by the yellow rectangle is selected manually only in the first frame of the left camera, which is used as a 2D template. Normalized cross correlation based template matching is performed in the corresponding right image and following frames to locate the ROIs. 2D contours of the front teeth within the ROIs in the stereo images are then extracted with sub-pixel accuracy. For each point on the left contour, the corresponding point on the right contour is obtained by epipolar constraint searching (they are supposed to have the same y image coordinate). The 3D contour is finally reconstructed using stereo triangulation. The algorithm also can apply to the upper teeth. By this way, the 3D contour is tracked in real-time.

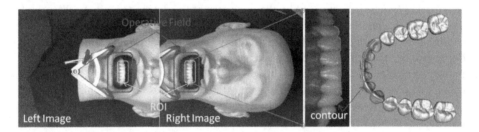

Fig. 3. Simulated surgical scene and 3D contour of teeth

3.2   3D Contour Matching

We have so far explained the intra-operative acquisition of the teeth's geometric data. Next, this intra-operative data will be registered to the preoperative one. As the teeth are rigid objects, there is a high fidelity between their intra-operative shapes and the model created from the preoperative CT image. We first obtain the same contour on the model preoperatively and then match the two contours intra-operatively.

Model Contour Extraction. The triangle mesh model of the lower tooth crowns is created by an iso-surface extractor and is rendered by OpenGL as shown in Fig. 4(a). The OpenGL camera is adjusted to prepare a view for front tooth edge extraction shown in Fig. 4(b). The foreground and background of rendered image (b) are segmented using the OpenGL z-buffer as shown in Fig. 4(c). Those pixels whose z-buffer value is -1 are classified as background (white), otherwise they are classified as foreground (black). Then the edge detection of the front teeth could be easily carried out to obtain the 2D contour indicated by the red curve. Finally, 3D coordinates of the extracted 2D contour is reconstructed according to the additional z-buffer values held in the OpenGL frame buffer. The recovered 3D contour (red points) is shown in Fig. 4(d). Note that the above procedure needs to be done only once preoperatively.

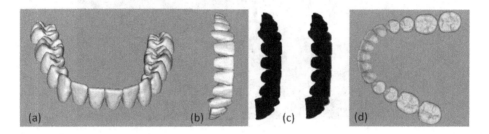

Fig. 4. (a) Surface rendering of lower tooth crowns (b) Prepared view for contour extraction (c) Binary z-buffer image and edge extraction (d) Recovered 3D contour

ICP Matching. The intra-operatively tracked tooth contour is registered to the preoperative one using the iterative closest point (ICP) algorithm [12]. To avoid converging to local minima, the principal axes of the two point sets are calculated which are used together with their centers for initial match. The initial match is easily achieved by transforming the frame consisting of the center and the three orthogonal principal directions of the tracked contour to that of the extracted model contour. After the initial match, the ICP algorithm is applied to further refine the alignment between the two contours. By this way, the transformation from the model frame to the stereo camera frame is obtained, which is used to map the surgical instrument to the atlas for surgical navigation. The above procedure is carried out just after the intra-operative tooth contour is successfully tracked.

4   Experiments and Results

All experiments were performed using a computer with an Intel Core i7-3960 CPU@3.30GHz and 16GB memories. The stereo camera worked in a monochrome mode with 60 fps and was connected to the computer workstation by USB3.0 interface. C++ and OpenGL4.3 were adopted for algorithm implementation.

4.1   Instrument Tracking Evaluation

The experimental setup is shown in Fig. 5. The instrument with the tool marker is fixed on a 3D stage whose step resolution is 0.01mm.

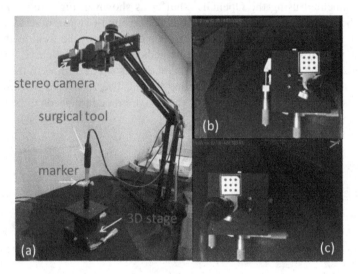

Fig. 5. (a) Experimental setup (b) /(c) Left/right image of instrument tracking

Tracking Precision Evaluation. The tool tip frame (represented by the origin x, y, z and the XYZ type Euler angles α, β, γ) was tracked while keeping stationary. 6400 samples were acquired to evaluate the tracking precision statistically and the results are shown in Table 1, where the range is defined as the absolute difference between the maximum and the minimum; std represents the standard deviation. The average tracking time was 18 milliseconds.

Table 1. tracking precision evaluation

	x(mm)	y(mm)	z(mm)	α(deg)	β(deg)	γ(deg)
range	0.305	0.340	0.098	0.199	0.188	0.031
std	0.043	0.044	0.013	0.026	0.026	0.004

Tracking Accuracy Evaluation. For accuracy evaluation, the stage was moved every 10 mm along its x, y axis and 5 mm along the z axis. The tool tip position was recorded at each position to create a 5×5×5 spatial dot array which would be registered to the ground truth using a point-based registration algorithm. The FRE (fiducial registration error) was used to evaluate the tracking accuracy which is given by

$$FRE = \sqrt{\frac{\sum_{i=1}^{N} \left\| y_i - (\hat{R}x_i + \hat{t}_i) \right\|^2}{N}} \tag{1}$$

Where x_i and y_i are corresponding points; $\hat{R}$ and $\hat{t}$ are the estimated transformation to transform the recorded dot array to the ground truth; N is the number of points (equal to 5×5×5). The alignment result is shown in Fig. 6 and the FRE was 0.15 mm.

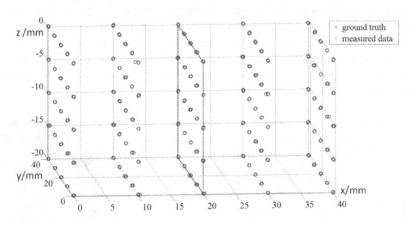

Fig. 6. Tracking accuracy evaluation

4.2   Patient Tracking and Matching Evaluation

Tooth models (lower and upper teeth) were created using a 3D printer from the segmented CT data of a patient and were assembled with a head phantom, which aimed to simulate the real surgical scene. The phantom was moved with different position and orientation. The stereo camera tracked the teeth and matched them to the preoperative model in real-time. The tracking and matching results of upper teeth are shown in Fig. 7. The average time cost was 35 milliseconds for one pair of frames.

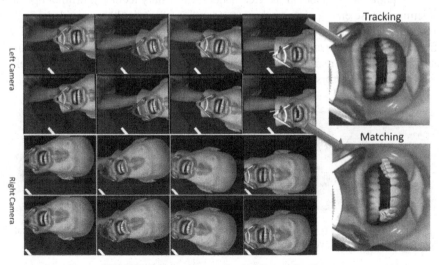

Fig. 7. Patient tracking and matching evaluation

4.3   Image-Based Navigation Evaluation

Dental navigation experiments were carried out to evaluate the overall error of the proposed method, which includes the device tracking error, the real-time registration error (further including the patient tracking error and the ICP matching error) and the manual error caused by hand tremor. For each frame pair of the stereo camera, both patient tracking and instrument tracking are performed. The former is to update the registration matrix and the latter is to map the surgical tool into the CG model space for visualization. Fig. 8 shows the navigation interface demonstrating a drilling process between adjacent tooth roots.

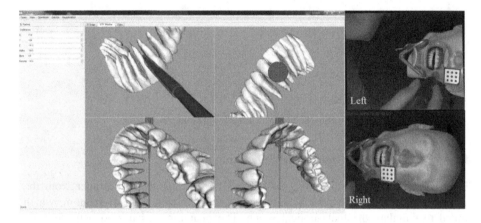

Fig. 8. Image-based navigation

A post evaluation method was used for accuracy evaluation.   As shown in Fig. 9, 10 entry points were made on the CG model of maxillary teeth (a); drilling operation targeting at those entry points on the corresponding phantom (b) was guided using our proposed method; 3D scan (c) of the phantom after drilling were obtained and was aligned with the preoperative CG model (d). The deviation between the preplanned entry points and the real drilled points were measured on the overlaid CG models as overall navigation errors. The results are summarized in Table 2.

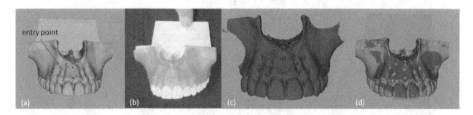

Fig. 9. Post evaluation (a) CG model with entry points (b) Model for drilling (c) 3D scan of the model after drilling (d) Overlay of the CG model and the post-3D scan

Table 2. error measurement

point index	1	2	3	4	5	6	7	8	9	10	mean
error (mm)	0.67	0.89	0.28	1.08	0.75	0.66	0.88	0.86	0.62	0.44	0.71

5   Conclusion

An image-based navigation method using stereovision for dental surgery without invasive and/or cumbersome patient registration procedures has been presented. The stereo camera has stable tracking precision and satisfactory accuracy of less than 0.2 mm. The proposed registration scheme works in a tracking-matching way which can deal with the patient movement. The total time cost of the instrument tracking and the patient registration is less than 60 milliseconds which is fast enough for clinical use. Benefitting from the real-time registration, it is free to adjust the stereo camera or move the patient intra-operatively, in which case the registration matrix can be accordingly updated within less than 1 second. Surgeons would not feel the existence of the registration procedure, although it indeed exists. Experimental evaluations on the stereo tracking device, the real-time registration and the overall accuracy of navigation were carried out and an overall navigation error of 0.71 mm was achieved. Note that the overall error also includes the manual error during drilling. That is why we chose to evaluate the error at entry points. Even though the navigation system gives correct current position and orientation, the drilling path may deviate owing to the hand tremor. A robotic arm or holder may help in reducing the manual error.

Acknowledgements. This work was supported in part by Grant for Translational Systems Biology and Medicine Initiative (TSBMI) from the Ministry of Education, Culture, Sports, Science and Technology of Japan.

References

1. Hassfeld, S., Muhling, J.: Computer Assisted Oral and Maxillofacial Surgery - A Review and an Assessment of Technology. Int. J. Oral. Maxillofac. Surg. 30, 2–13 (2001)
2. Li, C., Wang, D., Zhang, Y.: iFeel3: A Haptic Device for Virtual Reality Dental Surgery Simulation. In: Proceedings of 2011 International Conference on Virtual Reality and Visualization (ICVRV), pp. 179–184 (2011)
3. Pohlenz, P., Grobe, A., Petersik, A., et al.: Virtual Dental Surgery as A New Educational Tool in Dental School. J. Cranio. Maxill. Surg. 38, 560–564 (2010)
4. Wang, D., Zhang, Y., Wang, Y.H., et al.: Cutting on Triangle Mesh: Local Model Based Haptic Display for Dental Preparation Surgery Simulation. IEEE Trans. Vis. Comput. Graph. 6, 671–683 (2005)
5. Casap, N., Nadel, S., Tarazi, E., Weiss, E.: Evaluation of a Navigation System for Dental Implantation as a Tool to Train Novice Dental Practitioners. J. Oral. Maxil. Surg. 69(10), 2548–2556 (2011)

6. Casap, N., Laviv, A., Wexler, A.: Computerized Navigation for Immediate Loading of Dental Implants with a Prefabricated Metal Frame: A Feasibility Study. J. Oral. Maxil. Surg. 69(2), 512–519 (2011)

7. Casap, N., Wexler, A., Persky, N., et al.: Navigation Surgery for Dental Implants: Assessment of Accuracy of the Image Guided Implantology System. J. Oral. Maxil. Surg. 62(2), 116–119 (2004)

8. Ewers, R., Schicho, K., Truppe, M., et al.: Computer-aided Navigation in Dental Implantology: 7 Years of Clinical Experience. J. Oral. Maxil. Surg. 62(3), 329–334 (2004)

9. Tsuji, M., Noguchi, N., Shigematsu, M., et al.: A New Navigation System Based on Cephalograms and Dental Casts for Oral and Maxillofacial Surgery. Int. J. Oral. Max. Surg. 35(9), 828–836 (2006)

10. Bouchard, C., Magill, J.C., Nikonovskiy, V., et al.: Osteomark: A Surgical Navigation System for Oral and Maxillofacial Surgery. Int. J. Oral. Max. Surg. 41, 265–270 (2012)

11. Nijmeh, A.D., Goodger, N.M., Hawkes, D., et al.: Image-guided Navigation in Oral and Maxillofacial Surgery. Brit. J. Oral. Max. Surg. 43(4), 294–302 (2005)

12. Rusinkiewicz, S., Levoy, M.: Efficient Variants of the ICP Algorithm. In: Proceedings of Third International Conference on 3-D Digital Imaging and Modeling, pp. 145–152 (2001)

Segmentation of 3D Transesophageal Echocardiograms by Multi-cavity Active Shape Model and Gamma Mixture Model

Alexander Haak[1], Gonzalo Vegas-Sanchez-Ferrero[2], Harriët H. Mulder[4],
Hortense A. Kirisli[3], Nora Baka[3], Coert Metz[3], Stefan Klein[3], Ben Ren[1],
Gerard van Burken[1], Antonius F.W. van der Steen[1], Josien P.W. Pluim[4],
Theo van Walsum[3], and Johan G. Bosch[1]

[1] BME, Erasmus MC, Dr. Molewaterplein 50, 3015 GE Rotterdam, The Netherlands
[2] Image Processing Laboratory - Valladolid University, 47011 Valladolid, Spain
[3] BIGR, Erasmus MC, Dr. Molewaterplein 50, 3015 GE Rotterdam, The Netherlands
[4] ISI, UMC Utrecht, Utrecht, The Netherlands
j.bosch@erasmusmc.nl

Abstract. Segmentation of three-dimensional (3D) transesophageal ultrasound (TEE) is highly desired for intervention monitoring and guidance, but it is still a challenging image processing task due to complex local anatomy, limited field of view and typical ultrasound artifacts. We propose to use a multi-cavity active shape model (ASM) derived from Computed Tomography Angiography (CTA) segmentations in conjunction with a blood/tissue classification by Gamma Mixture Models to identify and segment the individual cavities simultaneously. A scheme that utilized successively ASMs of the whole heart and the individual cavities was used to segment the entire heart. We successfully validated our segmentation scheme with manually outlined contours and with CTA segmentations for three patients. The segmentations of the three patients had an average distance of 2.3, 4.9, and 2.1 mm to the manual outlines.

Keywords: TEE, ASM, Gamma Mixture Model, ultrasound, segmentation, heart.

1 Introduction

Three-dimensional transesophageal echocardiography (3D TEE) is an excellent modality for cardiac imaging and live monitoring of interventions. It allows direct visualization of the complex 3D anatomy of the different heart cavities and valves and the relative position of catheters, closure devices, and artificial valves. The position of the ultrasound probe within the esophagus allows high-resolution, unobstructed visualization of structures in the atrial and valvular regions of the heart, and a stable viewpoint for sustained imaging with much higher image quality than from the chest. Orientation, interpretation and automated segmentation of the 3D TEE images, however, can still be challenging, since only a

C.A. Linte et al. (Eds.): MIAR/AE-CAI 2013, LNCS 8090, pp. 19–26, 2013.
© Springer-Verlag Berlin Heidelberg 2013

small part of the cardiac anatomy can be covered at once, and manipulation of the probe requires considerable operator skill.

Current segmentation methods for cardiac 3D ultrasound (US) aim either at undifferentiated blood/tissue separation (e.g. for 3D anatomical visualization) or at segmentation of a single structure such as the mitral valve [1] or the left ventricle. Most are based on generic approaches such as level sets [2] which do not combine naturally with shape priors, multi-object concepts and incomplete cavity separations (e.g. open valves or wall dropout).

Here, we propose a novel segmentation method for 3D TEE aiming at complete segmentation of the different cardiac cavities in the sector view, by use of a multi-cavity Active Shape Model (ASM), based on a full-heart statistical shape model derived from Computed Tomography Angiography (CTA) images, in combination with TEE tissue/blood classification based on Gamma Mixture Models (GMM). Such a model can provide full anatomical context for the partial TEE view, and may accommodate multi-view TEE fusion, multimodal image registration and tracking of interventional devices within the reconstructed anatomy. Even when only small parts of different cavities are included in the image sector, the full model context may still provide the proper clues to identify and correctly segment the partial cavities.

2   Methodology

We use a statistical shape model derived from 151 atlas CTA based segmentations [3]. The three patients of this study were not included in the ASM. The model includes the left ventricle (LV), right ventricle (RV), left atrium (LA), right atrium (RA), and the aorta (Ao). An ASM describes a shape (s) by a linear combination of a mean shape ($\bar{s}$) and the modes of shape variation derived by principal component analysis [4]. A shape can therefore be expressed as

$$s = \bar{s} + \Phi b, \tag{1}$$

where Φ are the eigenvectors of the shape variation and b is the shape parameter vector containing the linear combination coefficients. ASM of all cavities, ASM_{total}, and individual cavities, ASM_{part}, were built according to Cootes et al. [4]. For the ASM_{total} 90% and for the ASM_{part} 98% of the shape variation were kept. The ASM is updated by blood/tissue interface detection exploiting a probabilistic characterization of speckle proposed in [5].

New update points (r') for the ASM are found along the normals of the model surface for each model point (r). The new points are selected by minimizing an objective function as proposed by van Ginneken et al. [6], which gives a robust estimator of the blood-tissue transition point. New shape instances are computed using a weighted back projection. Each selected updated point is assigned a weighting factor, w, consisting of a GMM based edge probability, $w_{GMM}(r')$, a model distance term, $w_{ASM}(r')$, and a term disqualifying points outside the pyramidal TEE volume, $w_{US}(r')$. The weighting factor is computed as follows:

$$w(r') = w_{ASM}(r') \, w_{US}(r') \, w_{GMM}(r'), \tag{2}$$

where

$$w_{ASM}(r') = \exp\left(-\frac{(r - r')^2}{\sigma^2}\right), \tag{3}$$

and σ is set to 20 (stage 1 and 2) and 10 (stage 3). The term, $w_{US}(r')$, is derived by convolving the binary TEE mask with a Gaussian kernel with a variance of 20 voxel^2.

The term $w_{GMM}(r')$ accounts for the probabilistic characterization of speckle, enhancing voxels at the blood tissue border (see below). In this case, we consider the gamma distribution as a good candidate to characterize the speckle for both blood and myocardial tissue [7,8]. Consequently, we model the intensity distribution of US images with a two-component GMM with one component for blood and one for myocardial tissue [5]. The voxel intensities of an ultrasound image region ($X = \{X_i\}$, $1 \leq i \leq N$) can be considered a set of identically distributed random variables. The probability density function of X_i is given by

$$p(x|\Theta) = \sum_{j=1}^{2} \pi_j f_X(x|\alpha_j, \beta_j), \tag{4}$$

where Θ describes the parameters of the GMM ($\pi_1, \pi_2, \alpha_1, \beta_1, \alpha_2, \beta_2$), and f_X is the gamma probability density function (PDF) [7]. The condition $\sum_{j=1}^{2} \pi_j = 1$ must hold to ensure a well defined probability $p(x|\Theta)$. The expectation maximization (EM) algorithm [9] is used to estimate the GMM parameters [5]. The probability maps of voxels belonging to blood or tissue ($k = 1, 2$) are computed by the Bayes Theorem:

$$p_k(x|\Theta) = \frac{\pi_k f_X(x|\alpha_k, \beta_k)}{\sum_{j=1}^{2} \pi_j f_X(x|\alpha_j, \beta_j)}. \tag{5}$$

An example slice of a GMM map of blood and tissue is shown in Fig. 1. Then, the GMM term, $w_{GMM}(r')$, is defined as

$$w_{GMM}(r') = 1 - \frac{|p_2(I(r')|\Theta) - 0.5|}{0.5}, \tag{6}$$

where $I(r')$ stands for the intensity in the US image at r'.

The schematic layout of the segmentation algorithm is shown in Fig. 2 and comprises the following stages:

First Stage. In the first step the ASM of the entire heart containing all cavities (ASM_{total}) are used. The mean shape ($\bar{X}_{total}$) of this ASM is initially transformed to the TEE image by a similarity transform T_{init} which was derived by manually indicating three landmark points in the TEE image (center of mitral valve, center of aortic valve, and LV apex (or a long axis point)). The optimal pose ($T_{\bar{X}_{total}}$) of the $\bar{X}_{total}$ is found by extending the methods from Arun et al. [10] to a weighted least square sense.

To prevent pose jumps by erroneous edge responses, all estimates of newly found transforms (T') are constrained to the transform (T'') of the previous

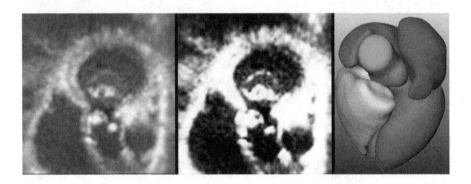

Fig. 1. Slice of a 3D TEE image (left) and the corresponding GMM map of blood (middle). Mean shape of the used statistical shape model (right). Red: LA, green: RA, yellow: RV, blue: LV, light green: Ao.

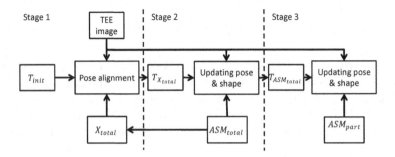

Fig. 2. Segmentation scheme

stage of the segmentation scheme by $T' = \alpha T'' + (1 - \alpha) T'$, where α weights the resulting transform. The transform weighting factor, α, is set to 0.0 for estimating T_{init}, and to 0.4 for estimating $T_{\bar{X}_{total}}$.

Second Stage. After the initial pose estimation the pose and shape of ASM_{total} are iteratively updated. New shape parameters, b, are computed from the update points (r') and b is limited to a hyper-ellipsoid with radii up to 1.5 times the shape variance [4].

Third Stage. In the last stage of the segmentation for each cavity a separate shape model covering 98% of the shape variation is used. The pose updates of each ASM are more strongly constrained by setting α to 0.8. The shape updates are again limited to a hyper-ellipsoid with radii up to 1.5 times the shape variance.

3   Experiments and Results

The segmentation method was validated in three datasets (TEE1, 2, and 3) obtained from different patients (2 male, 1 female; mean age: 74) undergoing a Transcatheter Aortic Valve Implantation (TAVI) were selected for this work. All TAVI patients had 3D TEE data acquired with a matrixTEE probe (X7-2t, Philips Healthcare, The Netherlands) during the preparation of the intervention. The patients were anesthetized and in a supine position. The image volumes of varying image quality were acquired during one heart cycle and the end diastolic time-frame was manually selected. All patients underwent a CTA for preoperative planning. The end diastolic time frame was manually selected and the CTA images were cropped so that only the heart was in the image volume.

To provide a segmentation ground truth, 2D contours of all visible cavities in multiple short and long axis views were manually annotated by two independent observers in all TEE images. First, one observer indicated four landmark points on the mitral valve (MV) annulus, one on the aortic valve (AV), and one at the apex of the left ventricle. The center of the four MV points, AV, and apex points were then used to compute an initial similarity transform for the mean shape of the total heart model($\bar{X}_{total}$). The mean shape was overlaid with the TEE image and small adjustments could be made to the landmark points to obtain an optimal initial pose of the model. Using this transformation as a starting point, the manual outlining was, performed by two observers, in ten equally distributed 2D short axis views and 4 long axis views, obtained by slicing the TEE image and the mean shape model. The 2D contours of $\bar{X}_{total}$ were interpolated by B-splines and the control points were interactively manipulated by the observers to adapt the contours to the correct borders of the different cavities.

Additionally, CTA images were obtained from the same patients and were segmented using the multi-atlas based approach introduced in [11]. The obtained CTA cardiac chamber segmentations were first manually registered to the TEE segmentations, and subsequently automatically registered rigidly using Elastix [12]. The Dice coefficients of TEE and CTA segmentations were calculated for all data sets within the pyramidal TEE image.

All ASM results were compared to the average manual observer outline, which was constructed from the mean delineations of both human observers. The mean points were computed by iterating through the contour points of observer 1 and finding the point with the smallest Euclidean distance of observer 2. This was done for all contour points lying within the pyramidal image volume. The average point-to-point distance (PTPD) was computed and served as a baseline for the segmentation performance of the ASM.

The average point-to-surface (P2S) distance between the average observer and the initial mean shape model ($\bar{X}_{total}$) and the final segmentations of the ASM were calculated (Dinit and Dasm respectively) to assess the automatic segmentation quality.

The average inter observer variabilities for all sets and heart cavities are shown in the boxplot of Fig. 3. The average point-to-surface distance of the average observer to $\bar{X}_{total}$ and to the final segmentation result are also shown in Fig. 3. The average Dasm was 2.3, 4.9, and 2.1 mm for TEE1, 2, and 3 respectively.

Note that the TEE 1 data set (Fig. 3, top) shows a good initial overlap of the cavities (more than 75%), though the distance between average observer

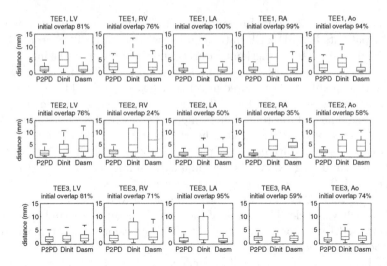

Fig. 3. Boxplots of interobserver variability of manual ground truth (P2PD), P2S distance of initial model to ground truth (Dinit) and P2S distance of final segmentation to ground truth (Dasm) for the three patients (rows) per cavity (column). Initial overlap specifies overlap of $\bar{X}_{total}$ with the pyramidal TEE image.

Table 1. Dice Coefficient CTA to TEE segmentations

heart cavity	LV	RV	LA	RA	Ao	total
TEE1	0.88	0.80	0.84	0.81	0.76	0.85
TEE2	0.73	0.78	0.68	0.74	0.74	0.80
TEE3	0.81	0.76	0.74	0.79	0.84	0.80

and the initial mean shape is far from the inter-observer range. In that case, the proposed segmentation scheme obtains a segmentation which lays within the inter-observer range. The same behavior is observed for the TEE 3 data set (Fig. 3, bottom), where the mean distance of the final ASM segmentation lays in the inter-observer range even for an initial overlap of 71%. For the TEE 2 dataset (Fig. 3, middle), the performance of the segmentation is decreased due to the very low initial overlap of cavities, which is less than a 35% in some cases.

The TEE segmentations were also validated with CTA segmentations. The obtained Dice coefficients between TEE and CTA segmentations are listed in Tab. 1 and a qualitative example of the TEE1 segmentation overlaid with the original TEE image and transformed to the CTA image is shown in Fig. 4. Note that these results show a very substantial overlap, even though correspondence between the separately acquired CTA and TEE will be compromised.

4   Discussion

In this paper, we introduced a novel multi-cavity ASM segmentation method for 3D TEE, capable of handling the complex anatomy, varying image quality,

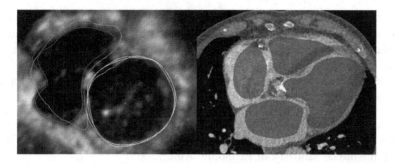

Fig. 4. Qualitative example of TEE1 segmentation of RV (green) and LV (cyan) over-laid with the manual outlines (red: RV, yellow: LV) of observer 1 and 2 (left). Final segmentation of TEE1 transformed into the CTA image (right). Structures detected in TEE overlap well with those in the CTA image.

and the narrow field of view. The GMM approach provides a solid estimation of blood/tissue membership probability which, in combination with the multi-cavity statistical model, creates a robust segmentation scheme with automatic identification of the different cavities in the complex TEE images.

The accuracy of the segmentation for the different cavities was comparable to the interobserver variability of the manual segmentations that served as ground truth. Accuracy was highest for TEE1 which had the best image quality and the highest overlap of the pyramidal image volume with the heart cavities. The lowest accuracy was obtained for TEE2 which had the lowest image quality and the lowest image overlap with the heart cavities. The manual segmentation for TEE2 was also harder to perform accurately and due to the small overlap less contour points were used. Nevertheless, this confirms the relative robustness of our method.

TEE3 had worse image quality than TEE1 but comparable overlap of the heart cavities with the image volume. For RV, LA, and Ao segmentation accuracy gains up to 76% could be achieved compared to the initial model. This indicates that our approach is quite robust to image noise and artifacts but needs sufficient overlap of the cavities to perform well.

The patients used in our study were quite different from the normal population with a rather abnormal anatomy and reduced TEE image quality. Although this may form a challenge for the ASMs statistical shape model coverage, still very acceptable segmentations were achieved.

Similarly, comparison to automatically segmented CTA of the same patients showed very good correspondence which is strongly supported by the obtained Dice coefficients. The good agreement of the TEE segmentations with the real anatomical structure can be qualitatively inspected by overlaying the trans-formed TEE segmentations with the CTA image (see Fig. 4).

Several extensions of the current approach are foreseen. Especially, an iterated estimation of blood/tissue probability based on prior knowledge of blood and tissue from the previous model estimate seems to be a promising approach. Further evaluation on additional datasets is desired and additionally we would like to investigate the optimization of a range of ASM parameters. Also, the pose constraint (α) was set to a constant value for each segmentation stage which may have been suboptimal for some cases. Relaxing this parameter with the amount of overlap of the cavity with the image sector and for the last iterations may improve the accuracy further.

This whole-heart model segmentation method will provide excellent opportunities for multi-view fusion and instrument tracking in procedure guidance.

Acknowledgments. This research is supported by the Dutch Technology Foundation STW, which is the applied science division of NWO, and the Technology Programme of the Ministry of Economic Affairs.

References

1. Schneider, R.J., Tenenholtz, N.A., Perrin, D.P., Marx, G.R., del Nido, P.J., Howe, R.D.: Patient-specific mitral leaflet segmentation from 4D ultrasound. In: Fichtinger, G., Martel, A., Peters, T. (eds.) MICCAI 2011, Part III. LNCS, vol. 6893, pp. 520–527. Springer, Heidelberg (2011)
2. Burlina, P., Mukherjee, R., Juang, R., Sprouse, C.: Recovering endocardial walls from 3D TEE. In: Metaxas, D.N., Axel, L. (eds.) FIMH 2011. LNCS, vol. 6666, pp. 284–293. Springer, Heidelberg (2011)
3. Metz, C., Baka, N., Kirisli, H., Schaap, M., Klein, S., Neefjes, L., Mollet, N., Lelieveldt, B., de Bruijne, M., Niessen, W., van Walsum, T.: Regression-based cardiac motion prediction from single-phase cta. IEEE Trans. Med. Imag. 31(6), 1311–1325 (2012)
4. Cootes, T., Cooper, D., Taylor, C., Graham, J.: Active shape models - their training and application. Comput. Vis. Image Und. 61(1), 38–59 (1995)
5. Vegas-Sánchez-Ferrero, G., Tristán-Vega, A., Aja-Fernández, S., Martín-Fernández, M., Palencia, C., Deriche, R.: Anisotropic LMMSE denoising of MRI based on statistical tissue models. In: ISBI, pp. 1519–1522 (2012)
6. van Ginneken, B., Frangi, A., Staal, J., ter Haar Romeny, B., Viergever, M.: Active shape model segmentation with optimal features. IEEE Trans. Med. Imag. 21(8), 924–933 (2002)
7. Vegas-Sánchez-Ferrero, G., Martín-Martinez, D., Aja-Fernández, S., Palencia, C.: On the influence of interpolation on probabilistic models for ultrasonic images. In: ISBI, pp. 292–295 (2010)
8. Nillesen, M., Lopata, R., Gerrits, I., Kapusta, L., Thijssen, J., de Korte, C.: Modeling envelope statistics of blood and myocardium for segmentation of echocardiographic images. Ultrasound Med. Biol. 34(4), 674–680 (2008)
9. Moon, T.: The expectation-maximization algorithm. IEEE Signal Process. Mag. 13(6), 47–60 (1996)
10. Arun, K.S., Huang, T.S., Blostein, S.D.: Least-squares fitting of two 3-d point sets. IEEE Trans. Pattern Anal. Mach. Intell. PAMI-9(5), 698–700 (1987)
11. Kirişli, H., Schaap, M., Klein, S., Papadopoulou, S., Bonardi, M., Chen, C., Weustink, A., Mollet, N., Vonken, E.P.A., van der Geest, R., van Walsum, T., Niessen, W.: Evaluation of a multi-atlas based method for segmentation of cardiac cta data: A large-scale, multi-center and multi-vendor study. Medical Physics 37(12), 6279–6292 (2010)
12. Klein, S., Staring, M., Murphy, K., Viergever, M., Pluim, J.: elastix: A toolbox for intensity-based medical image registration. IEEE Trans. Med. Imag. 29(1), 196–205 (2010)

Automatic and Real-Time Identification of Breathing Pattern from Ultrasound Liver Images

Jiaze Wu[1], Yanling Chi[1], Cheng Li[2], Bien Soo Tan[3],
London Lucien Ooi[4], Satheesh Ramamurthy[3], and Jimin Liu[1]

[1] Singapore Bioimaging Consortium, Agency for Science, Technology and Research, Singapore
{wu_jiaze,liujm}@sbic.a-star.edu.sg
[2] Department of Bioengineering, National University of Singapore, Singapore
[3] Department of Diagnostic Radiology, Singapore General Hospital, Singapore
[4] Department of Surgery, Singapore General Hospital, Singapore

Abstract. In respiratory motion modeling for the liver, the breathing pattern is usually obtained by using special tracking devices from skin or diaphragm, and subsequently applied as input to a 4D motion model for motion estimation. However, due to the intrinsic limits and economical costs of these tracking devices, the identification of the breathing pattern directly from intra-operative ultrasound images is a more attractive option. In this paper, a new method is proposed to automatically track the breathing pattern from 2D ultrasound image sequences of the liver. The proposed method firstly utilizes a Hessian matrix-based 2D line filter to identify the liver boundary, then uses an adaptive search strategy to in real-time match a template block centered inside the identified boundary, and consequently extract the translational motion of the boundary as the respiratory pattern. The experiments on four volunteers demonstrate that the respiratory pattern extracted by our method is highly consistent to those acquired by an EM tracking system with the correlation coefficient of at least 0.91.

Keywords: ultrasound images, breathing pattern tracking, Hessian matrix-based filtering, adaptive search strategy.

1 Introduction

Image-guided robot-assisted surgery and intervention are now used in more and more hospitals to overcome limitations of traditional open and minimally invasive procedures. The most successful and established surgical robot system is the Da Vinci® operating system by Intuitive Surgical Inc. The issues with the Da Vinci system, however, are high cost of system and consumables, long set-up time for use and the absence of built-in intelligence. Despite these issues, it plays an established role in complex surgeries because of the value-added benefits but its use in simple procedures is conversely limited. To address the use of robots for simple procedures, a new trend in the medical devices is to develop simple image-guided, dedicated, low cost and easy-to-use robotic systems for specific surgical and/or interventional procedures.

C.A. Linte et al. (Eds.): MIAR/AE-CAI 2013, LNCS 8090, pp. 27–34, 2013.
© Springer-Verlag Berlin Heidelberg 2013

Enlightened by the success of the prostate robot [1], we are developing an ultrasound (US) guided robot to achieve quantitatively targeted liver tumor biopsy and ablation, which requires accurate registration of pre-operative 3D computational tomography (CT) or magnetic resonance (MR) liver models to 2D intra-operative ultrasound images. However, the registration is challenging due to the movement and deformation of the liver soft tissue mainly caused by the respiration.

In order to compensate the respiration-induced motion, a possible solution is to track the targets using a 3D US probe [2], but the 3D US has limited scanning range, and produces large image data which causes the problems of processing, storing and transferring. Another potential scheme is to utilize a 2D US probe to track the target's in-plane motion, and move the probe swiftly to derive the out-of-plane motion [3]. The limitation of this method is that only a very thin slice near the plane is scanned, and the vibration of the probe can also reduce the imaging quality.

Therefore, at present, more attention is focused on model-based approach for the motion compensation [4]. With this approach, a pre-operative 4D whole liver motion model [5-7] or target-specific motion model [8, 9] is first created. During the intra-operative stage, a set of external or internal landmarks are tracked as the surrogate of respiratory pattern to drive the models to predict the liver motion. The external landmarks, applied on the abdomen or chest, are usually tracked using special optical or electromagnetic (EM) devices [8, 9]. These devices, however, create certain restrictions for the surgical robots. For example, there should be no optical or magnetic obstructs along the path of optical or electromagnetic tracker. On the other hand, as internal landmarks, the implanted fiducials [6] has the issue of invasiveness, and the diaphragm [7] requires an extra imaging device to track it. To overcome these problems, and particularly, to further reduce the cost of our surgical robot, and make it simple and portable, we wish to automatically identify the respiratory pattern from intra-operative US liver images.

Since the liver motion is strongly related to the respiration [10] and the liver boundary has relatively high contrast in 2D US images. Visually, the translational motion of the liver boundary in a fixed US imaging plane is quite related to the respiration pattern. In previous work [12], we discussed a manual way to select the liver boundary and extract the respiration pattern from the boundary. In this paper, we mainly present an automatic method to identify the liver boundary and extract its translational motion as respiratory pattern.

2   Materials and Methods

2.1   Overview

The main framework of our method is shown in Fig. 1, which is roughly divided into three main stages: 1) acquisition of US image sequences; 2) automatic identification of the liver boundary; 3) fast extraction of the breathing pattern. The experiment settings for acquiring the US images are elaborated in subsection 2.2.

After acquired, the first image of the image sequence is selected as the reference image for the following identification. The liver boundary will be recognized by a serial of consecutive processes (Fig. 1), namely filtering (enhancing the liver boundary and removing other parts in the reference image), masking (eliminating the periphery of the filtered image), thresholding (removing the weak non-boundary part), and finding the largest connected part (i.e. the liver boundary). Subsection 2.3 will describe the Hessian-based 2D line filter, which plays a key role in recognizing the liver boundary.

After the liver boundary is recognized, a template block (65×65 pixels by experiments), whose center is located inside the liver boundary, is automatically selected from the reference image of the image sequence. Using this template block, a frame-by-frame matching process, based on the normalized correlation (NC) similarity metric and adaptive search range, is executed to extract the breathing pattern. The search range on the current frame is adaptive because its center is updated as the optimally matched position of the former frame. Subsection 2.4 gives a detailed explanation on this search strategy, which makes use of the inter-frame dependency.

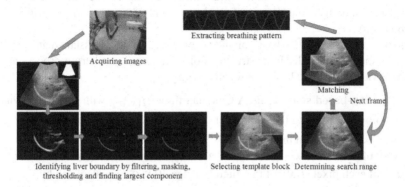

Fig. 1. The processing flow of our method for identifying and extracting the breathing pattern. It consists of three basic consecutive stages: 1) acquisition of image sequences; 2) identification of the liver boundary; 3) extraction of the breathing pattern.

2.2   Data Acquisition

The US image sequences (image resolution of 640 × 480 pixels, pixel size of about 0.37 × 0.37 mm and temporal resolution of 10 FPS) for analysis are acquired from four healthy volunteers (male, average age 36, ranged 25-46), and each sequence consists of 256 frames. The used US imaging system is the Terason t3000 with a 5C2 transducer. In order to validate the breath pattern identified by our method, a NDI Aurora electromagnetic (EM) tracking system is used to track an EM sensor on the umbilicus of the volunteers while acquiring the US images. The motion of umbilicus is selected as the reference breathing pattern for evaluation because the umbilicus on the abdominal surface is usually a good position to monitor the abdominal respiration [4]. By using the dynamic libraries from NDI and Terason, we implemented a module in our software platform to synchronously record the US images and EM signals, each US frame corresponding to an EM position. Actually, each EM position has 3 components (x, y, z), but we only need to choose one of them, which changes highly correspond to the movement of the skin marker. In order to avoid the tremor of the US probe by hands, a robotic arm is designed to fix the probe, which can stably acquire the images.

2.3   Hessian-Based 2D Line Filter

We introduce a 2D line filter to selectively enhance the line-like structures (mainly the liver boundary) in US liver images and filter out other non-line structures. This filter is inspired by Frangi's multi-scale line filter [11], which was designed to enhance the vessels of different sizes in 2D digital subtraction angiography (DSA) and 3D magnetic resonance angiography (MRA) images. In this paper, the liver boundary, which we are interested in, may be regarded as a vessel-like structure of strong contrast, which is observed in the US images of Fig. 1. However, compared to the multi-scale nature of Frangi's filter simultaneously considering the vessels of various sizes in images, our filter is of single scale only dependent on the width of the liver boundary.

Our line filter is on the basis of the eigenvalues of the Hessian matrix, which represents the second-order local structures of an image. The filtering process can be roughly divided into three basic consecutive steps:

1) **Gaussian-based smoothing.** A Gaussian filter $G(x;\sigma)$ with standard deviation σ is employed to smooth the each pixel $I(x)$ of the 2D image I, where $x = (x, y)$ denotes a pixel location in the image;

2) **Calculation of Hessian matrix and its eigenvalues.** The Hessian matrix $H(x;\sigma)$ of each pixel $I(x)$ of the filtered image $I(x;\sigma)$ is calculated by

$$H(x;\sigma) = \nabla I(x;\sigma) = \begin{bmatrix} I_{xx}(x;\sigma) & I_{xy}(x;\sigma) \\ I_{yx}(x;\sigma) & I_{yy}(x;\sigma) \end{bmatrix}, \tag{1}$$

where partial second-order derivatives of the filtered image $I(x;\sigma)$ at the pixel location x are denoted by $I_{xx}(x;\sigma)$, $I_{xy}(x;\sigma)$ and so on. Assume that $\lambda_1(x;\sigma)$ and $\lambda_2(x;\sigma)$ are the eigenvalues of the Hessian matrix $H(x;\sigma)$, and satisfy $|\lambda_1(x;\sigma)| \le |\lambda_2(x;\sigma)|$;

3) **Resulting filtering.** By combination of both eigenvalues, the resulting response is calculated by [11]

$$V(x;\sigma) = \begin{cases} 0 & \text{if } \lambda_2(x;\sigma) > 0 \\ \exp\left(-\dfrac{R^2(x;\sigma)}{2\beta^2}\right)\left(1 - \exp\left(-\dfrac{S^2(x;\sigma)}{2c^2}\right)\right) & \text{otherwise,} \end{cases} \tag{2}$$

where $R(x;\sigma) = \lambda_1(x;\sigma)/\lambda_2(x;\sigma)$ measures the blobness of each pixel in the image, $S(x;\sigma) = \sqrt{\lambda_1^2(x;\sigma) + \lambda_2^2(x;\sigma)}$ defines the local second-order structureness of each pixel, and β and C decide the sensitivity of the line filter to both measures $R(x;\sigma)$ and $S(x;\sigma)$.

The blobness measure will gain small values in the blob-like structures or background, but large values in the line-like structures, for instance the liver boundary. On the other hand, the structureness measure will be fairly low in the background where no outstanding objects are present, but in regions with high contrast, the measure will be comparatively high. Therefore, both measures are glued together to achieve the selective response of this filter on the line structures, and ignore the blob structures or background. In all the experiments of this paper, β is fixed to 0.5. The value of C depends on the grey-scale range of the image and half the value of the maximum Hessian norm has proven to work in most cases [11].

2.4   Adaptive Search Strategy

Due to the quasi-periodicity of the normal respiration, the liver tissue also moves in an approximately periodical way. Therefore, the liver tissue repeatedly appears in a relatively fixed extent (the maximal motion appears in the superior-inferior direction with the range of 5-25 mm [10]) in a normal or even deep breathing cycle, and the search range can be restricted as a medium extent. Our experiment shows that a region of 129×129 pixels is required to find the optimal match. During the frame-by-frame matching process, the traditional search strategy is to fix the center of the search range according to the position of the template region on the reference image, which is called as *center-fixed search strategy*, which is time-consuming and cannot satisfy the real-time requirement for the motion tracking.

Motivated by this problem, we present a new *adaptive search strategy* [12], which defines a serial of small center-variant search ranges along the frame-by-frame matching process. Our search strategy makes full use of the inter-frame dependency of the US image sequence, which assumes that the motion extent of the liver tissue is small for two successive frames. Therefore, any specified image block on the former frame should appear inside the small neighbor region of the same position on current frame. The optimal matching position of the former frame can be used as the center of the search range of the current frame. Based on this principle, a serial of relatively small search ranges (17×17 pixels), whose centers are automatically updated according to the former matched result, are formed along the image sequence. Here, we call center-variant search range as *adaptive search range*. Using the adaptive search strategy, we may quickly extract the respiratory pattern from the liver boundary.

3   Results

Fig. 2 shows the gradually varying filtering responses by tuning the smooth scale parameter in Eq. (2). The results show that this filter gains strongest response near the scale $\sigma = 11$ where the filtered boundary is maximally close to that in the original image. The experiments on various US images from four volunteers also support this conclusion. Therefore, in all the following experiments of this paper, the smooth scale is fixed to 11. These experiments also prove the scale parameter is roughly proportional to the width of the liver boundary.

Fig. 3 shows the selectivity characteristic of the Hessian matrix-based line filter, where four sample images scanned from four corresponding volunteers are filtered. It is observed that the response has high value at the liver boundary and other line structures of high contrast. Since the smooth scale is set to fit the liver boundary and the boundary has higher contrast than other line-like structures, the response is strongest near the boundary. Therefore, as expected, the liver boundary can always be selectively preserved by the subsequent thresholding and largest-region-selection.

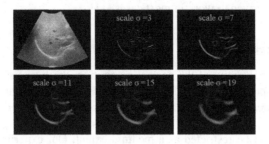

Fig. 2. Responses of our line filter under different smoothing scales. The strongest response on the liver boundary is gained at the scale $\sigma = 11$, which simultaneously most approximates the boundary in the original image.

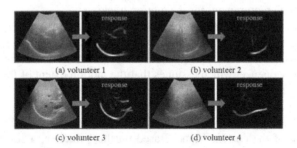

Fig. 3. The sample images (left one of each image pair) from four volunteers are processed by the line filter, and the response is strongest near the liver boundary

In order to validate our method, we chose the movement of the umbilicus on the abdominal skin as the reference breathing pattern. Four image sequences from three corresponding volunteers were used for processing, and, for each image sequence, two exemplary image blocks centered inside the recognized liver boundary were selected as matching templates. The extracted breathing patterns (Fig. 4, plotted in red) were visually compared to the reference breathing patterns of the umbilicus (Fig. 4, in green). A visual inspection on both patterns shows that the extracted breathing patterns are highly consistent with the reference ones. For convenience of visual inspection, all motion curves, including the reference ones, were normalized to the interval of 0 to 1. Using the correlation coefficient (CC) metric, the extracted breathing patterns by our method were quantitatively compared to the reference ones. The results from Table 1 show high relevance between both kinds of breathing patterns, which can be explained by that the motions of the liver and the abdominal skin are all induced by the respiration.

In addition, we also performed a quantitative analysis on the computation efficiency of our method, which is listed in Table 2. It is noticed that our adaptive search method can extract the breathing patterns in about 5 seconds for an image sequence of 256 frames, whereas the traditional search method takes nearly 6 minutes. These experiments were executed on a Dell workstation with Intel Xeon CPU E5620 2.4 GHz and 12G RAM, and the single-thread programming mode was used.

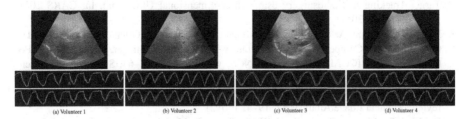

(a) Volunteer 1   (b) Volunteer 2   (c) Volunteer 3   (d) Volunteer 4

Fig. 4. Consistency is visually compared between the breathing patterns (in red), identified by our method, and the EM-tracked reference patterns of the umbilicus (in green). 8 template blocks from 4 volunteers' image sequences of 256 frames are used.

Table 1. The consistency between the extracted breathing patterns and the reference breathing patterns is analyzed using the correlation coefficient (CC). The image sequences are the same as Fig. 4.

	Volunteer 1		Volunteer 2		Volunteer 3		Volunteer 4	
Blocks	A	B	C	D	E	F	G	H
Relevance	0.9559	0.9541	0.9511	0.9379	0.9844	0.9784	0.9172	0.9206

Table 2. The computation time between the traditional search strategy and our adaptive strategy is compared. The image sequences are the same as Fig. 4, and the time unit is second.

		Volunteer 1		Volunteer 2		Volunteer 3		Volunteer 4	
Blocks		A	B	C	D	E	F	G	H
Time (s)	Traditional	301.4	299.6	260.0	278.0	299.4	299.7	290.8	291.7
	Adaptive	5.19	5.22	5.17	5.19	5.22	5.14	5.07	5.05

4   Conclusion

We have introduced an efficient Hessian matrix-based 2D line filter to automatically identify the liver boundary from the ultrasound image sequences, and then proposed an adaptive block matching method to extract the translation motion of the liver boundary as the respiratory pattern. The experiments have also demonstrated that our method can automatically and precisely recognize the liver boundary, and in several seconds extract the breathing pattern, which is in phase comparable to that of the EM tracking system. This will be of great help for US-guided surgical robots to have a build-in respiratory signal tracking system, resulting in a more compact and flexible design at low cost.

References

1. Ho, H., Yuen, J.S.P., Cheng, C.W.S.: Robotic prostate biopsy and its relevance to focal therapy of prostate cancer. Nature Reviews Urology 8, 579–585 (2011)
2. Bruder, R., Ernst, F., Schlaefer, A., Schweikard, A.: A Framework for Real-Time Target Tracking in Radiosurgery using Three-dimensional Ultrasound. In: CARS 2011, pp. S306–S307 (2011)
3. Nadeau, C., Krupa, A., Gangloff, J.: Automatic Tracking of an Organ Section with an Ultrasound Probe: Compensation of Respiratory Motion. In: Fichtinger, G., Martel, A., Peters, T. (eds.) MICCAI 2011, Part I. LNCS, vol. 6891, pp. 57–64. Springer, Heidelberg (2011)
4. McClelland, J.R., Hawkes, D.J., Schaeffter, T., King, A.P.: Respiratory motion models: A review. Medical Image Analysis 17, 19–42 (2012)
5. Rohlfing, T., Maurer, C.R., O'Dell, W.G., Zhong, J.: Modeling liver motion and deformation during the respiratory cycle using intensity-based nonrigid registration of gated MR images. Medical Physics 31, 427–432 (2004)
6. Preiswerk, F., Arnold, P., Fasel, B., Cattin, P.C.: Robust tumour tracking from 2D imaging using a population-based statistical motion model. In: IEEE Workshop on Mathematical Methods in Biomedical Image Analysis, pp. 209–214 (2012)
7. Rijkhorst, E.-J., Rivens, I., ter Haar, G., Hawkes, D., Barratt, D.: Effects of Respiratory Liver Motion on Heating for Gated and Model-Based Motion-Compensated High-Intensity Focused Ultrasound Ablation. In: Fichtinger, G., Martel, A., Peters, T. (eds.) MICCAI 2011, Part I. LNCS, vol. 6891, pp. 605–612. Springer, Heidelberg (2011)
8. Khamene, A., et al.: Characterization of Internal Organ Motion Using Skin Marker Positions. In: Barillot, C., Haynor, D.R., Hellier, P. (eds.) MICCAI 2004. LNCS, vol. 3217, pp. 526–533. Springer, Heidelberg (2004)
9. Ernst, F., Martens, V., Schlichting, S., Beširević, A., Kleemann, M., Koch, C., Petersen, D., Schweikard, A.: Correlating Chest Surface Motion to Motion of the Liver Using ε-SVR – A Porcine Study. In: Yang, G.-Z., Hawkes, D., Rueckert, D., Noble, A., Taylor, C. (eds.) MICCAI 2009, Part II. LNCS, vol. 5762, pp. 356–364. Springer, Heidelberg (2009)
10. von Siebenthal, M.: Analysis and modelling of respiratory liver motion using 4DMRI. Ph.D. thesis, ETH Zurich (2008)
11. Frangi, A.F., Niessen, W.J., Vincken, K.L., Viergever, M.A.: Multiscale vessel enhancement filtering. In: Wells, W.M., Colchester, A.C.F., Delp, S.L. (eds.) MICCAI 1998. LNCS, vol. 1496, pp. 130–137. Springer, Heidelberg (1998)
12. Wu, J., Li, C., Huang, S., Liu, F., Tan, B.S., Ooi, L.L., Yu, H., Liu, J.: Fast and robust extraction of surrogate respiratory signal from intra-operative liver ultrasound images. International Journal of Computer Assisted Radiology and Surgery (publish online, 2013)

Simultaneous Tracking, 3D Reconstruction and Deforming Point Detection for Stereoscope Guided Surgery

Bingxiong Lin[1], Adrian Johnson[1], Xiaoning Qian[1],
Jaime Sanchez[2], and Yu Sun[1,*]

[1] Computer Science and Engineering, University of South Florida, Tampa FL, USA
[2] Department of Surgery, University of South Florida, Tampa FL, USA
yusun@cse.usf.edu
http://rpal.cse.usf.edu

Abstract. Tissue deformation is one of the major difficulties in the registration of pre-operative and intra-operative data. Vision based techniques have shown the potential to simultaneously track the endoscope and recover a sparse 3D structure of the tissue. However, most of such methods either assume a static environment or require the tissue organ to have a periodic motion such as respiration. To deal with the general tissue deformation, a new framework is proposed in this paper with the ability of simultaneous stereoscope tracking, 3D reconstruction and deforming point detection in the Minimally Invasive Surgery (MIS) environment. First, we adopt a Parallel Tracking and Mapping (PTAM) framework and extend it for the use of stereoscope in MIS. Second, this newly extended framework enables the detection of deforming points without restricted periodic motion model assumptions. Our proposed method has been evaluated on a phantom model, and *in vivo* experiments demonstrate its capability for accurate tracking in nearly real time speed as well as 3D reconstruction with hundreds of 3D points. Those experiments have shown that our method is robust towards tissue deformation and hence have promising potential for information integration by registration with pre-operative data.

1 Introduction

Real-time on-site simultaneous endoscope localization and 3D structure recovery are important tasks for Minimally Invasive Surgery (MIS). First of all, vision cues and interpolation methods have been exploited to obtain semi-dense or dense tissue structure, such as stereo [1], shadow [2] and thin plate spline [3]. Based on the endoscope localization results, those recovered tissue structures from past and current endoscope locations can be merged together to obtain a larger field of view [4]. Secondly, most current registration methods of intra-operative and pre-operative data in abdominal MIS are global and static and therefore the

---

* Corresponding author.

C.A. Linte et al. (Eds.): MIAR/AE-CAI 2013, LNCS 8090, pp. 35–44, 2013.

registration becomes inaccurate when tissue organs shift and deform. Endoscope localization and tissue structure recovery based on the intra-operative video can be used to refine the global registration and reduce the errors from organ movements. To achieve the benefits mentioned above, general tissue deformations, which can be caused by tool interaction as well as patients' respiration and heartbeats, should be carefully taken care of during the endoscope localization and structure recovery procedure.

Many existing endoscope localization methods in different anatomical settings typically assume a static scene. For example, in the monocular Simultaneous Tracking and Mapping (SLAM) system introduced in [5,6] for sinus surgery, the endoscope's pose was estimated by two successive frames based on the static assumption. Mountney et al. [7] applied and extended the monocular Extended Kalman Filter SLAM (EKF-SLAM) framework from Davison [8] to stereoscope in MIS environment. Combining the stereo EKF-SLAM framework and Stoyanov et al.'s semi-dense reconstruction [1], Totz et al. [4] presented a method to recover a large and dense abdominal tissue surface. For periodic liver deformation, Mountney and Yang [9] proposed to learn the parameters of the periodic motion first and then use it to improve the SLAM estimation. For non-periodic deformation, Giannarou and Yang [10] presented a work to detect deforming points using monocular Structure From Motion (SFM) framework, whose speed is unclear and doesn't seem to be fast.

This paper aims to simultaneously track the stereoscope and recover the 3D structure accurately in an environment with small and non-periodic deformations, such as the MIS environment in abdomen cavity. To obtain accurate 3D structure, we adopt the Parallel Tracking and Mapping (PTAM) framework [11], which is able to recover more 3D points than the commonly used EKF-SLAM system. We first extend the PTAM framework for stereoscope and apply it in MIS environment. Later, a method is introduced to remove deforming points and robustly track the stereoscope's position and orientation based on rigid points only. By removing deforming points, our system is able to simultaneously track the stereoscope and recover the 3D structure in a non-periodic deforming environment.

2   Methods

We first briefly review the PTAM framework and then explain how we extend it for stereoscope and describe how we detect deforming points.

2.1   PTAM Basics

PTAM was originally designed for monocular cameras. Instead of updating the 3D map in each frame as EKF-SLAM does, tracking and mapping have been separated into two parallel threads and the mapping thread has much lower priority. The two threads run in parallel and communicate with each other through the 3D map. The tracking thread estimates the camera pose based on the 3D map generated from mapping thread. The mapping thread receives new well-tracked frames from the tracking thread and updates the 3D map accordingly. There are three major steps in tracking. First, a decaying velocity motion model is used to predict the current camera's pose. Second, 3D points are reprojected on the current frame and a fixed-range search is applied to find the reprojected points. Third, the identified 3D points and their stereo measurements are used for pose estimates. On the other hand, mapping also requires three important steps. First, user is required to translate the camera and the obtained "stereo" pair and the tracked features are used for map initialization. Second, when exploring a new area, a frame will be saved in the map for 3D reconstruction purpose. The saved frame is called keyframe. Third, local and full bundle adjustment [12], which is a standard routine to simultaneously optimize the 3D points and camera poses, are run to refine the map. The major advantage of PTAM is its ability to recover a large number of 3D points. However conventional PTAM is difficult to be directly applied in MIS setting because a static environment is assumed.

2.2   Stereoscope PTAM

In order to accurately track the scope in MIS and reconstruct the deforming surgery scene in real-time, we adopt PTAM to utilize the stereo cameras on a stereoscope and develop both stereo tracking with deforming point detection and stereo mapping in our new stereoscope PTAM. First of all, MIS images have abundant specular reflections, whose boundaries can easily be picked up as feature points, which would cause large error to the pose estimation due to their view dependent property. Before further processing, specular reflections should be detected and removed. For efficiency, bright pixels with intensities larger than 180 (0 for black and 255 for white as in standard grayscale image) are simply detected as specular reflection as well as their 5-by-5 neighbors.

For stereo tracking, we design two modes: static tracking mode and deforming tracking mode. The static tracking mode is very similar as the conventional PTAM except that the 3D points are reprojected and found in both left and right images from stereoscope. In the deforming tracking mode, the system detects deforming points and only rigid points are used for pose estimation. Our tracking system does not detect deforming points in each frame due to two reasons. The first is for efficiency to get nearly real time performance. Second, not all tissue organs in abdomen have deformations all the time. For stereo mapping, the original bundle adjustment is extended for stereo images. The outline of our system is shown in Figure 1 and the components are detailed in the following sections respectively.

2.3   Deforming Point Detection

As static tracking mode is similar to PTAM, we only describe deforming tracking mode in detail. The deforming tracking mode is triggered based on two conditions: 1) whether the tracking quality is poor; and 2) whether the speed of the camera is slow, which is designed to allow the stereoscope to explore a deforming

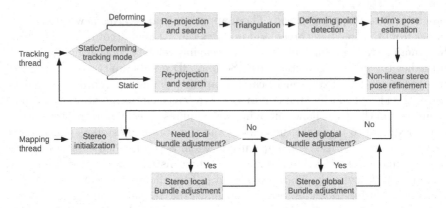

Fig. 1. Outline of our stereoscope PTAM, which contains two parallel threads: stereo tracking and stereo mapping. Stereo tracking has two modes: static tracking and deforming tracking.

area. The measure of poor tracking quality in [11] is adopted here. The camera pose update is a 6D vector, when the L2 norm of this vector is smaller than 0.1, the camera motion is considered as slow.

When the deforming tracking mode is triggered, both the tissue deformation and the stereoscope movement can contribute to the pixel displacement. To detect deforming points, each stored 3D map points that are visible in the current camera's field of view is projected on the image and a square area with width of 50 pixels centered at the projected position is searched. The set of 3D map points that are found in both left and right images is called the first point set, which may contain deforming, rigid and mismatched points. To remove the mismatched points from the first point set, each pair of points found in the left and right images is further required to be a stereo correspondence, namely, their corresponding patches should be similar and their sum of square distance (SSD) should be small. After the above removal, the rest of the mismatched points, if any, will be treated as deforming ones. On the other hand, with calibrated stereo cameras, triangulation is applied to calculate the 3D coordinates of points in the first set which leads to a second set of 3D points represented in the left camera's coordinate. The first set of 3D map points is denoted as $\{p_i\}_{i=1}^{n}$ and the second one as $\{p_i'\}_{i=1}^{n}$.

From these two point sets, we can estimate the stereoscope's pose and identify the rigid points based on the fact that only rigid points will follow a global Euclidean transformation while deforming or mismatched points do not. We apply RANSAC to select rigid points as inliers. During each RANSAC iteration, 3 pairs of corresponding 3D points are randomly selected to calculate the Euclidean transformation, which minimizes the following objective function:

$$min \sum_{i=1}^{n} ||p_i - (R * p_i' + T)||, \tag{1}$$

where R is a rotation matrix and T denotes translation. A closed-form solution of Equation (1) is obtained using Horn's absolute orientation algorithm [13]. With the derived transformation, we can identify rigid points as inliers and deforming points as outliers. The threshold of the residual error using in the RANSAC iteration is 2mm in this paper.

The above classification of rigid and deforming points is based on a single frame. However, as claimed in [14], the most significant property of deforming points is that they will continuously deform and hence their 3D registration errors in Equation (1) will always be large. Therefore, the 3D registration error for each point is accumulated and the average registration error is used to classify whether a point is deforming or not. The average registration error contains temporal information and is therefore very robust to detect deforming points. It is worth noting that once the deforming points are detected, they will not be used in the following non-linear pose refinement and stereo bundle adjustment procedure. Therefore, the error caused by tissue deformation can be significantly reduced.

2.4 Non-linear Stereo Pose Refinement

An initial estimate of the stereoscope pose can be obtained from previous information for each tracking mode: motion updated pose from previous frame in static tracking mode and pose from RANSAC in deforming tracking mode. The initial pose estimation is further refined by minimizing the reprojection error, which is a non-linear least square optimization problem. Different parameterizations are available for this problem and we follow the $SE(3)$ parameterization used in [11], which is claimed to give better results than others [15]. Since we assume that the stereo cameras are well synchronized, the extrinsic transformation between the left camera and right camera should be fixed during the pose estimation procedure. Therefore, the stereo pose update optimization problem is given in Equation (2) and 3. The calculation of Jacobian matrices of Equation (3) can be found in [15].

$$\mu' = \underset{\mu}{argmin} \sum_{i=1}^{n} \rho(||e_i||_2) \tag{2}$$

where $e_i = [e_{1i}^T, e_{2i}^T]^T$ is the reprojection error from both cameras.

$$\begin{cases} e_{1i} = \begin{pmatrix} \hat{u}_{1i} \\ \hat{v}_{1i} \end{pmatrix} - ProjCam_1(exp(\mu) \oplus E_{LW} \oplus p_j)) \\ e_{2i} = \begin{pmatrix} \hat{u}_{2i} \\ \hat{v}_{2i} \end{pmatrix} - ProjCam_2(exp(\mu) \oplus E_{RL} \oplus E_{LW} \oplus p_j)) \end{cases} \tag{3}$$

in which subscripts 1 and 2 represent left and right camera respectively; $(u, v)^T$ represents the measured 2D feature point location; $\rho(\cdot)$ is Tukey biweight objective function; $\mu \in SE(3)$ denotes a 6D vector parameterization of Euclidean transformation; and $exp(\cdot)$ is an exponential map, which maps a 6D vector to an element in $SE(3)$. Further, $E_{LW}, E_{RL} \in SE(3)$ and $\oplus$ are the pose-pose and pose-point compositions [15]. Subscript LW denotes the transformation from the world coordinate to the left camera and RL for the transformation from the left camera to the right camera. $ProjCam(\cdot)$ represents the camera perspective projection. Due to real-time performance requirement, only multiple iterations of re-weighted least square are applied to refine the pose.

2.5 Map Initialization

With calibrated stereoscope, no user cooperation is required for map initialization and the coordinates of 3D points are in mm. Since the created 3D points are used for tracking purpose, we do not perform classic stereo matching [1], which is likely to generate more 3D points but not necessarily good for tracking. Instead, similar as PTAM, we detect FAST feature points in both images and keep the ones that are easy to track. To speed up stereo matching procedure, prior information of the tissue environment is exploited. Since our target application is abdominal MIS, we accordingly set the minimum and maximum distance of stereoscope to the target as $20mm$ and $400mm$ respectively when performing epipolar search.

2.6 Stereo Bundle Adjustment

To incorporate calibrated external information to the local and full bundle adjustment, we minimize the following objective function:

$$\{\{\mu'\}, \{p'\}\} = \underset{\{\{\mu\}, \{p\}\}}{argmin} \sum_{i,j} \rho(||e_{ji}||_2) \tag{4}$$

where $e_{j,i} = [e_{1ji}^T, e_{2ji}^T]^T$ is the reprojection error of the j-th point in the i-th keyframe. μ represents the poses of keyframes and p 3D map points.

3   Experimental Results

3.1 Tracking Accuracy

To show the tracking performance of our method, we quantitatively analyze the camera tracking accuracy using a non-deforming intestine phantom. The ground truth is obtained from OptiTrack system (NaturalPoint Inc.), whose tracking accuracy is within $0.01mm$ and tracking speed is $100fps$. In this experiment, the intestine phantom is shown in Figure 2 a) with dimension $19cm * 14cm * 6cm$. The stereo cameras used in this phantom experiment has been introduced in [16,17]. Four optical trackers are attached on the stereo system's back, as shown in Figure 2 b). The stereo vision system is designed for evaluation purpose only, and therefore the system is not a miniature one. The stereo cameras are first placed at a distance of about $11cm$ to the phantom. They are then manually moved at a speed of about $10mm/s$ and held still at four locations.

It should be noted that our tracking system selects the first frame of the left camera as the world coordinate and the OptiTrack system has a different world coordinate. To enable the comparison of trajectories from these two different coordinate systems, the Euclidean transformation between them need to be calculated. To achieve this, the stereo cameras are held still for a couple of seconds at four different locations during the movement, which results in four line segments in the trajectories in Figure 3. These four point pairs in the two trajectories can be used to calculate the Euclidean transformation using Horn's absolute orientation algorithm. The two 3D trajectories are represented in OptiTrack's coordinate system and shown in Figure 3 a). The tracking accuracies in each dimension are also displayed in Figure 3 b), c), and d). The numerical tracking accuracy is available in Table 1. Notice that the tracking error along the X axis is much larger than the others. One contributing factor is that the stereo system's viewing direction is mostly parallel with the X axis.

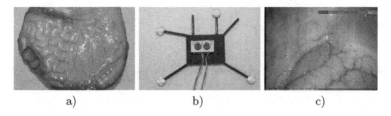

a)   b)   c)

Fig. 2. Phantom experiment setup. a) The intestine phantom. b) The stereo cameras attached with four optical markers. c) One example of detected deforming points shown as white.

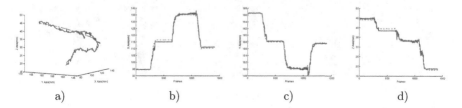

a)   b)   c)   d)

Fig. 3. Comparison of stereo tracking accuracy with ground truth. Tracking results of our method are shown in solid red and ground truths are shown in dotted blue. The recovered 3D trajectory and ground truth are shown in a) and their projection in X b), Y c) and Z axis d).

Table 1. Mean error and variance of the tracking results

	3D Trajectory	X Axis	Y Axis	Z Axis
Mean error (mm)	1.29	1.52	0.15	0.66
Variance (mm^2)	0.66	8.37	0.13	0.65

3.2 Evaluation with *In Vivo* Data

We further show the tracking results of our system on three *in vivo* videos. The first two stereo videos are from Hamlyn Center [18]: Dataset1, Dataset6. The last video was recorded while the surgeon was performing a colon surgery. Our system is able to run at speed of $15 \sim 20fps$ with a desktop computer (3.2GHz×4 cores, 3.7GB memory). Since no ground truth of the trajectories of those videos is available, we only show the 3D trajectories from our methods in Figure 4. The number of recovered 3D points for the three datasets are about

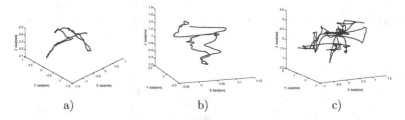

Fig. 4. 3D trajectories of the stereoscope tracked by our method over three videos: a) Dataset1, b) Dataset6 and c) Colon surgery

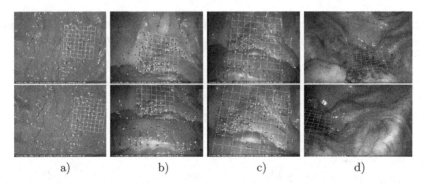

Fig. 5. Typical 3D feature points detected in one frame (zoom in for detail). Each frame has four pyramid levels and the color of each point indicates at which level it is detected [11]. Each column shows two random frames from one experiment. a) Intestine phantom, b) Dataset1, c) Dataset6 and d) Colon surgery.

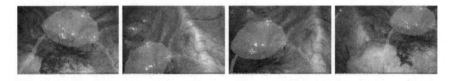

Fig. 6. A bladder model reconstructed from Computerized Tomography (CT) was augmented in the colon surgery video

600, 900, and 1600 respectively. As an example, the detected deforming points are shown as white in Figure 2 a). The typical feature points detected in each frame among different videos are shown in Figure 5, where a virtual white grid is mounted at a fixed position in the real scene to indicate the tracking accuracy. In the colon surgery video, to demonstrate the stereoscope tracking accuracy, a virtual bladder was manually registered in the first frame and was successfully tracked and augmented through out the whole video. Four frames are randomly picked to show the augmented results in Figure 6. Videos are provided in the supplemental materials to illustrate the feature point tracking procedure and organ augmented effect.

4   Conclusions

In this paper, we have introduced a new stereoscope PTAM for abdominal MIS. Our method is able to simultaneously track the stereoscope, perform 3D reconstruction and detect deforming points. The method has been tested on both phantom model and *in vivo* data, which shows our method's advantages in speed, tracking accuracy, 3D reconstruction and robustness towards deformation. The major weakness of the current system is that the stereoscope is only allowed to move slowly and smoothly. This is because the PTAM's feature point matching in MIS environment is not robust towards view angle changes. To solve this problem, in the near future, we plan to build a hybrid feature tracking method, which combines FAST feature points, vessel branch points and vessel segments.

References

1. Stoyanov, D., Scarzanella, M.V., Pratt, P., Yang, G.-Z.: Real-time stereo reconstruction in robotically assisted minimally invasive surgery. In: Jiang, T., Navab, N., Pluim, J.P.W., Viergever, M.A. (eds.) MICCAI 2010, Part I. LNCS, vol. 6361, pp. 275–282. Springer, Heidelberg (2010)
2. Lin, B., Sun, Y., Qian, X.: Dense surface reconstruction with shadows in mis. IEEE Transactions on Biomedical Engineering (2013)
3. Lin, B., Sun, Y., Qian, X.: Thin plate spline feature point matching for organ surfaces in minimally invasive surgery imaging. In: SPIE Medical Imaging (2013)
4. Totz, J., Mountney, P., Stoyanov, D., Yang, G.-Z.: Dense surface reconstruction for enhanced navigation in MIS. In: Fichtinger, G., Martel, A., Peters, T. (eds.) MICCAI 2011, Part I. LNCS, vol. 6891, pp. 89–96. Springer, Heidelberg (2011)
5. Burschka, D., Li, M., Ishii, M., Taylor, R.H., Hager, G.D.: Scale-invariant registration of monocular endoscopic images to ct-scans for sinus surgery. Medical Image Analysis 9, 413–426 (2005)
6. Mirota, D., Wang, H., Taylor, R.H., Ishii, M., Gallia, G.L., Hager, G.D.: A system for video-based navigation for endoscopic endonasal skull base surgery. IEEE Trans. Med. Imaging 31(4), 963–976 (2012)
7. Mountney, P., Stoyanov, D., Davison, A.J., Yang, G.-Z.: Simultaneous stereoscope localization and soft-tissue mapping for minimal invasive surgery. In: Larsen, R., Nielsen, M., Sporring, J. (eds.) MICCAI 2006, Part I. LNCS, vol. 4190, pp. 347–354. Springer, Heidelberg (2006)

8. Davison, A.J.: Real-time simultaneous localisation and mapping with a single camera. In: ICCV, pp. 1403–1410 (2003)
9. Mountney, P., Yang, G.-Z.: Motion compensated SLAM for image guided surgery. In: Jiang, T., Navab, N., Pluim, J.P.W., Viergever, M.A. (eds.) MICCAI 2010, Part II. LNCS, vol. 6362, pp. 496–504. Springer, Heidelberg (2010)
10. Giannarou, S., Yang, G.-Z.: Tissue deformation recovery with gaussian mixture model based structure from motion. In: Linte, C.A., Moore, J.T., Chen, E.C.S., Holmes III, D.R. (eds.) AE-CAI 2011. LNCS, vol. 7264, pp. 47–57. Springer, Heidelberg (2012)
11. Klein, G., Murray, D.W.: Parallel tracking and mapping for small ar workspaces. In: ISMAR, pp. 225–234 (2007)
12. Hartley, R.I., Zisserman, A.: Multiple View Geometry in Computer Vision, 2nd edn. Cambridge University Press (2004) ISBN: 0521540518
13. Horn, B.K.P.: Closed-form solution of absolute orientation using unit quaternions. Journal of the Optical Society of America 4, 629–642 (1987)
14. Lladó, X., Bue, A.D., Oliver, A., Salvi, J., de Agapito, L.: Reconstruction of non-rigid 3d shapes from stereo-motion. Pattern Recognition Letters 32(7), 1020–1028 (2011)
15. Blanco, J.L.: A tutorial on se(3) transformation parameterizations and on-manifold optimization. Technical report, University of Malaga (September 2010)
16. Sun, Y., Anderson, A., Castro, C., Lin, B., Gitlin, R., Ross, S., Rosemurgy, A.: Virtually transparent epidermal imagery for laparo-endoscopic single-site surgery. In: EMBC, pp. 2107–2110 (2011)
17. Castro, C.A., Alqassis, A., Smith, S., Ketterl, T., Sun, Y., Ross, S., Rosemurgy, A., Savage, P.P., Gitlin, R.D.: A wireless robot for networked laparoscopy. IEEE Transactions on Biomedical Engineering 60(4), 930–936 (2013)
18. Giannarou, S., Stoyanov, D., Noonan, D., Mylonas, G., Clark, J., Visentini-Scarzanella, M., Mountney, P., Yang, G.-Z.: Hamlyn centre laparoscopic / endoscopic video datasets, http://hamlyn.doc.ic.ac.uk/vision/

Hybrid Multimodal Deformable Registration with a Data-Driven Deformation Prior

Yongning Lu[1,2], Ying Sun[2], Rui Liao[4], and Sim Heng Ong[1,2,3]

[1] NUS Graduate School for Integrative Sciences and Engineering, NUS, Singapore
[2] Department of Electrical and Computer Engineering, NUS, Singapore
[3] Department of Bioengineering, NUS, Singapore
[4] Siemens Corporation, Corporate Research and Technology

Abstract. Deformable registration for images with different contrast-enhancement and hence different structure appearance is extremely challenging due to the ill-posed nature of the problem. Utilizing prior anatomical knowledge is thus necessary to eliminate implausible deformations. Landmark constraints and statistically constrained models have shown encouraging results. However, these methods do not utilize the segmentation information that may be readily available. In this paper, we explore the possibility of utilizing such information. We propose to generate an anatomical correlation-regularized deformation field prior by registration of point sets using mixture of Gaussians based on a thin-plate spline parametric model. The point sets are extracted from the segmented object surface and no explicit landmark matching is required. The prior is then incorporated with an intensity-based similarity measure in the deformable registration process using the variational framework. The proposed prior does not require any training data set thus excluding any inter-subject variations compared to learning-based methods. In the experiments, we show that our method increases the registration robustness and accuracy on 12 sets of TAVI patient data, 8 myocardial perfusion MRI sequences, and one simulated pre- and post- tumor resection MRI.

1 Introduction

Image registration helps the clinicians to combine the image information acquired from different modalities, different time points, or pre- and post- contrast-enhancement for better evaluation. Many of the medical applications rely on the technique of image registration, ranging from examination of disease progression, to the usage of augmented reality in the minimal-invasive interventions. For some cases, rigid/affine registration may be sufficient; however, in many cases, deformable registration is needed to compensate for local movements.

Deformable registration is inherently ill-posed and under-constrained from the mathematical point of view. It becomes more challenging when dealing with different structure appearances due to different levels of contrast-enhancement between two images. This problem widely exists in the field of medical image registration, e.g., registration of the perfusion cardiac image in the wash

C.A. Linte et al. (Eds.): MIAR/AE-CAI 2013, LNCS 8090, pp. 45–54, 2013.
© Springer-Verlag Berlin Heidelberg 2013

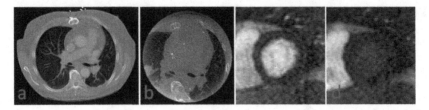

Fig. 1. Structure appearance may be largely different due to different levels of contrast-enhancement. (a) and (b) is a pair of images from pre-operative contrast-enhanced CT and intra-operative non-contrast-enhanced C-arm CT for TAVI procedure. (c) and (d) is a pair of images from a perfusion cardiac sequence at different phases.

in/out phases, and 3D/3D registration of pre-operative contrast-enhanced CT and intra-operative non-contrast-enhanced C-arm CT images. In these cases, purely relying on the intensity information produces anatomically implausible deformation. To facilitate the deformable registration process, landmark constraints were proposed to increase the registration accuracy and robustness [1,2,3]. These methods added a penalty term to penalize the correspondence pairs from moving too far apart, therefore, accurate correspondence matching is crucial. Incorporating the knowledge of statistical analysis on shape and displacement field variability to the image registration process is another popular approach [4,5]. Xue et al. [6] tackled the problem of high dimensional statistical deformation models (SDMs) using wavelet based decompositions. Despite the promising results, training the SDMs suffers from the curse of dimensionality, and how to select the training data to represent the population remains unclear. Recently, Lu et al. proposed the structural-encoded mutual information (SMI) [7] which emphasizes the structures that commonly exist in both images. And they further incorporated the rigid spine motion into their proposed application. Incorporating the rigid motion of spine movement is clearly adhoc: it cannot be applied to images which do not contain spine and/or have deformable motion. Among the aforementioned methods, one important and potentially readily available information is missing and may be utilized — the segmentation of some dominant and common objects in the images. The motion of these segmented objects could be modeled and may greatly improve the registration accuracy. In addition, from the clinical workflow perspective, this segmentation may be needed for diagnosis and guidance purpose alone, and as a result, utilization of the available segmentation results does not impose additional requirement for the purpose of image registration.

In this paper, we propose a novel hybrid deformable registration framework for multimodal image registration. The proposed method targets at image pairs that have different structure appearance. Theoretically it is a generalization of the method in [7] to deal with general structures containing deformable motion by utilizing available segmentations. A data-driven anatomical correlation-regularized deformation field prior is generated by registration of the point sets from the segmented objects using mixture of Gaussians based on a TPS model. The proposed cost function combines the high-level knowledge from the anatomical correlation-regularized deformation field and low-level intensity statistical information. Therefore, the segmentation does not need to be complete, and may focus only on the dominant structures to provide regularization on the deformation field. The fine-level registration is largely driven by the image intensity, which leads to a much more accurate registration compared to simple warping using the segmentation results alone.

2   Method

2.1   Anatomical Correlation-Regularized Deformation Field Prior

Despite the popularity of landmark-based image registration techniques, for many applications, it is very difficult to find exact/accurate landmark correspondences from the images automatically due to the poor image quality. However, relatively good segmentation of some dominant objects in these image is still possible. In our work, we assume that the segmentation of some dominant objects is given *a priori*, and the point sets are extracted from the object surfaces. The distribution of the points were modeled using mixture of Gaussians. Then we use the method in [8] to register the sampled point sets efficiently without establishing explicit point correspondences. We generate an anatomical correlation-regularized deformation field prior v using TPS model by optimizing:

$$E_{TPS}(v) = \int (f_v - g)^2 dx + \lambda E_{bend}(v), \qquad (1)$$

where f_v is the distribution representing the transformed point set warped by v, and g is the distribution of the reference point set. A small λ ensures that the TPS approximate local deformations well [9]. In our work, we choose λ to be 0.001. $E_{bend}(v)$ is the bending energy of the TPS. We refer the readers to [10] for more details of the TPS warping.

TPS is chosen to represent the underlying transformation model due to its nice properties, including its smoothness, no free parameters to tune manually, closed-form solutions for both warping and parameter estimation, and physical explanation for its energy function [3,11]. Moreover, the point sets are modeled using mixture of Gaussians for the purpose of efficient and robust registration [8]. Registration of models of mixtures of Gaussians may not be highly accurate at the edges, compared to other computationally-expensive landmark-based registration methods that focus on point-to-point matching. However, the deformation prior generated from the point sets registration results is sufficient to provide a high-level knowledge of the plausible deformation field. Note that, different from spline-based optimization schemes in other hybrid methods, we only used TPS to approximate the segmentation-based registration results. Furthermore, the distribution of the point sets obtained from segmentation are modeled as mixture of Gaussians, thus no iterative volume intensity interpolation is involved which leads to much higher computation efficiency. In our hybrid registration method, the registration will be largely driven by image intensity in regions where structural information is rich. In contrast, in regions where the structures do not match (e.g. due to different levels of contrast enhancement), the registration will be mainly regularized by the generated prior deformation field.

2.2   Cost Function

The proposed cost function E combines a data term E_s and a penalty term E_p, and the weight α balances the influences of the two terms:

$$E(u) = E_s(u) + \alpha E_p(u), \tag{2}$$

where u is the deformation field. The data term E_s aims to maximize the low-level intensity statistical dependency of the two images, whereas the penalty term E_p discourages certain implausible deformations deviated from the prior deformation field, and the weight term α is set to 0.1.

Data Term. Intensity-based similarity measures are widely reported. Popular similarity measures include mutual information, normalized mutual information, correlation ratio, and cross correlation etc. As the main focus of our paper is to introduce a prior deformation field into the deformable registration framework, we would not specify the intensity-based similarity measure. The readers are free to choose any of the intensity-based similarity measures which varies by different applications, and can then be combined with the proposed prior deformation field.

Penalty from Prior Deformation Field. Optimizing (1) provides a data-driven prior deformation field v, and we want the prior deformation field v to guide the deformable registration process. The penalty term is defined as:

$$E_p(u) = -\int_\Omega w(x)||u(x) - v(x)||^2 dx. \tag{3}$$

x is the location of the pixel/voxel. A local weight term $w(x)$ is included in the penalty term. $w(x)$ is assigned to be large at the structure mismatching area, and small at the area where structure information is rich and corresponds well in the two images.

2.3   Optimization

To optimize the cost function, we follow the variational framework proposed by Hermosillo et al. [12], which exhibits nice properties in terms of accuracy, capture range, and computational efficiency compared to the parametric deformable models. In particular, following the notation in [12], the gradient for variational minimization of the cost function is derived as:

$$\frac{\partial u}{\partial t} = -\frac{\partial E(u)}{\partial u} = -\frac{\partial E_s(u)}{\partial u} - \alpha\frac{\partial E_p(u)}{\partial u}. \tag{4}$$

As $\frac{\partial E_s}{\partial u}$ varies according to the choice of the data term, in this section, we only provide the derivation of $\frac{\partial E_p(u)}{\partial u(x)}$.

$$\frac{\partial E_p(u)}{\partial u(x)} = 2w(x)(u(x) - v(x)), \tag{5}$$

The use of the weight term $w(x)$ leads to desirable properties while updating the deformation field at each iteration. Specifically, at the locations with mismatching structures, $w(x)$ is large. These areas usually produce large registration error when solely relying on the data term, so we highly rely on the penalty term (i.e. the deformation prior) to guide the registration process in these areas. On the other hand, at the locations where the structures appear in both images, $w(x)$ is small, therefore, the registration process relies more on the data term. Fast Gaussian filtering [13] is applied at each iteration to regularize the registration process.

2.4 Implementation

Our implementation is advanced with efficient filtering and fully parallelized. A multi-resolution scheme is deployed to speed up the registration process and reduce the chance of the optimization being trapped in the local minimum during the energy minimization process. For a typical 3D volume of $512 \times 512 \times 100$, the entire registration process takes around 4 minutes for a dual core CPU, compared to 105 minutes for a B-spline based implementation reported in EMPIRE10 Challenge [14].

3   Experiments

3.1 Pre-operative CT and Non-contrast-enhanced C-arm CT

Registration of pre-operative contrast-enhanced CT and non-contrast-enhanced C-arm CT eliminates the need for acquiring contrast-enhanced C-arm CT, which is harmful to trans-catheter aortic valve implantation (TAVI) patients with kidney impairments. Our first experiment is performed on 12 TAVI patients who had undergone both CT and contrast-enhanced C-arm CT scans.

Experimental Setup. Following the same procedure in [7], we create non-contrast-enhanced C-arm CT volumes from the contrast-enhanced C-arm CT. The contrasted aortic area in the C-arm CT is replaced by intensities generated from a Gaussian distribution with mean equal to the heart area. The generated volume is visually indifferent from real non-contrast-enhanced C-arm CT volume acquired clinically. Thus we are essentially matching the CT with the non-contrast-enhanced C-arm CT with known ground truth. In this experiment, lung segmentation and rough spine segmentation can be obtained using the

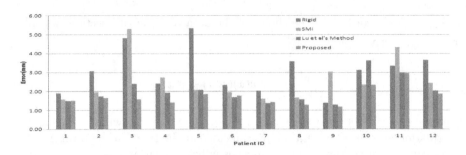

Fig. 2. Mesh-to-mesh error for 12 patients, using different registration methods

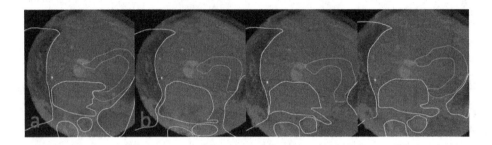

Fig. 3. Registration results, (a) Rigid (b) Deformable using SMI (c) Lu et al.'s method (d) The proposed method

methods from [15] and [16]. The point sets are sampled from the lung surface and the spine area with equal spacing. $w(\boldsymbol{x})$ is defined as:

$$w(\boldsymbol{x}) = \exp(-(\frac{d_{\text{spine}}(\boldsymbol{x})}{W})) + (1 - \exp(-(\frac{d_{\text{lung}}(\boldsymbol{x})}{W}))), \qquad (6)$$

where d_{lung} and d_{spine} are the distance maps to the surfaces of the lung and spine respectively. W is set to 2.25 cm to control the effective confidence region. $w(\boldsymbol{x})$ gives higher weight to the region away from the lung surface because in these textureless regions, the deformation prior is the main driving force. Similarly, in the spine region, the derived prior is more reliable and thus a higher weight is given. We use SMI as the data term as proposed in [7].

Results. We measure the mesh-to-mesh distance by calculating the distance between the points on surface mesh of the aortic root from CT to the closest point on the ground truth mesh from the C-arm CT (Fig. 2). We validate on the aortic root because it is the most important anatomical feature for guidance purpose during TAVI. The errors are 3.08 ± 1.17 mm, 2.59 ± 1.15 mm, 2.01 ± 0.69 mm and 1.74 ± 0.50 mm for rigid-body registration, deformable registration using SMI, Lu et al.'s method [7] and our proposed method, respectively. The results show that deformable registration is necessary to compensate for the residual motion after rigid registration. Compared to the intensity-based SMI, our method and Lu et al.'s method show the importance of incorporating anatomical knowledge into the deformable registration framework. Clinically, a registration error below 2.5 mm is deemed acceptable. Compared to Lu et al.'s method, we improve the result for patient 3 from borderline acceptable to very accurate, and furthermore, the result for patient 10 is improved from clinically not acceptable to applicable. We further perform a paired t-test between these two methods, and the two-tailed P value equals to 0.0411, showing that the proposed method is statistically significantly better than Lu et al.'s method. This is largely attributed to the proposed deformation prior, which is able to model the deformable heart motion, instead of simple rigid-body motion in the spine area as proposed in [7]. One registration example is shown in Fig. 3. The proposed method produces the most accurate registration result at the targeted area – the aortic root (red contours). Furthermore, the anatomical structure at the heart area is nicely preserved, thanks to the incorporated deformation prior. We can see that intensity-based method fails badly because of the large area of mismatched structures. Although Lu et al.'s method performs well around the spine and heart surface (yellow contours), the registration result at the heart area is not clinically meaningful, e.g. the myocardium (green contours) is badly distorted.

3.2 Myocardial Perfusion MRI

We perform our second set of experiment on 8 myocardial perfusion MRI sequences. Due to the intensity change caused by the contrast enhancement, registration of myocardial perfusion MRI is considered as multimodal.

Experimental Setup. We select a floating frame which has the best contrast in the sequence, and the selected floating frame is registered to every frame of the sequence. In this experiment, we can obtain the epicardium segmentation

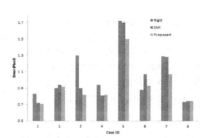

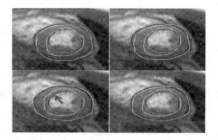

Fig. 4. Quantitative comparison of the registration errors (in *pixel*) obtained by rigid registration, SMI and the proposed method.

Fig. 5. Registration results (a) Rigid. (b) SMI. (c) Simple warping using the deformation prior. (d) Proposed method. Yellow and blue lines are the propogated and the ground truth contour.

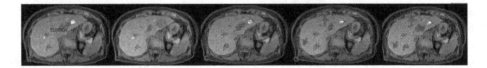

Fig. 6. (a) Pre-operative MRI. (b) Simulated post-operative MRI. (c), (d) and (e) are the registration results obtained by SMI, simple warping using the deformation prior, and the proposed method, respectively.

using [17]. The point sets are sampled from the epicardium outline with equal spacing. Similar to (6), $w(x)$ is a distance function to the segmented epicardium. The information of epicardium segmentation is thus implicitly embedded into the registration process. Again, SMI is used as the data term.

Results. For our data set, myocardial contours (epicardium and endocardium) of all the slices were drawn by a cardiologist. These contours serve as the ground truth. We calculated the root mean square distance from the ground truth to the propagated contours. The comprehensive comparison of each sequence can be found in Fig. 4. The paired t-test indicates that our hybrid method is statistically significantly better than the intensity-based method with P value equaling to 0.0263. We demonstrate the result using an example shown in Fig. 5, the main deficiency of the intensity-based and simple warping is emphasized using the red arrows. It is shown that intensity-based registration does not perform well in the homogeneous area because of the lack of structure information, while simple warping using the deformation prior results in noticeable registration errors at the structure-rich areas as the intensity information is ignored. In comparison, by combining the strength of both intensity-based and segmentation-based methods, our hybrid method produecs the best result. Note that Lu et al's method [7] is not applicable to this data due to the fact that there is no spine and the motion prior is non-rigid.

3.3   Simulated Pre- and Post- liver Tumor Resection MRI

The proposed hybrid method could be potentially applied to another category of registration problems with mismatching structures, i.e., registration between volumes of pre- and post- tumor resection. In this experiment, the registration is performed on pre-operative MRI and simulated post-operative MRI.

Experimental Setup. We simulated a post tumor resection image based on the pre-operative MRI. Then we artificially deform the pre-operative MRI, and registration is performed between the deformed pre-opeartive MRI and the simulated post-operative MRI. $w(x)$ is one at the resected area and zero otherwise. SMI is used as data term, where we do not count the statistics in the resected area. The deformation of the resected area solely relies on the regularization.

We assume the liver segmentation is available, and the point set is extracted from the liver surface.

Results. Here we get the qualitative preliminary results using one data set as shown in Fig. 6. Again, we use the arrows to emphasize the regions where intensity-based and simple warping using segmentation do perform well. Qualitatively, intensity-based registration does not perform well in the resected area, and simple warping using the liver segmentation does not preserve the detailed structures well. The proposed hybrid method guides the registration using the deformation prior at the resected area, while at the rest of the area, intensity-based method dominates. By combining the strength of both, the hybrid method achieves the best registration result as demonstrated in Fig. 6.

4   Discussion and Conclusion

In this paper, we present a hybrid multimodal deformable registration framework with a data-driven deformation prior. The proposed method addresses registration of images with different structure appearance due to different levels of contrast medium, and is validated on both TAVI and perfusion MR data. In addition, preliminary results show that the proposed method can also be applied to registration of pre- and post- tumor resection images. The experimental results demonstrate the superiority of the proposed method compared to intensity-based method and simple warping using segmentation. Furthermore, we derived the analytical solution for optimization under the variational framework which is computationally efficient. The main limitation of our method is the availability of the segmentation information. For our algorithm, we do not require very accurate segmentation result to generate the deformation prior to guide the registration process. Therefore, we can make use of the available segmentation algorithms to achieve the rough segmentation. Our algorithm is not applicable to images that no segmentation is available. In the future, we plan to apply the algorithm to more clinical data sets. We will also study how different segmentations will affect the registration results.

References

1. Sorzano, C.O., Thevenaz, P., Unser, M.: Elastic registration of biological images using vector-spline regularization. TBME 52, 652–663 (2005)
2. Papademetris, X., Jackowski, A., Schultz, R., Staib, L., Duncan, J.: Integrated intensity and point-feature nonrigid registration. In: Barillot, C., Haynor, D.R., Hellier, P. (eds.) MICCAI 2004. LNCS, vol. 3216, pp. 763–770. Springer, Heidelberg (2004)
3. Mitra, J., Kato, Z., Martí, R., Oliver, A., Lladó, X., Sidibé, D., Ghose, S., Vilanova, J., Comet, J., Meriaudeau, F.: A spline-based non-linear diffeomorphism for multimodal prostate registration. MIA (2012)
4. Wang, Y., Staib, L., et al.: Physical model-based non-rigid registration incorporating statistical shape information. MIA 4, 7–20 (2000)

5. Rueckert, D., Frangi, A., Schnabel, J.: Automatic construction of 3-D statistical deformation models of the brain using nonrigid registration. TMI 22, 1014–1025 (2003)
6. Xue, Z., Shen, D., Davatzikos, C., et al.: Statistical representation of high-dimensional deformation fields with application to statistically constrained 3D warping. MIA 10, 740–751 (2006)
7. Lu, Y., Sun, Y., Liao, R., Ong, S.H.: Registration of pre-operative CT and non-contrast-enhanced C-arm CT: An application to trans-catheter aortic valve implantation (TAVI). In: Lee, K.M., Matsushita, Y., Rehg, J.M., Hu, Z. (eds.) ACCV 2012, Part II. LNCS, vol. 7725, pp. 268–280. Springer, Heidelberg (2013)
8. Jian, B., Vemuri, B.: A robust algorithm for point set registration using mixture of Gaussians. In: IEEE ICCV 2005, vol. 2, pp. 1246–1251 (2005)
9. Rohr, K., Stiehl, H., Sprengel, R., Buzug, T., Weese, J., Kuhn, M.: Landmark-based elastic registration using approximating TPS. TMI 20, 526–534 (2001)
10. Bookstein, F.L.: Principal warps: Thin-plate splines and the decomposition of deformations. IEEE Transactions on Pattern Analysis and Machine Intelligence 11, 567–585 (1989)
11. Richa, R., Poignet, P., Liu, C.: Efficient 3D tracking for motion compensation in beating heart surgery. In: Metaxas, D., Axel, L., Fichtinger, G., Székely, G. (eds.) MICCAI 2008, Part II. LNCS, vol. 5242, pp. 684–691. Springer, Heidelberg (2008)
12. Hermosillo, G., Chefd'Hotel, C., Faugeras, O.: Variational methods for multimodal image matching. IJCV 50, 329–343 (2002)
13. Chefd'hotel, C., Hermosillo, G., Faugeras, O.: Flows of diffeomorphisms for multimodal image registration. In: IEEE ISBI 2002, pp. 753–756 (2002)
14. Murphy, K., Van Ginneken, B., Reinhardt, J., Kabus, S., Ding, K., Deng, X., Cao, K., Du, K., Christensen, G., Garcia, V., et al.: Evaluation of registration methods on thoracic CT: The empire10 challenge. IEEE TMI 30, 1901 (2011)
15. Wang, J., Li, F., Li, Q.: Automated segmentation of lungs with severe interstitial lung disease in CT. Medical Physics 36, 4592 (2009)
16. Miao, S., Liao, R., Pfister, M.: Toward smart utilization of two X-ray images for 2-D/3-D registration applied to abdominal aortic aneurysm interventions. In: IEEE ISBI 2011, vol. 1, pp. 550–555 (2011)
17. Li, C., Jia, X., Sun, Y.: Improved semi-automated segmentation of cardiac CT and MR images. In: IEEE ISBI 2009, pp. 25–28 (2009)

Planning of Middle Hepatic Vein-Guided Hemihepatectomy: Resection Pathway Construction and Optimization

Wenyu Chen[1], Jiayin Zhou[1], Weimin Huang[1], Yanling Chi[2], Wei Xiong[1],
Sudhakar Kundapur Venkatesh[3], Stephen Kin Yong Chang[4],
Jimin Liu[2], and Qi Tian[2]

[1] Institute for Infocomm Research, A*STAR, Singapore
[2] Singapore BioImaging Consortium, A*STAR, Singapore
[3] Department of Radiology, Mayo Clinic, Rochester, Minnesota, USA
[4] National University Hospital, Singapore

Abstract. Hemihepatectomy is a regular way to resect the liver graft for living donor liver transplantation. Middle hepatic vein (MHV)-guided precise hemihepatectomy demands high-quality pre-surgery planning. This paper presents a pre-operative planning system to assist surgeons in risk assessment and planning the resection pathway with a desired safety margin to MHV. Our algorithm is able to automatically construct a smooth resection pathway according to a few user-input control points and the desired safety margin. Moreover, the resection pathway is optimized by minimizing the resection area for less liver impair. Experiment of planning MHV-guided hemihepatectomy on six healthy livers was conducted and the blood-free liver parenchyma volumes of the graft and the remnant were computed for risk assessment. The comparison between the planning results using the proposed system and the results from the conventional 2D slice-based planning suggests that the proposed planning system is more convenient and provides a better planning result.

1 Introduction

Living donor liver transplantation (LDLT) is an ultimate but effective method to treat liver failure caused by late-stage liver cirrhosis and liver cancer [1,2]. In this operation, a portion of a donor's healthy liver will be resected and transplanted to a patient (recipient), whose entire liver is to be removed. Hemihepatectomy, with the desired outcome of splitting a liver into 2 portions with nearly equal volumes, is the regular way to resect the donor's liver into graft, which is for the recipient, and remnant, which remains for the donor. Pre-operative surgical planning is important to determine the surgical proposal, define the resection pathway, and calculate the volumes of liver parenchyma in both of the graft and the remnant, to guarantee 1) the safety of the donor and the recipient during the operation, and 2) there is enough liver parenchyma in both the remnant and the graft to support the lives of the donor and the recipient after the operation.

C.A. Linte et al. (Eds.): MIAR/AE-CAI 2013, LNCS 8090, pp. 55–64, 2013.
© Springer-Verlag Berlin Heidelberg 2013

The liver has a set of complex vascular systems, including hepatic artery (HA), hepatic vein (HV), portal vein (PV) and bile duct (BD). In the planning of hemi-hepatectomy, middle hepatic vein (MHV) and gallbladder fossa are important landmarks to define the resection pathway (Fig.1). The traditional recommendation for right or left hemihepatectomy is to transect the liver approximately 1 cm to the right or left side of MHV to avoid damage to MHV. Fan [3] proposed MHV-guided precise hemihepatectomy. Briefly, the precise liver transection plan is obtained by exposing the MHV early in the phase of liver transection and following its course to the inferior vena cava. Compared with traditional hepatectomy, precise hepatectomy can minimize the liver injury, ensure intact blood supply, venous drainage, and biliary drainage of the remnant liver, and preserve the greatest functional hepatic tissue through accurate preoperative evaluation and individual operation planning [3,4].

The structure, branching and confluence pattern of MHV is highly variable among individuals, hence planning MHV-guided hemihepatectomy on the basis of individual donor is essential. Conventional planning by tracking MHV and drawing the transection plane on a stack of 2D computed tomography (CT) slices is tedious and time-consuming. In addition, if a safety margin from the resection plane to MHV is required, it is not easy for 2D slice-based planning to guarantee the exact safety margin required.

There is no gold standard to define a resection surface. It is subjectively defined by surgeons. Thus, even a fully automated planning is subjected to further revision. Commercialized systems such as MeVisLab [5,6], Mint Liver [7], and Scout Liver [8] can be used to interactively define the resection surface for hemihepatectomy. However, they may require lots of user iterations to define a proper resection plan in order to guarantee the safety margin to MHV. In this paper, a semi-automatic 3D liver surgery planning system is proposed. Surgeons only need to modify a few control points, then the system will automatically construct the resection surface fulfilling the required safety margin. The system has the following features.

- Simple and friendly user interaction. To modify a resection surface, users only need to simply edit a few control points of the resection surface or change the safety margin to the MHV. As such, re-planning is easy and fast.
- Automatic construction and optimization of the resection surface. Based on the control points and the safety margin, an algorithm has been developed to construct a resection surface from the control points, guaranteeing the safety margin. The algorithm also optimizes the resection surface by reducing its surface area to reduce the potential impair and bleeding.

2   Interactive Planning System

As presented in Fig.2, the proposed planning system consists of 4 parts.

CT data pre-processing segments the liver objects and extracts the major branch of MHV.

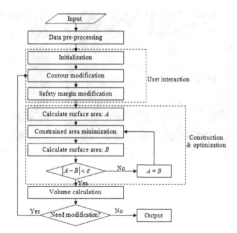

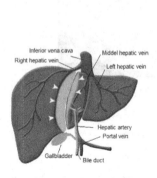

Fig. 1. Resection pathway of hemihepatectomy (arrow head)

Fig. 2. The flowchart of the resection planning

User interaction enables users to interactively edit the resection surface and select a desired safety margin.

Surface construction and optimization automatically creates the resection surface, guaranteeing the safety margin while minimizing the resection area.

Volume calculation provides the blood-free volumes of the two lobes to support risk assessment and clinical decision making.

After volume calculation, the safety margin is guaranteed. Thus, users only need to assess whether the volumes are enough for both of the donor and the recipient. If not, user can keep refining the resection plan by further editing the resection surface. The proposed algorithm will update the resection surface and present the corresponding lobe volumes. The following sections will detail each part.

2.1 Representation of the Resection Surface

A resection surface is used to resect the liver into the left lobe and the right lobe (Fig.3(a)). In the developed planning system, the resection surface depends on its contour, which is a closed 3D polygon (Fig.3(b)). Our algorithm constructs a smooth surface interpolating the contour while using the contour as its boundary. As such, the vertices of the contour act as the control points, which are used to control the shape of the resection surface. Users only need to modify the control points without considering the interior portion of the resection surface.

2.2 CT Data Pre-processing

Contrast-enhanced abdominal CT scans in PV phase were used in this study. A 3D flipping-free mesh deformation algorithm [9] was employed on the CT

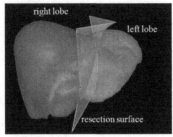
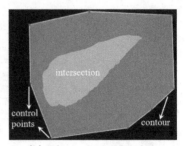
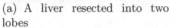

(a) A liver resected into two lobes

(b) The resection surface

Fig. 3. Two lobes and the resection surface

scan after an anisotropic diffusion filtering, for the segmentation of the 3D gross liver as the volume-of-interest (VOI, Fig.4(a)) . Then hepatic vasculatures were segmented from the VOI and grouped into the trees of PV and HV accordingly, by a context-based voting scheme which utilized region-based vessel features [10]. In short, it represents vessels in terms of shape and intensity within a local region using vessel context, and segments and separates vessels hierarchically based on vessel context and its derived features (Fig.4(b)). After that, the major branch of MHV was traced and extracted from HV tree, using a semi-automated vessel tracking algorithm from VMTK (www.vmtk.org) (the blue vessel in Fig.4(b)). The major branch of MHV is a polygon S with a sequence of points S_i, and it is approximated using a set of cylinders $C_i(S_i, S_{i+1}, r_i)$, each of which is a cylinder between S_i and S_{i+1} with radius r_i. Fig.4(c) is a MHV approximated by 12 cylinders. For any vertex V_i on the resection surface, its distance to the cylinder C_i is denoted as $d(V_i, C_i)$, and its distance to MHV is taken as

$$d_{\mathbf{MHV}}(V_i) = \min_i\{d(V_i, C_i)\}. \tag{1}$$

After this, guaranteeing the safety margin α to MHV is equivalent to guaranteeing that $d_{\mathbf{MHV}}(V_i) \geq \alpha$.

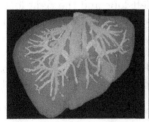
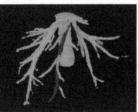
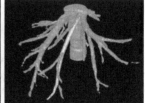

(a) Segmentation of liver, PV and HV

(b) Extract of MHV

(c) Cylinder approximation

Fig. 4. Input CT data pre-processing

2.3   User Interactions

User interaction in the proposed planning system is simple, that only the following three basic operations are required.

Initialization requires users to manually click two points on the screen (two red points in Fig.5(a)). A plane perpendicular to the screen is created interpolating the two points. The contour of the resection is initialized as the intersection between the plane and the bounding box of the liver.

Contour modification enables users to interactively edit the contours by either re-positioning a control vertex or inserting/removing a control vertex.

Safety margin modification allows users to input any required safety margin to MHV. As an example, the safety margin can be changed from 0 mm (Fig.5(b)) to 10 mm (Fig.5(c)).

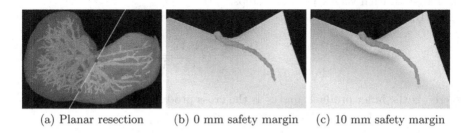

(a) Planar resection   (b) 0 mm safety margin   (c) 10 mm safety margin

Fig. 5. User interactions

2.4   Surface Construction and Optimization

The resection surface is initialized as a planar surface. After its contour is modified, the resection surface should be updated accordingly. To make the resection surface surgically resectable, the updating of the resection surface should guarantee that

- The resection surface should be smooth,
- Each vertex on the resection surface should keep the safety margin to MHV, and
- The area of the resection surface is minimized so as to reduce the potential impair and bleeding.

The local minimization algorithm [11] provides a method to construct a surface of minimal area. However, planning directly using this algorithm can lead to an unacceptable result that is too close to MHV or cuts through MHV. In this section, we will extend the algorithm to guarantee the safety. Such extension is not trivial. Since the MHV surface and the resection surface are triangular meshes, directly extending the local area minimization algorithm to guarantee the safety margin to MHV surface involves lots of point-mesh-distance calculations. When the surface resolutions for the resection surface and the MHV surface are high, the algorithm will not be fast enough for realtime applications. In our algorithm, we adopt a cylinder approximation to MHV during preprocessing and turn the complex calculation into simple point-cylinder-distance.

The resection surface is constructed as a triangular mesh R consisting of a set of vertices V and a set of triangles T. Each triangle (i, j, k) is defined by three vertices V_i, V_j and V_k. The area A of the mesh R is the sum of all triangles' areas. With the contour fixed, A is a function of interior vertices V_i. The process of area minimizing is to find appropriate positions for V_i such that A is minimized.

$$\min A = \min \sum_{(i,j,k)\in T} \tfrac{1}{2}|V_iV_j \times V_iV_k|$$
$$\text{s.t. } d_{\mathbf{MHV}}(V_i) \geq \alpha, V_i \in V. \tag{2}$$

The resection surface will be updated iteratively. In each iteration, all interior vertices of the resection surface are updated one-by-one. A new position is to be calculated for each vertex V_i in two steps.

Firstly, for each vertex V_i, $\bar{V}_i$ is obtained following Chen's method [11] as

$$\bar{V}_i = -C^{-1} \sum_{(i,j,k)\in NT(i)} \frac{(V_jV_k \cdot V_j)V_jV_k - (V_jV_k)^2V_j}{\sqrt{(V_jV_k \times V_jV_i)^2}}, \tag{3}$$

where $\cdot$ is the inner product, and $\times$ is the cross product, and $NT(i) \subseteq T$ is the subset of all the triangles that contain vertex V_i, and

$$C = \sum_{(i,j,k)\in NT(i)} \frac{(V_jV_k)^2 \begin{pmatrix} 1 & 0 & 0 \\ 0 & 1 & 0 \\ 0 & 0 & 1 \end{pmatrix} - (V_jV_k)(V_jV_k)^{\perp}}{\sqrt{(V_jV_k \times V_jV_i)^2}}.$$

Secondly, check the distance from $\bar{V}_i$ to MHV. If $d_{\mathbf{MHV}}(\bar{V}_i) \geq \alpha$, V_i is updated to be $\bar{V}_i$. Otherwise, extend the radius of each cylinder by α, and project $\bar{V}_i$ to the the nearest cylinder. Updating the V_i as the projection point will guarantee that $d_{\mathbf{MHV}}(\bar{V}_i) = \alpha$.

In one iteration, all interior vertices are updated once and each vertex satisfies $d_{\mathbf{MHV}}(\bar{V}_i) \geq \alpha$. As shown in Fig.2, the process continues until the area change in one iteration is smaller than the prescribed tolerance ε. Experimental results have shown that the resection surface converges.

2.5   Volume Calculation

The lobe volumes are very important in hemihepatectomy planning. In our system, once the resection surface is defined, the volume portions of PV and HV in the left and right lobes can be calculated. Thus, the blood-free volume for each lobe and its ratio to the whole liver can be provided. Users can refine the resection pathway to achieve the desired volume ratio for the remnant and the graft.

3   Experiments and Results

This section shows the planning of right hemihepatectomy, that the left lobe is remnant for the donor and the right lobe is the graft for the recipient. Contrast-enhanced abdominal CT scans in PV phase from six human subjects with health livers were included in the experiment. CT images were reconstructed into the image matrix of 512x512, with in-plane resolution of 0.65-0.73 mm and slice thickness of 1 mm. The resection pathway of MHV-guided right hemihepatec-tomy with MHV PRESERVATION (preserved for the donor) was planned in two scenarios: 1) the resection pathway was kept next to the major branch (or the right major branch) of MHV, and 2) a 10-mm safety margin was kept from the resection pathway to the major branch (or the right major branch) of MHV. The planning procedure was performed jointly by a surgeon and a scientist using 1) the developed 3D interactive planning tool, and 2) 2D slice-based planning on ImageJ (http://rsb.info.nih.gov/ij/) with the support from maximal intensity projection volume rendering for the original CT data.

3.1   Hemihepatectomy

Whether MHV should be harvested or not remains one point of debate in hemi-hepatectomy. Using our planning system, users can easily plan harvesting MHV for the recipient or preserving MHV for the donor, and compare the results to make the final decision. Fig.6 shows the planning result for a case with 5 mm safety margin. The ratio of remnant for the donor is only 29% if MHV is har-vested (Fig.6(a)). On the other hand, the figure is 55% if MHV is preserved for the donor. In this case, MHV can not be harvested.

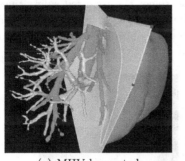
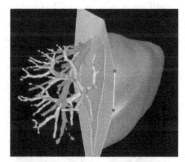

(a) MHV harvested   (b) MHV preserved

Fig. 6. Harvest or preserve MHV

3.2   Automatical Planning vs Manual Planning

Table 1 collects the blood-free volumes of the planning for the six cases. In all cases, MHVs are preserved in remnants. Conventionally, the surgeon will plan

Table 1. Right hemihepatectomy planning results

Case	3D sliced-based planning				Planning using the proposed system			
	0 mm		10 mm		0 mm		10 mm	
	Graft	Remnant	Graft	Remnant	Graft	Remnant	Graft	Remnant
1	718(57%)	533(43%)	626(50%)	625(50%)	574(46%)	677(54%)	586(47%)	665(53%)
2	710(63%)	416(37%)	639(57%)	487(43%)	539(48%)	587(52%)	530(47%)	596(53%)
3	1199(64%)	671(36%)	1111(59%)	759(41%)	897(48%)	973(52%)	895(48%)	975(52%)
4	958(60%)	636(40%)	835(52%)	759(48%)	774(49%)	820(51%)	760(48%)	834(52%)
5	1232(71%)	496(29%)	1100(64%)	628(36%)	838(48%)	890(52%)	822(48%)	906(52%)
6	861(56%)	669(44%)	813(53%)	717(47%)	718(47%)	812(53%)	700(46%)	830(54%)

* The unit is mL.

the resection pathway on each slice with a safety margin to MHV. The planned resection pathway can only keep the safety margin to the MHV on this slice but may not keep the safety margin to MHV on other slices, thus such operations may not guarantee the safety margin to MHV in 3D. Moreover, the planning result may not guarantee enough liver parenchyma volumes in both the remnant and the graft. As such, the obtained surgical proposal may not be operable. For example, in Cases 2, 3, 4 and 5, during the slice-based planning, as the surgeon planed the resection with a 0 mm safety margin slice-by-slice, the final graft volumes are much greater than the remnant volume. It means the remnant volume is significantly smaller than half of the whole liver volume. The same situation occurs for Cases 2, 3, 5 with a 10 mm safety margin. A re-planning will be required. However, it is time-consuming to re-plan in 2D slices with a prescribed safety margin. It requires even more time to plan for different safety margins.

Re-planning using the proposed system is easy and fast. The surgeon only need to modified a few control points and select the required safety margin to perform a re-planning. For the six cases, better surgical plans which preserve 51-55% of the whole liver volumes for donors were obtained by using the proposed

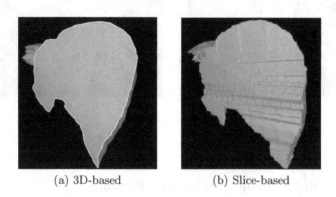

(a) 3D-based　　　　　　(b) Slice-based

Fig. 7. Semi-automatical planning VS manual planning in the smoothness of the resection surface

system. With our system, surgeons only need to adjust a few control points to achieve any ratio of graft-remnant partition for the donor, but the acceptable ratio and the actual surgical proposal is decided by surgeons.

As presented in Fig.7(b), slice-based planning result may not provide a smooth resection surface. On the other hand, the resection surface constructed by the proposed system is a smooth surface, which can be integrated for intra-operative application. During the actual operation, there are many ways to help surgeons to follow the smooth resection surface, such as augmented reality.

4   Conclusions and Future Work

For the planning of hemihepatectomy, the resection plan is subjectively defined by surgeons. In this paper, a semi-automatic system is developed to help surgeons to plan MHV-guided hemihepatectomy. Surgeons only need to interactively adjust a few control points and select the desired safety margin. Our algorithm can automatically construct a smooth resection pathway according to the control points and guaranteeing the safety margin. In parallel, area minimization is adopted to optimize the resection surface to reduce the potential impair and bleeding in the operation. Blood-free volumes of the graft and the remnant are calculated based on the planning result to support the users' decision making. Users can decide whether to harvest MHV or not by trying different resection pathways. As the user interactions to define the resection path way is very simple, re-planning is therefore very fast. Compared with the conventional 2D slice-based planning, the proposed system is faster and provides better planning results, which are surgically resectable thus can be integrated for intra-operative application. As a future work, we will adopt augmented reality to help surgeon to follow the planned pathway during the operation.

Acknowledgements. This work is partially supported by a research grant (JCOAG03-FG05 2009) from A∗STAR of Singapore.

References

1. Müller, S.A., Mehrabi, A., Schmied, B.M., Welsch, T., Fonouni, H., Engelmann, G., Schemmer, P., Weitz, J., Schmidt, J.: Partial liver transplantation-living donor liver transplantation and split liver transplantation. Nephrology Dialysis Transplantation 22(suppl. 8), viii13–viii22 (2007)
2. Singh, A.K., Cronin, C.G., Verma, H.A., Boland, G.W., Saini, S., Mueller, P.R., Sahani, D.V.: Imaging of preoperative liver transplantation in adults: What radiologists should know. Radiographics 31(4), 1017–1030 (2011)
3. Fan, S.T.: Precise hepatectomy guided by the middle hepatic vein. Hepatobiliary & Pancreatic Diseases International 6(4), 430–434 (2007)
4. Qiu, Y., Zhu, X., Zhu, R., Zhou, J., Zhou, T., Wang, Y., Ding, Y.: The clinical study of precise hemihepatectomy guided by middle hepatic vein. World Journal of Surgery, 1–8 (2012)

5. Bourquain, H., Schenk, A., Link, F., Preim, B., Prause, G., Peitgen, H.: HepaVision2-A software assistant for preoperative planning in living-related liver transplantation and oncologic liver surgery. In: Proceedings of CARS, pp. 341–346 (2002)
6. Konrad-Verse, O., Preim, B., Littmann, A.: Virtual resection with a deformable cutting plane. In: Proceedings of Simulation und Visualisierung, pp. 203–214 (2004)
7. Pianka, F., Baumhauer, M., Stein, D., Radeleff, B., Schmied, B., Meinzer, H., Müller, S.: Liver tissue sparing resection using a novel planning tool. Langenbeck's Archives of Surgery 396(2), 201–208 (2011)
8. DuBray Jr., B., Levy, R., Balachandran, P., Conzen, K., Upadhya, G., Anderson, C., Chapman, W.: Novel three-dimensional imaging technique improves the accuracy of hepatic volumetric assessment. HPB 13(9), 670–674 (2011)
9. Zhou, J., Ding, F., Xiong, W., Huang, W., Tian, Q., Wang, Z., Venkatesh, S.K., Leow, W.K.: Segmentation of liver and liver tumor for the liver-workbench. In: Proceeding of SPIE, vol. 7962, p. 88 (2011)
10. Chi, Y., Liu, J., Venkatesh, S.K., Huang, S., Zhou, J., Tian, Q., Nowinski, W.L.: Segmentation of liver vasculature from contrast enhanced ct images using context-based voting. IEEE Transactions on Biomedical Engineering 58(8), 2144–2153 (2011)
11. Chen, W., Cai, Y., Zheng, J.: Constructing triangular meshes of minimal area. Computer-Aided Design and Applications 5(14), 508–518 (2008)

Cascaded Shape Regression for Automatic Prostate Segmentation from Extracorporeal Ultrasound Images

Jierong Cheng, Wei Xiong, Ying Gu, Shue Ching Chia, and Yue Wang

Institute for Infocomm Research
1 Fusionopolis Way, #21-01 Connexis (South Tower)
Singapore 138632

Abstract. Prostate segmentation from extracorporeal ultrasound (ECUS) images is considerably challenging due to the prevailing speckle noise, shadow artifacts, and low contrast intensities. In this paper, we proposed a cascaded shape regression (CSR) method for automatic detection and localization of the prostate. A sequence of random fern predictors are trained in a boosted regression manner. Shape-indexed features are used to achieve invariance against geometric scales, translation, and rotation of prostate shapes. The boundary detected by CSR is used as the initialization for accurate segmentation by using a dynamic directional gradient vector flow (DDGVF) snake model. DDGVF proves to be useful to distinguish desired edges from false edges in ECUS images. The proposed method is tested on both longitudinal- and axial-view ECUS images and achieves Root Mean Square Error (RMSE) under 1.98 mm (=4.95 pixels). It outperforms the active appearance model in terms of RMSE, failure rate, and area error metrics. The testing time of CSR+DDGVF is less than 1 second per image.

Keywords: Cascaded regression, prostate segmentation, random ferns, dynamic directional gradient vector flow.

1 Introduction

High Intensity Focused Ultrasound (HIFU) is being used throughout the world as a therapeutic procedure for prostate cancer and benign prostate hyperplasia (BPH). An important component in BPH removal using HIFU is to position and focus on the targeted prostate tissue. Extracorporeal ultrasound (ECUS) images are usually noisier than the transrectal ultrasound (TRUS) images. Therefore, accurate automatic prostate segmentation from ECUS images faces considerable challenges. Numerous prostate segmentation methods have been developed in literature, either for TRUS, MR, or CT images (see [1] for an extensive review).

According to the information used to guide the segmentation, the prostate segmentation methods can be classified into four groups [1]: contour and shape based method, region based methods, supervised and un-supervised classification methods, and hybrid methods. Since edge information is unreliable and edges

C.A. Linte et al. (Eds.): MIAR/AE-CAI 2013, LNCS 8090, pp. 65–74, 2013.

are even broken in ultrasound images, the use of the first group of methods, e.g. active contour model (ACM) [6], [5], and curve fitting [7], [8] alone are often ineffective. Region based methods such as graph partitioning [10] and regional level set [9], solve the segmentation problem in an energy minimization framework. The popular regional level set [11] relies on region homogeneity, which is often violated due to artifacts and dropouts in ultrasound images, and generates fragmented regions. Classification methods cluster [12] or classify [13] the pixels into the prostate or the background based on feature vectors. To produce accurate segmentations, the above methods are often combined into hybrid methods so that the segmentations are more robust to artifacts and noises.

A widely used approach is to match statistical shape models to images to locate points on deformable objects. Cootes et al. proposed the active shape model (ASM) [14] which maintains the principal modes of shape variations in a deformable model framework. The later active appearance models (AAM) [15] combine models of both shape and texture using an efficient parameter update scheme. One of the limitations of parametric shape model approaches is that minimizing model parameter errors in the training set is indirect and suboptimal [3]. Moreover, ACM and AAM based methods need good initialization since they are local optimization. The linear regression used in the original AAM may be insufficient to capture the variance of shape and appearance of the prostate in ECUS images. Non-linear regression based matching methods have been introduced using boosted regression [17], [18] and random forest regression [19]. Zhou proposed shape regression machine (SRM) which uses image-based boosting regression for left ventricle segmentation from echocardiogram [16]. Sequences of random fern predictors have been used in a cascaded way for face alignment [2], [3]. Recently, regression based voting approaches [20], [21] show efficiency in locating facial feature points accurately.

In this work, we propose a cascaded shape regression (CSR) method for efficient prostate detection and localization with the shape being represented by a sequence of sampled points on the prostate contours. The advantages of the CSR are:

– The alignment error is explicitly minimized during the training of regressors, instead of minimizing model parameters which is indirect.
– The regressed shapes are constrained by the linear subspace constructed by all training shapes. We need no parameter tuning to estimate the variation of shapes in the regression model.
– The initialization is fully automatic. We use the average of all training shape and the true shape of other training samples to initialize the CSR for training, assuming that the training samples well represent the possible location, rotation and scale of the prostate shapes. Afterwards, the CSR is simply initialized by the average of all training shapes during testing.

To achieve accurate prostate segmentation, the CSR results have to be refined. Following the CSR, the dynamic directional gradient vector flow (DDGVF) snakes [23] is adopted to optimize the detected shape boundary. DDGVF is a type of external force model which endows the snake/active contour model the ability to discern edges of different orientations dynamically during the contour deformation. This property is very useful to distinguish desired edges from false edges in noisy images such as ECUS images efficiently [23]. Furthermore, DDGVF snake is faster than other existing methods such as contour or region based level set, mesh, and atlas.

2   Methodology

In this section, we present the cascaded shape regression method which is used for estimating the prostate shape and position, given a set of training data. The regressed shape is then used to initialize dynamic directional gradient vector flow snakes for accurate boundary segmentation.

2.1   Cascaded Shape Regression (CSR)

A prostate shape is represented by a sequence of M landmark points: $S = [x_1, y_1, ..., x_M, y_M]^T$. A training sample, $\{(I_i, \hat{S}_i)\}$, consists of an image I_i and a true shape $\hat{S}_i$, $i = 1, 2, ..., N$. As a landmark-based shape model, an essential requirement is that landmarks on all training samples are located at corresponding positions. Because of the ellipsoidal shape of the prostate, it is not an easy task to label the same points. To find these landmarks, we first fit the manually drawn prostate boundary in the image to an ellipse. Starting from the orientation of fitted ellipse, equally-distanced landmarks are selected automatically from the prostate boundary.

A cascaded regressor $R = (R^1, R^2, ..., R^T)$ consists of T weak regressors. Given an image I and an initial prostate shape S^0, each regressor generates a shape increment vector δS to update the previous shape:

$$S^t = S^{t-1} + R^t(I, S^{t-1}), \text{with } \delta S^t = R^t(I, S^{t-1}), t = 1, 2, ..., T. \qquad (1)$$

The output of regressors depends on image I and the previous shape S^{t-1}, using random fern and shape-indexed features which will be described in the following sections. Each regressor is trained to minimize the difference between the true shape and the new shape updated by the regressor, i.e.,

$$R^t = \arg \min_R \sum_{i=1}^{N} \|\hat{S}_i - (S_i^{t-1} + R(I_i, S_i^{t-1})\|_2. \qquad (2)$$

Random Fern Regressors. We use random ferns as weak regressors in the cascade. The fern was firstly introduced for classification [4] and later used for regression [2], [3]. A fern regressor is created by randomly selecting s features from a vector of F features and comparing them with s thresholds randomly selected. In this way, each input feature vector is divided into one of 2^s bins. Each bin b is associated with a regression output δS_b that minimizes the alignment error of training samples Ω_b that fall into the bin:

$$\delta S_b = \arg\min_{\delta S} \sum_{i \in \Omega_b} \|\hat{S}_i - (S_i + \delta S)\|_2. \tag{3}$$

Eqn. (3) is solved by simply taking the mean of all shape differences,

$$\delta S_b = \frac{\sum_{i \in \Omega_b}(\hat{S}_i - S_i)}{|\Omega_b| + \rho N}, \tag{4}$$

where ρ is a regularization term to overcome over-fitting when the number of training samples in the bin is insufficient. The exact solution of Eqn. 3 is given by Eqn. 4 when $\rho = 0$. At each stage in the cascaded regression, a pool of K ferns are randomly generated and the one with the lowest regression error is chosen.

In [2], single-variate regressors are trained separately for individual pose parameters. We train multi-variate regressors for all the M landmark points simultaneously: they either fall into a bin or not. As shown in Eqn. 4, each shape increment is a linear combination of certain training shapes $\{\hat{S}_i\}$. We choose the average of all training shapes as the initial estimate of shape S^0 for regression. Therefore, all intermediate shapes in the regression and the final regressed shape are always a linear combination of all training shapes [3]. Therefore, no extra constraint is used to impose smoothness on the output shape. In contrast, if we train separate single-variate regressors for each individual component of S, then the shape will become more and more irregular after each regression.

Shape-Indexed Features. We used simple shape-indexed features to learn each regressor. Shape-indexed features mean that a pixel is indexed relative to the currently estimated shape rather than the original image coordinates. Since the prostate shapes are mostly elliptical, we can estimate the best fit to an ellipse from a given prostate shape S, using the least-square criterion. The ellipse is parameterized by its location (t_x, t_y), major/minor axis a, b, and the orientation φ. Therefore, the current shape is reflected by the translation, scale, and rotation of the fitted ellipse.

These features are computed as the intensity difference between two pixels in the image. To compute F shape-indexed features from the current estimated shape, we first randomly sample $2F$ pixels within a circle of radius r centered at $(0, 0)$. Then F of them are randomly selected as p_1^n, and the rest of them as $p_2^n, n = 1, ..., F$. So p_1^n and p_2^n are not correlated. These points are then undergone a similarity transform according to the parameters of the best-fit ellipse $H(t_x, t_y, a, b, \varphi)$. The intensity differences at the transformed $2F$ pixels result in F shape-indexed features $I(H(p_1^n)) - I(H(p_2^n))$, which are invariant against the geometry scale, translation, and rotation of different prostate shapes. As any ellipse may be construed as an affine transformation of a circle, we use similarity transform as an approximate in order to generate randomly sampled pixel pairs nearby and within the prostate shape.

Training for CSR. The training process for CSR is summarized in Algorithm 1. For each training sample S_i, we use the average of all training shape $\left(S^0 = \frac{\sum_{j=1}^{N} \hat{S}_j}{N}\right)$ and the true shape of the rest of training samples $\{\hat{S}_j | j = 1, 2, ..., N, j \neq i\}$ to initialize the CSR. The CSR is trained to move the shape to the true shape $\hat{S}_i$ even if the initial positions are far from $\hat{S}_i$. For each testing sample, CSR is only initialized for once by the average shape because it is the single shape estimate that minimize the training error before regression starts.

Algorithm 1. Training for cascaded shape regression

Require: $\{(I_i, \hat{S}_i)\}, i = 1, 2, ..., N$

   begin initialize $S_i^0 = \frac{\sum_{j=1}^{N} \hat{S}_j}{N}$ or $S_i^0 = \left\{\hat{S}_j | j = 1, 2, ..., N, j \neq i\right\}, i = 1, 2, ..., N$ for data augmentation

   for $t = 1$ to T **do**

        for $i = 1$ to N **do**

            Fit the current shape S_i^{t-1} to an ellipse and compute shape-indexed features

        end for

        Train K random ferns on all N current shapes and select the best fern which gives the lowest training error

        Apply Eqn. (4) to compute $\delta S_b = R_b^t$ for each bin b in the best fern

        for $i = 1$ to N **do**

            $S_i^t = S_i^{t-1} + \delta S_b$, suppose the features of S_i^{t-1} fall into bin $b, b \in \{1, 2, ..., 2^s\}$

        end for

   end for

return $R = (R^1, R^2, ..., R^T)$

2.2   Dynamic Directional Gradient Vector Flow

In CSR, the prostate shape is represented by a sequence of landmark points. Overfitting will occur if a large set of landmark points is used but the number of training data is limited. If using less number of landmark points, the regressed shape may miss the curvature change in prostate boundary. Given the CSR result as an initialization for the snake, we adopt the DDGVF [23] method to detect the prostate boundary more accurately in noisy and low-contrast ECUS images.

To compute DDGVF, an edge map $\mathbf{f} = [f_x^+(x,y), f_x^-(x,y), f_y^+(x,y), f_y^-(x,y)]$ is generated from image I, where f_x^+, f_x^-, f_y^+, and f_y^- are the gradients of positive step edges in x, $-x$, y, and $-y$ directions respectively. Accordingly, the DDGVF field $\mathbf{v}(x,y) = [u^+(x,y), u^-(x,y), v^+(x,y), v^-(x,y)]$ has four components, which are found by solving the following partial differential equations separately:

$$\mathbf{v}_t = \mu \nabla^2 \mathbf{v} - (\mathbf{v} - \mathrm{d}\mathbf{f})\mathrm{d}\mathbf{f}^2, \text{ initialized by } \mathbf{v}_0 = \mathrm{d}\mathbf{f} \qquad (5)$$

where t is the time and $\mathbf{df} = [df_x^+, df_x^-, df_y^+, df_y^-]$. Finally, the snake is deformed under the external force $F_{ext} = [F_x, F_y]$, defined by

$$F_x = u^+ * \max\{\cos(\theta), 0\} - u^- * \min\{\cos(\theta), 0\} \tag{6}$$

$$F_y = v^+ * \max\{\sin(\theta), 0\} - v^- * \min\{\sin(\theta), 0\} \tag{7}$$

where θ is the contour's normal directional at a certain snaxel.

3   Experiments

We validate the performance of our method (CSR+DDGVF) on two datasets: 74 longitudinal view and 76 axial view ECUS images of the prostate. The resolution of the images is 488×744 pixels and (0.40 mm/pixel). 50 images are randomly selected from each dataset as the respective training sets and the rest as the testing sets respectively. Each prostate shape is described by $M = 20$ landmarks. The parameters of the CSR are set as follows: number of training data $N = 50$, number of phases in the cascade $T = 512$, fern depth $s = 5$, number of ferns $K = 128$, radius $r = 1.5$, and number of features $F = 64$.

We use average Root Mean Square Error (RMSE), failure rate, precision, recall, and Dice coefficient (DSC)[1] to evaluate the segmentation result. To calculate the failure rate, two thresholds on RMSE ($\phi = 2.4$ or 3 mm) are used, which corresponds to 6.5% and 8.1% of average prostate length in longitudinal view images. The precision, recall, and DSC are averaged respectively only for those images where the segmentation result and the ground truth are at least overlapped. The results are compared with the original AAM proposed by Cootes et al. [15] using the optimized C++ implementation from [22].

During the testing of CSR, we use the average of all training shapes as the initialization by simply overlaying it on the testing image domain. In our ECUS prostate segmentation application, because the training data are from the same imaging setting as those for the testing data, their scales are considered the same. As long as the training data are representative for the size, shape and position variations, there is no need to invoke transformations in terms of scale and translation. As for rotation, the orientation of the prostate is estimated by fitting an ellipse to determine the correspondence of landmarks in the model and the object in the test image. Similarly, AAM was initialized by putting the mean shape (up to a scale factor) in the test image domain. The DSC of the average shape against true shapes is 0.79 ± 0.13 and 0.66 ± 0.24 for longitudinal and axial images respectively. In Fig. 1, the position of prostate shape at different stages is illustrated. The two initial shapes used for the two datasets respectively are shown in the first column (t=0) and the final regression results are shown in the last column (t=512).

---

[1] precision= $\frac{TP}{TP+FP}$, recall= $\frac{TP}{TP+FN}$, and DSC= $\frac{2TP}{2TP+FP+FN}$, where TP, FP, and FN are the number of true positive, false positive, and false negative pixels, respectively.

Table 1. Quantitative comparison of segmentation results for the two datasets. RMSE_ϕ: average RMSE in mm under ϕ mm, f_ϕ: failure rate ($\text{RMSE} > \phi$ mm).

Dataset	Method	$\text{RMSE}_{2.4}$	$f_{2.4}$	RMSE_3	f_3	Precision	Recall	DSC
Longi-tudinal	AAM	2.00±1.42	84.1%	2.29±0.11	72.8%	0.76±0.20	0.83±0.15	0.78±0.15
	CSR	1.89±0.17	27.0%	1.98±0.19	17.5%	0.88±0.14	0.93±0.06	0.90±0.10
	CSR+DDGVF	-	-	-	-	0.91±0.13	0.90±0.08	0.90±0.09
Axial	AAM	1.85± 0.44	96.0%	2.05±0.44	94.7%	0.87±0.11	0.82±0.06	0.84±0.08
	CSR	1.73 ±0.11	9.1%	1.75±0.14	6.5%	0.90±0.11	0.93±0.10	0.91±0.10
	CSR+DDGVF	-	-	-	-	0.94±0.11	0.89±0.10	0.91±0.10

Table 2. Training and testing time

Method	Training (50 images)	Testing (per image)
AAM	10.9 sec	51 sec
CSR	22 min	0.11 sec
CSR+DDGVF	22 min	0.92 sec

For the experiment, we use 5-fold cross validation (4 for training and 1 for testing) to avoid bias in such a splitting. All metrics are first averaged within each fold and the mean/standard deviation among the 5-fold are shown Table 1. It can be observed that the AAM has a much higher fail rate due to its sensitivity to initialization. The CSR achieves an average RMSE (under 3 mm) of 1.98 and 1.75 mm for the two datasets respectively. The CSR also outperforms the AAM for other performance metrics when only successful segmentation cases are counted. Our method is implemented in Matlab R2012a on a Windows machine with 3.2GHz CPU and 12GB RAM. The training and testing time is compared in Table 2. With an unoptimized Matlab code, the CSR requires 22 minutes to train 50 images, which is relatively long. However, our testing speed is only 0.92 seconds per image which is much faster than the AAM. This is desirable for real-time applications such as in-vivo experiments of BPH removal. The segmentation results of the CSR and the AAM is compared in Fig. 2.

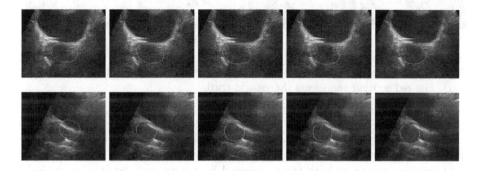

Fig. 1. Regressed shapes at different stages (from left to right) t=0, t=1, t=3, t=7, and t=512 respectively. First row is longitudinal view and the second row is axial view.

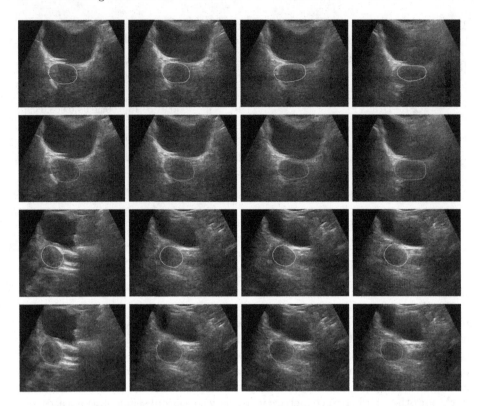

Fig. 2. Prostate segmentation results by active appearance model (first and third row) and cascaded shape regression (second and forth row). The red contour represents the ground truth and the green/yellow contour represents the segmentation results.

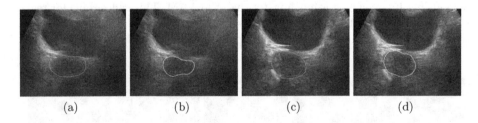

      (a)   (b)   (c)   (d)

Fig. 3. Segmentation results of CSR (green contour) and CSR+DDGVF (yellow contour). The red contour represents the ground truth.

Fig. 3 displays the final segmentation results. The prostate boundary after snake deformation using DDGVF is closer to the ground truth. We interpolate the landmark points on both the segmented boundary and the ground truth so that the distance between two neighboring points is between 0.5 to 1.5 pixels. The overlap ratios in the results of CSR+DDGVF are also shown in Table 1.

4   Conclusion and Future Work

A novel approach has been proposed for prostate segmentation from ECUS images. By using cascaded shape regression, our approach is able to efficiently locate the prostate boundary against shape, position, and orientation variations in ECUS images. With the help of DDGVF, efficient and accurate segmentation is achieved. Future work includes developing CSR+DDGVF into a real-time prostate tracking framework.

Acknowledgments. The project is supported by SERC Grant No. 1211480001, A*STAR, Singapore. Henry Ho and Tay Kae Jack for domain knowledge, Zhou Yufeng and Wilson Gao for experiment device, Huang Weimin and Zhou Jiayin for experiments and data.

References

1. Ghose, S., Oliver, A., Marti, R., Llado, X., Vilanova, J.C., Freixenet, J., Mitra, J., Sidibé, D., Meriaudeau, F.: A Survey of Prostate Segmentation Methodologies in Ultrasound, Magnetic Resonance and Computed Tomography Images. Comput. Methods Programs Biomed. 108(1), 262–287 (2012)
2. Dollar, P., Welinder, P., Perona, P.: Cascaded pose regression. In: CVPR, pp. 1078–1085 (2010)
3. Cao, X., Wei, Y., Wen, F., Sun, J.: Face Alignment by Explicit Shape Regression. In: CVPR (2012)
4. Ozuysal, M., Calonder, M., Lepetit, V., Fua, P.: Fast keypoint recognition using random ferns. IEEE Trans. Pattern Analysis and Machine Intelligence 32(3), 448–461 (2010)
5. Zaim, A., Jankun, J.: An Energy-Based Segmentation of Prostate from Ultrasound Images Using Dot-Pattern Select Cells. In: IEEE International Conference on Acoustics, Speech and Signal Processing, pp. 297–300 (2007)
6. Ladak, H.M., Mao, F., Wang, Y., Downey, D.B., Steinman, D.A., Fenster, A.: Prostate Segmentation from 2D Ultrasound Images. In: Proceedings of the 22nd Annual International Conference of the IEEE Engineering in Medicine and Biology Society, pp. 3188–3191 (2000)
7. Gong, L., Pathak, S.D., Haynor, D.R., Cho, P.S., Kim, Y.: Parametric Shape Modeling Using Deformable Superellipses for Prostate Segmentation. IEEE Transactions on Medical Imaging 23, 340–349 (2004)
8. Badiei, S., Salcudean, S.E., Varah, J., Morris, W.J.: Prostate Segmentation in 2D Ultrasound Images Using Image Warping and Ellipse Fitting. In: Larsen, R., Nielsen, M., Sporring, J. (eds.) MICCAI 2006. LNCS, vol. 4191, pp. 17–24. Springer, Heidelberg (2006)
9. Fan, S., Voon, L.K., Sing, N.W.: 3D Prostate Surface Detection from Ultrasound Images Based on Level Set Method. In: Dohi, T., Kikinis, R. (eds.) MICCAI 2002, Part II. LNCS, vol. 2489, pp. 389–396. Springer, Heidelberg (2002)
10. Zouqi, M., Samarabandu, J.: Prostate Segmentation from 2D Ultrasound Images Using Graph Cuts and Domain Knowledge. In: Canadian Conference on Computer and Robot Vision, pp. 359–362. IEEE Computer Society Press, USA (2008)

11. Chan, T.F., Vese, L.A.: Active contours without edges. IEEE Transactions on Image Processing 10(2), 266–277 (2001)
12. Richard, W.D., Keen, C.G.: Automated Texture Based Segmentation of Ultrasound Images of the Prostate. Computerized Medical Imaging and Graphics 20, 131–140 (1996)
13. Mohamed, S.S., Youssef, A.M., El-Saadany, E.F., Salama, M.M.A.: Prostate Tissue Characterization Using TRUS Image Spectral Features. In: Campilho, A., Kamel, M.S. (eds.) ICIAR 2006. LNCS, vol. 4142, pp. 589–601. Springer, Heidelberg (2006)
14. Cootes, T.F., Taylor, C.J., Cooper, D., Graham, J.: Active shape models - their training and application. Computer Vision and Image Understanding 61, 38–59 (1995)
15. Cootes, T.F., Edwards, G.J., Taylor, C.J.: Active appearance models. IEEE Trans. Pattern Analysis and Machine Intelligence 23, 681–685 (2001)
16. Zhou, S.: Shape regression machine and efficient segmentation of left ventricle endocardium from 2D B-mode echocardiogram. Medical Image Analysis 14, 563–581 (2010)
17. Friedman, J.H.: Greedy function approximation: A gradient boosting machine. The Annals of Statistics 29(5), 1189–1232 (2001)
18. Duffy, N., Helmbold, D.P.: Boosting methods for regression. Machine Learning 47(2-3), 153–200 (2002)
19. Breiman, L.: Random forests. In: Machine learning (2001)
20. Valstar, M., Martinez, B., Binefa, X., Pantic, M.: Facial point detection using boosted regression and graph models. In: CVPR (2010)
21. Cootes, T.F., Ionita, M.C., Lindner, C., Sauer, P.: Robust and Accurate Shape Model Fitting Using Random Forest Regression Voting. In: Fitzgibbon, A., Lazebnik, S., Perona, P., Sato, Y., Schmid, C. (eds.) ECCV 2012, Part VII. LNCS, vol. 7578, pp. 278–291. Springer, Heidelberg (2012)
22. Open source C++ AAM implementation, `http://www2.imm.dtu.dk/~aam/`
23. Cheng, J., Foo, S.: Dynamic directional gradient vector flow for snakes. IEEE Transactions on Image Processing 15(6), 1563–1571 (2006)

Evaluation of Endoscopic Image Enhancement for Feature Tracking: A New Validation Framework

Faïçal Selka[1,2], Stephane A. Nicolau[2], Vincent Agnus[2], Abdel Bessaid[1], Jacques Marescaux[2,3], and Luc Soler[2,3]

[1] Biomedical Engineering Laboratory, Abou Bekr Belkaid University-Algeria
[2] IRCAD 1 place de l'Hopital, Strasbourg-France
[3] IHU 1 place de l'Hopital, Strasbourg-France
selka.faical@gmail.com

Abstract. Feature tracking for endoscopic images is a critical component for image guided applications in minimally invasive surgery. Recent work in this field has shown success in acquiring tissue deformation, but it still faces issues. In particular, it often requires expensive algorithms to filter outliers. In this paper, we firstly propose two real-time pre-processes based on image filtering, to improve feature tracking robustness and thus reduce outlier percentage. However the performance evaluation of detection and tracking algorithms on endoscopic images is still difficult and not standardized, due to the difficulty of ground truth data acquisition. To overcome this drawback, we secondly propose a novel framework that allows to provide artificial ground truth data, and thus to evaluate detection and feature tracking performances. Finally, we demonstrate, using our framework on 9 different *in-vivo* video sequences, that the proposed pre-processes significantly increase the tracking performance.

1 Introduction

Minimally Invasive Surgery (MIS) gets more and more common nowadays. In comparison to open surgery, there are many advantages for the patient: less trauma, faster recovery, aesthetic reasons... However, important disadvantages arise for the surgeon: restricted vision, difficult hand-eye coordination, no tactile perception, loss of depth perception. Extensive research work in the field of computer vision, which attempts to provide 2D or 3D preoperative or intraoperative information to the surgeon [2], has been performed to reduce these disadvantages. For example, image mosaicing [19], 3D depth recovery [17,11] and augmented reality view [14] can assist surgeons to increase intervention safety. For these technologies to be successful, feature tracking of tissues must be robust and accurate. In addition, depending on the applications, it is desirable that the tracked features span the whole field of view.

The ability to successfully track a feature depends on its representation which usually includes colors, edges, corners, intensities, textures or gradients. Unlike

C.A. Linte et al. (Eds.): MIAR/AE-CAI 2013, LNCS 8090, pp. 75–85, 2013.
© Springer-Verlag Berlin Heidelberg 2013

synthetic scenes and outdoor environments, MIS images exhibit considerable drawbacks: specular reflection, shadow effects, dynamic lighting conditions, non-rigid deformation due to patient motion (heartbeat, breathing) and interactions with surgical instruments. These conditions may result in tracking failure. Several research studies attempt [13,21,20,16] to identify the best features to track from endoscopic images using optical flow and/or feature descriptor methods. Nevertheless, they have not yet resulted in a routinely used clinical application due to MIS image properties. In particular, no quantitative work has been conducted to evaluate the benefit of a pre-processing step based on image filtering to enhance image quality (dynamic range, contrast, noise response), which can improve feature tracking performance and avoid supplementary techniques to remove outliers [8] and/or to recover tracking failure [5] which can be time consuming. We believe that an adapted pre-processing step in **real-time** for MIS images is important to increase the tracking performance.

In this paper we investigate the influence of pre-process in tracking performance and show rigorously and quantitatively their improvement on detection and tracking steps using our proposed framework for feature tracking validation.

2   Related Work

Improving the identification of robust features using pre-processing methods in MIS images is not common. Wu et. al.[20] use histogram equalization to emphasize the gradient intensity to avoid tracking failure. In [21], they perform a Gaussian smoothing to reduce the noise response. However, neither of them did perform a quantitative assessment to evaluate the benefits of the pre-process.

Regarding evaluation methodology, it usually depends on the type of feature tracking approach: recursive or descriptor based methods. In both cases, providing ground truth data is a problem to evaluate the tracking performance.

Evaluation of the Detection Quality: Previous work [21,13,16] usually compares the number of detected points for different detectors and reports the percentage of the robust ones. No quantitative analysis to measure the distribution of points is provided and it do not investigate the choice of algorithm parameter values. Up to now, there is no clear and recognized methodology to evaluate and to compare different methods.

Evaluation of the Tracking Quality: In [12,16], they visually assess whether the points are well tracked over the sequence and report the percentage of robust features. This method is tedious, time consuming, subjective and must be repeated for each new sequence. In addition, manual labelling could be only done on salient features, which is difficult for the liver due to its homogeneous surface texture. Other approaches [8,13,21] evaluate the tracking performance using a 3D rigid model or phantom. They compute the registration error between the reconstructed surface (using Structure From Motion or Stereo) from the tracked points and the scanned 3D model. Although this measure allows to evaluate the tracking quality, it is an indirect measure that does not provide the tracking pixel accuracy and the percentage of robust points.

The main problem for tracking performance validation is related to the lack of ground truth data. Recently, a method to detect tracking failure caused by motion, occlusion, and slowly drifting trajectory for recursive tracking was proposed [9]. It is based on the forward-backward tracking error of selected features. Features are tracked frame by frame as they move forward in time and then, the video is played on reversed frames and features are tracked backward until the beginning of the video. If a feature is perfectly tracked, it should go back to its location on the first frame. We highlight that the proposed method can be considered as an artificial ground truth for recursive tracking methods, since it allows to know where each selected feature should arrive on the last frame of the forward-backward sequence (initial frame). However, in [9] the tracking computation of a feature from frame t to $t+1$ is based on almost the same image window as from $t+1$ to t, therefore the forward and backward tracking are correlated causing the underestimation of the tracking error.

The main contributions of this paper are twofold. Firstly, we propose two pre-processes based on image filtering to improve feature detection and tracking. Secondly, we describe a novel framework for evaluating tracking efficiency (accuracy, robustness and distribution) for a recursive tracking method (as optical flow). This framework provides an artificial ground truth data based on an improved version of the forward-backward tracking that tackles the correlation issue mentioned above. This framework allows not only to evaluate the influence of pre-process, but also to compare different detection and tracking methods.

3   Pre-processing Methods

Because of varying illumination (shadows, reflections) and to the unique source of light located at the tip of the endoscope, dark areas in endoscopic images can be important (up to 40% of the image size) involving an underexposed histogram. It seems necessary to adaptively adjust the contrast on the dark area of the image and also to increase the gradient of the inner structure and vessels to improve feature detection and tracking. Our implementation uses GPU acceleration of OpenCV without a GPU parallelization and optimisation. Time computation per HD frame takes approximatively 0.01 seconds for Egal Smooth and 0.06 seconds for Top Hat on a PC core I7-3.4 GHz with Nvidia GTS 450 graphic card. Fig.1 shows an example on MIS images of the two pre-process methods we propose.

1. Egal Smooth : In order to enhance contrast of the images, histogram equalization (HE) seems well adapted since it will enlarge the dynamic of the gray level in the peak containing information on the dark area. A standard method to enhance contrast for color images applies HE to every channel of an RGB image independently. This technique may result in a higher concentration of bright pixels and can cause color artefact due to the combined encoding of intensity and chromaticity in the RGB images [6], which can cause undesirable effects for feature tracking. To overcome this problem, we convert the image to the HSV color space and enhance Saturation (S) and Value (V) independently and later re-transform to the RGB color space. We keep the chromaticity of the image

(Hue) unchanged. The HE of V (resp. S) makes the dark areas more contrasted (resp. the colors become more vivid). This technique gives better results for luminance distribution. We apply a Gaussian filter (G_σ) to the S and V channels after applying HE, with $\sigma = 1.5$ (and kernel size 5×5). The σ was adapted empirically for our specific image resolution so as not to erase the small inner structures (vessels). Applying a Gaussian filter to V (resp. S) reduces noise response and increases entropy of the histogram (resp. spreads out the color of dark edges like vessels and inner structures).

2. Top Hat : Another way to increase image contrast is to locally enhance details (edges, corners) in the image. A neighbourhood-based morphological contrast operator can be obtained by computing the white and black top hat of the image. The white top hat is then added to the original image to enhance bright objects and the black top hat is subtracted from the resulting image to enhance dark objects. In order to perform a morphological operator on color image, we use a vectorial order for the opening and closing [7]. We also apply a G_σ ($\sigma = 1.5$ and kernel size 5×5) to the output image to reduce the noise.

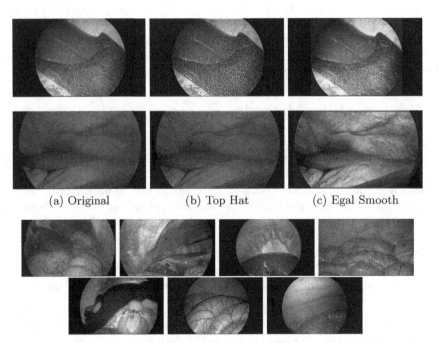

    (a) Original   (b) Top Hat   (c) Egal Smooth

Fig. 1. Example of the two pre-process results (2 first lines) and image samples of the various remaining sequences we used (2 last line).

4   Evaluation Methodology

In this section, we first explain our modified version of the forward-backward tracking to obtain artificial ground truth data. Secondly, we explain the two parts of our framework to evaluate feature tracking and feature detection performances.

4.1   Forward-Backward Tracking Based on Even-odd Frames

Our approach is based on the assumption that to evaluate the final drift error, the backward tracking should be decorrelated from the forward tracking. In other words, the feature should go back to the initial position with different frames than for the forward tracking. This decorrelation is done by making the forward tracking on the even frames and the backward tracking on the odd frames. Let $FB = (I_0, I_2, I_4, ..., I_{n-2}, I_n, I_{n-1}, ..., I_3, I_1, I_0)$ be the modified forward-backward sequence of $(n + 2)$ frames where I_t is the tth frame of the considered video sequence. For each feature we measure the Euclidean distance ϵ between its initial position and its final position of the FB sequence. This distance corresponds to the feature drift during the tracking step. In the case of an accurate feature tracking, ϵ should be less than 1 pixel. From the computation of ϵ for each feature, we firstly calculate the percentage of features, where ϵ is below a certain threshold. This percentage assesses **the robustness of tracking**. However, this threshold can be misleading because it does not indicate the accuracy of the properly tracked features. Indeed, two pre-processes may provide the same percentage of robust features, but the ϵ distances may be lower for one of the pre-processes. Thus, we also propose to provide the ϵ **histogram** of the set of tracked features, which gives the tracking accuracy.

4.2   Evaluation of Feature Tracking Performance

This first method evaluates the pre-process influence on the feature tracking robustness and accuracy (regardless of the feature detection method used). In fact, the number and robustness of features during the tracking step usually depends on a particular threshold. Varying the threshold could allow a supplementary detection of features but with doubtful tracking performance. Thus, to demonstrate the advantage of a pre-process, the percentage of robust points should be increased whatever the threshold used. Consequently, we propose the following methodology.

For a given threshold, we detect features in the first frame without pre-process. We then track the feature set over the forward/backward sequence with the pre-process and without it. We compare the **percentage of robust points** and the ϵ **histogram** with and without pre-process. This tracking is repeated for different threshold values that span the threshold range. Finally, we obtain a comparison of robustness and accuracy for the whole threshold range.

4.3   Evaluation of Feature Detection Performance

This second evaluation method assesses to what extent the pre-process improves the robustness, accuracy and distribution of the detected features. In fact, to compare two detection methods (or the benefit of a pre-process filter), the common approach is to provide the percentage of robust points only. However, the distribution and density of detected points in the first image are also important factors. Moreover, standard approaches compare the detection performance without evaluating the influence of detection threshold and use standard detection parameters provided by the available implementation [21,13,16]. The number of detected features can thus be totally different in the compared set. Finally, lowering the detection threshold causes the increase of the detected features but this does not necessarily mean they are robust and well distributed in the entire image. Therefore, we propose the following methodology.

In order to compare the quality of feature detection, we need to compare feature sets of the same size detected with and without pre-process. Hence, given a detector threshold for the sequence without pre-process, we choose a different threshold for pre-process sequence so that we get the same number of detected features. Then, we firstly compare the distribution of detected points with and without pre-process, using for each set 2 histograms: one for x-axis (image columns) and one for y-axis (image rows). Secondly, we compare tracking accuracy and robustness with and without pre-process, computed using the same method as in Sec. 4.2 (**percentage of robust points and ϵ histogram**). The process is repeated for different numbers of features (and so for different threshold values).

5   In-vivo Evaluation

We evaluate our approach on 9 *in-vivo* HD video sequences (1920×1080) $25 fps$, corresponding to a panning view of an abdominal exploration. Three of them contain a human liver and gallbladder and the others contain pig liver, spleen and bowels (cf Fig. 1). From top to bottom, then from left to right, the sequence contains respectively 109, 317, 185, 159, 111, 207, 429, 189, 105 frames. In this evaluation, we firstly evaluate the influence of pre-process during tracking with Shi-Tomasi (so called GFTT for good features to track) [18], FAST [15], BRISK [10] and SURF [3] detectors and Lucas-Kanade (LK) [1] tracking algorithm. Secondly, we show the influence of pre-process during detection. The OpenCV library was used with following parameters, which were used on all sequences: GFTT threshold was defined as: from 0.001 to 0.01 with a step of 0.001 and from 0.01 to 0.09 with a step of 0.01 to have a wide variation in the number of features detected. For BRISK: octave = 3, detection thresholds from 10 to 28 with a step of 1. For FAST: the default mask 9-16 was used, a non-maxima suppression set to true, and detection thresholds from 10 to 46 with a step of 2. For SURF: octave = 4, hessian thresholds from 50 to 900 with a step of 50. For LK: a window size of (25×25) and pyramid level of 3.

5.1   Evaluation of the Influence of Pre-process During Tracking

The evaluation was run for each sequence, we detect a set of points without preprocess, then track it in the 3 modes (no preprocess, Egal Smooth and Top Hat).

Table 1. Average percentage of robust features with and without pre-process

Detection		No pre-process	
Tracking	No pre-process	Top Hat	Egal Smooth
GFTT	77.7%	83.3%	81.1%
SURF	81.6%	90.4%	91.3%
BRISK	81.8%	85.6%	88.3%
FAST	77.5%	82.2%	84.8%

In Fig. 2 we show an example result for one sequence (pig bowels). Fig. 2a, 2b, 2c, 2d shows the percentage of robust features with a drift under 5 pixels (5 pixels correspond to the thinnest vessel width). One can clearly see that each proposed pre-process improves the robustness of tracking, whatever the detection threshold and the detector used. Fig. 2e, 2f, 2g, 2h shows the ϵ **distances histogram** for a fixed threshold to get 500 detected features with GFTT, SURF, BRISK and FAST detectors. We print the number of points with drift lower than one pixel. It appears clearly that pre-process also increases accuracy of the tracking. Tab.1 shows the percentage of average results of robust features for all threshold values and for the 9 sequences. The robustness is improved up to 9% for Top Hat and 10% for Egal Smooth. SURF detector performs with a better robustness than the other detectors as it has been already reported in [4].

5.2 Evaluation of the Influence of Pre-process During Detection

In this evaluation we adapt thresholds to get the same number of points detected using each pre-process and without as explained in Sec. 4.3. Fig. 3 shows the number and the distribution of detected features with and without pre-process on one example sequence (human liver 184 frames). One can see that for the same number of features detected, we provide a slightly better distribution. Tab. 2 provides the percentage of robust points for the example sequence and the average result over the 9 sequences. One can clearly see that each pre-process improves the robustness up to 8% for Top Hat and Egal Smooth with better results for SURF detector. On average the accuracy of tracking from the ϵ histogram is improved using Top Hat (resp. Egal Smooth) of 8.2% (resp. 9.4%).

Table 2. Percentage of robust features properly tracked with respect to the pre-process applied

Pre-processes	No pre-process		Top Hat		Egal Smooth	
Sequence	Liver	Average	Liver	Average	Liver	Average
GFTT	84.3%	78.7%	93.1%	82.1%	94.3%	83.8%
SURF	87.5%	76.4%	96.7%	84.3%	95.8%	84.5%
BRISK	84.1%	77.1%	91.3%	81.1%	93.5%	82.4%
FAST	83.1%	74.8%	88%	79.2%	91.3%	82%

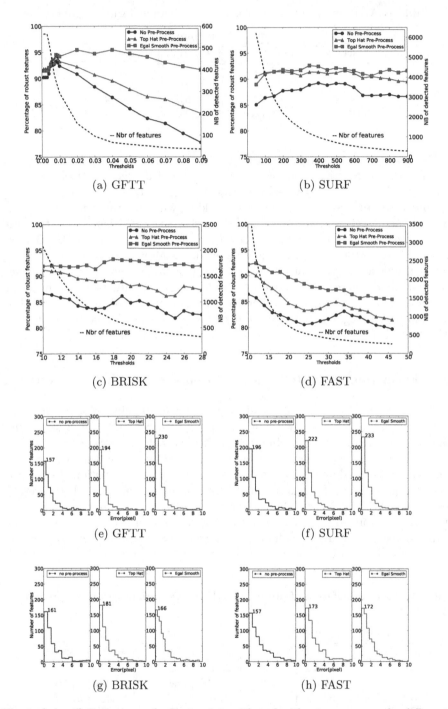

Fig. 2. (a,b,c,d) Percentage of robust points with and without pre-process for different thresholds. (e,f,g,h) ϵ histogram distance for 500 points.

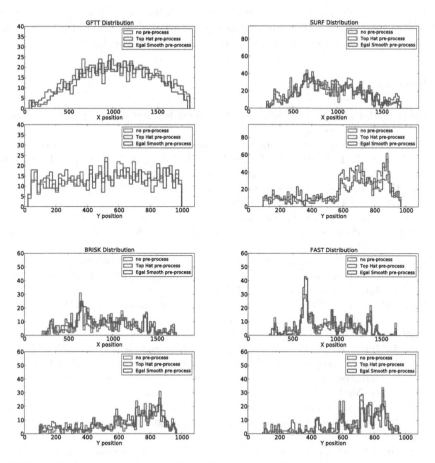

Fig. 3. Number of points and their distribution with and without pre-process

6 Conclusion

We have presented a novel methodology based on a revisited form of the forward backward error, for feature tracking and detection evaluation for endoscopic images. It allows to compare different detectors, tracking algorithms and
the influence of a pre-process step providing artificial ground truth. We highlight
that our framework requires a few seconds to evaluate tracking performance of
a triplet detector/tracker/parameters and thus can be applied in early intervention to find an adapted triplet to the current scene (provided that tracking is
required a few minutes after the intervention starts). We also show that including pre-process to improve image quality, can increase the efficiency of detector
and tracking algorithms. The pre-processes are designed to take the specificity
of endoscopic images into account, in particular the presence of vessels and their

noticeable characteristics (color and shape). Results showed an increase of feature robustness up to 10% and accuracy up to 9%. In the future, we will strengthen our evaluation on more organs (stomach, uterus, heart).

References

1. Baker, S.: Lucas-kanade 20 years on: A unifying framework. International Journal of Computer Vision 56(3), 221–255 (2004)
2. Bano, J., et al.: Simulation of pneumoperitoneum for laparoscopic surgery planning. In: Ayache, N., Delingette, H., Golland, P., Mori, K. (eds.) MICCAI 2012, Part I. LNCS, vol. 7510, pp. 91–98. Springer, Heidelberg (2012)
3. Bay, H., et al.: Speeded-up robust features (SURF). Computer Vision and Image Understanding 110(3), 346–359 (2008)
4. Elhawary, H., Popovic, A.: Robust feature tracking on the beating heart for a robotic-guided endoscope. The International Journal of Medical Robotics and Computer Asisted Surgery, 459–468 (July 2011)
5. Giannarou, S., Visentini-Scarzanella, M., Yang, G.-Z.: Probabilistic Tracking of Affine-Invariant Anisotropic Regions. IEEE Transactions on Pattern Analysis and Machine Intelligence, 1–14 (March 2012)
6. Han, J.H., et al.: A Novel 3-D Color Histogram Equalization Method With Uniform 1-D Gray Scale Histogram. IEEE Image Processing, 506–512 (2011)
7. Hanbury, A.: The morphological top-hat operator generalised to multi-channel images. In: International Conference on Pattern Recognition, pp. 672–675 (2004)
8. Hu, M., et al.: Reconstruction of a 3D surface from video that is robust to missing data and outliers: Application to minimally invasive surgery using stereo and mono endoscopes. Medical Image Analysis (December 2010)
9. Kalal, Z., et al.: Forward-Backward Error: Automatic Detection of Tracking Failures. In: International Conference on Pattern Recognition, pp. 2756–2759 (August 2010)
10. Leutenegger, S., Chli, M., Siegwart, R.Y.: BRISK: Binary Robust invariant scalable keypoints. In: 2011 International Conference on Computer Vision, pp. 2548–2555 (November 2011)
11. Mahmoud, N., Nicolau, S.A., Keshk, A., Ahmad, M.A., Soler, L., Marescaux, J.: Fast 3D structure from motion with missing points from registration of partial reconstructions. In: Perales, F.J., Fisher, R.B., Moeslund, T.B. (eds.) AMDO 2012. LNCS, vol. 7378, pp. 173–183. Springer, Heidelberg (2012)
12. Masson, N., et al.: Comparison of visual tracking algorithms on in vivo sequences for robot-assisted flexible endoscopic surgery. In: EMBC, pp. 5571–5576 (January 2009)
13. Mountney, P., Yang, G.-Z.: Context specific descriptors for tracking deforming tissue. Medical Image Analysis 16(3), 550–561 (2011)
14. Nicolau, S., et al.: Augmented reality in laparoscopic surgical oncology. Surgical Oncology 20(3), 189–201 (2011)
15. Rosten, E., Drummond, T.: Machine learning for high-speed corner detection. In: Leonardis, A., Bischof, H., Pinz, A. (eds.) ECCV 2006, Part I. LNCS, vol. 3951, pp. 430–443. Springer, Heidelberg (2006)
16. Selka, F., et al.: Performance evaluation of simultaneous RGB analysis for feature detection and tracking in endoscopic images. In: Medical Image Understanding and Analysis, pp. 249–254 (2012)

17. Stoyanov, D., Darzi, A., Yang, G.-Z.: Dense 3D depth recovery for soft tissue deformation during robotically assisted laparoscopic surgery. In: Barillot, C., Haynor, D.R., Hellier, P. (eds.) MICCAI 2004. LNCS, vol. 3217, pp. 41–48. Springer, Heidelberg (2004)
18. Tomasi, C.: Good features to track. In: Proceedings of IEEE Conference on Computer Vision and Pattern Recognition, CVPR 1994, pp. 593–600 (1994)
19. Vemuri, A.S., et al.: Endoscopic Video Mosaicing: Application to Surgery and Diagnostics. In: Living Imaging Workshop (December 2011)
20. Wu, C.-H.: Automatic extraction and visualization of human inner structures from endoscopic image sequences. In: Proceedings of SPIE, vol. 5369, pp. 464–473 (2004)
21. Yip, M., et al.: Tissue Tracking and Registration for Image-Guided Surgery. IEEE Transactions on Medical Imaging 31(11), 2169–2182 (2012)

Intensity-Based 3D-2D Mesh-to-Image Registration Using Mesh-Based Digitally Reconstructed Radiography

Shun Miao[1], Tri Huynh[1], Cyprien Adnet[1], Marcus Pfister[2], and Rui Liao[1]

[1] Siemens Corporation, Corporate Technology, Princeton, NJ, USA
[2] Siemens Healthcare, Erlangen, Germany

Abstract. Intensity-based 3D-2D registration is a well-established technique shown to be effective for many clinical applications. However, it is valid mainly for 3D Computed Tomography (CT) volume to 2D X-ray image registration because the computation of volume-based Digitally Reconstructed Radiography (DRR) relies on the linear relationship between CT's intensity and the attenuation coefficient of the underlying structure for X-ray. This paper introduces a mesh-based DRR renderer that simulates realistic-looking X-ray images from 3D meshes, which can be used to replace conventional volume-based DRR in intensity-based 3D-2D registration for 3D volumes from various image modalities. The proposed renderer calculates the travel distance of a given ray within the mesh, and computes X-ray attenuation based on the travel distance and the object's attenuation property. The proposed method also uses a novel ray-casting strategy that takes GPU architecture into consideration for high computational efficiency. Validation results show that the proposed mesh-based DRR simulates X-ray images with a high fidelity, and intensity-based 3D-2D registration using the resulting mesh-based DRR achieves satisfactory results on clinical data.

Keywords: 3D-2D Registration, Mesh Rendering, Digitally Reconstructed Radiography, Ray Tracing, Endovascular Aneurysm Repair.

1   Introduction

Registration of pre-operative 3D volumes and intra-operative 2D images is one of the enabling technologies widely used in image-guided therapy [1]. After being actively researched over a decade, intensity-based 3D-2D registration methods are shown to be effective for registering 3D Computed Tomography (CT) and 2D X-ray images. Specifically, volume-based Digitally Reconstructed Radiography (DRR) is produced to simulate 2D X-ray images from the 3D data and the pose of the 3D volume is iteratively optimized by maximizing the similarity between the DRR and X-ray images. However, volume-based DRR (volume-DRR) technique has two major limitations. First, the 3D image modality is largely limited to CT because the intensity of the 3D volume is assumed to be linearly correlated to the attenuation coefficient of the underlying structure for X-ray. Second, the speed of volume-DRR with large volumetric data (512x512x267) is relatively slow (184 ms/DRR) even on modern GPU (Geforce 8800

C.A. Linte et al. (Eds.): MIAR/AE-CAI 2013, LNCS 8090, pp. 86–96, 2013.

GTX) [2] due to the heavy computation of volume ray casting, which makes comprehensive optimization schemes using a large number of iterations less affordable.

To solve these limitations, some attempts have been made to use meshes of the target object to generate artificial 2D projection images to replace volume-DRR, and 3D-2D registration using meshes is referred to as mesh-to-image registration. In [3], Thivierge-Gaulin *et al.* proposed to render the mesh to a binary 2D mask, and classify the 2D pixels of the X-ray image into two groups: inside and outside the mask. Based on the extreme simplification by binarization of the mesh projection, a special similarity measure, i.e. the summation of the variance of intensities in each group, needs to be used for registration purpose. However, this similarity measure is relatively coarse and sensitive to outliers, and can only work under the assumption that intensities of the target object is homogeneous in the X-ray image. In addition, it is not sensitive to small movement and therefore may lead to deteriorated registration accuracy. Kaiser *et al.* proposed to divide the target object, a transesophageal echocardiogram probe, into two pieces according to the material's attenuation property [4]. Two binary masks are then rendered from the two meshes corresponding to the two pieces, and are blended using alpha values based on the material's attenuation coefficients to generate a DRR-like image. Although this method makes one step further comparing to [3], it still does not fully utilize the geometric information of the 3D mesh, and completely ignores the thickness of the object, which is in fact a key factor in the formation of real X-ray images.

In this paper, we introduce a novel mesh-based DRR (mesh-DRR) rendering algorithm that simulates the process of X-ray traveling through the object and getting attenuated. The proposed mesh-DRR takes both the attenuation property and the geometry of the object into consideration, and therefore can simulate real X-ray images with a high fidelity, similar to volume-DRR generated for CT. With the resulting mesh-DRR, almost all the existing intensity-based 3D-2D registration techniques can be directly applied on mesh-to-image 3D-2D registration, meaning that given the segmentation of the target objects it can register various 3D image modalities other than CT, e.g. Magnetic Resonance (MR), Positron Emission Tomography (PET), Computer-aid Design (CAD) model of medical devices and etc. In addition, rendering of mesh-DRR is much more computationally efficient than volume-DRR, which significantly speeds up the 3D-2D registration process and potentially enables more comprehensive optimization schemes.

2   X-ray Attenuation Model

When X-ray travels through an object, the attenuation can be described by

$$P = P_0 e^{\int_L \mu(x)dx}, \tag{1}$$

where P_0 and P are X-ray densities before and after attenuation, L is the path of X-ray in the target object, and $\mu(x)$ denotes the attenuation coefficients along the path of X-ray. When using a logarithm detector, the intensity of X-ray image is

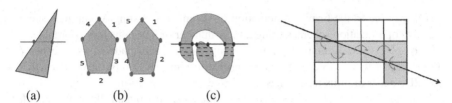

Fig. 1. (a) Calculation of intersection points and lines between a mesh triangle and a 2D slice. (b) Sorting and connection of the intersection lines in a 2D slice into 2D contours. (c) Row-by-row binarization by calculation of intersection points between a row and 2D contours.

Fig. 2. Voxel traversal for uniform grid space partitioning. The voxels can be naturally traversed in the front-to-back order.

$$I = \int_L \mu(x)dx. \tag{2}$$

For many objects, e.g. metal implants, contrast medium, bony structures, soft tissues, and etc., the attenuation coefficient is largely the same within the object. Assuming a uniform attenuation coefficient within the object, the X-ray image intensity becomes proportional to the distance the ray travels within the object:

$$I = \mu \cdot D. \tag{3}$$

If the target object is divided into several sub-objects with different attenuation coefficients, for example, bony structures versus soft tissues, the X-ray image intensity can be approximated as

$$I = \sum_i \mu_i \cdot D_i = \sum_i I_i. \tag{4}$$

where μ_i and D_i are the attenuation coefficient and travel distance in the i-th sub-object, respectively, and I_i is the mesh-DRR rendered for the i-th sub-object. In the rest of the paper, unless specified otherwise we focus on a mono-piece mesh-DRR for the simplicity of presentation, and the presented method can be directly extended to multi-piece cases following Eqn. 4.

3   Mesh-DRR Rendering

3.1   Mesh Cleaning

According to the X-ray attenuation model, the meshes used for mesh-DRR rendering must be non-overlapping, because otherwise the overlapping area will be counted multiple times. However, the segmentation of the target object can be presented in various forms for different applications, and might not meet the non-overlapping requirement. Therefore, we perform pre-processing on the input meshes to merge the multiple overlapping meshes corresponding to the same tissue property (i.e. attenuation coefficient) into a single closed mesh.

For a given mesh, we first convert it to a binary volume mask. For efficient computation, we perform the conversion slice by slice. In particular, for a given slice we calculate the intersection points and lines of the mesh with this slice (Fig.1(a)). The intersection lines for this slice are then sorted and connected to obtain one or multiple 2D contours (Fig.1.(b)). Finally, we calculate the intersection points between the 2D contours and each row in this slice. Those voxels between the odd and even intersection points are inside the mesh, and those voxels between the even and odd intersection points are outside the mesh (Fig. 1(c)). Conversion of the mesh into a binary mask for this slice is achieved by traversing all the rows in this slice, and the same process repeats for all the slices in this volume. Once the binary masks for all the meshes are created, they are classified into different groups according to their attenuation property, e.g. contrast agent, bone, soft tissue, air and etc. The binary masks in the same group are then merged to generate one binary mask with the same attenuation property. Marching cube algorithm [5] is applied on each of the merged binary masks to generate non-overlapping closed meshes, one for each group with a known attenuation coefficient. Note that the iso-surface of a binary mask tends to have aliasing artifacts; a pseudo distance map is thus built near the mask boundary and updated iteratively according to mean curvature flow [6]. The corresponding mesh is then extracted from the distance map as zero level set using marching cube algorithm.

3.2   Mesh Decimation

The meshes extracted from a high-resolution 3D binary volume by marching cube algorithm are usually very dense, providing details of the object that are typically not important for 3D-2D registration purpose. On the other hand, the rendering efficiency of mesh-DRR (will be described in details in the next section) is proportional to the number of triangles in the input meshes. Therefore, in most cases these meshes can be decimated dramatically without significantly affecting the appearance of mesh-DRR while significantly speeding up the rendering and in turn the registration process. In this paper, we use a mesh decimation algorithm similar to the algorithm described in [7], with some modifications to preserve the topology of the original mesh as well as increase the speed. Essentially the mesh decimation algorithm iteratively contracts one vertex pair into one point until the number of triangles is reduced to the target number. To determine which vertex pair to contract, a quadratic error is computed for each pair to measure the geometrical difference caused by contracting the pair, and the one with the smallest quadratic error is contracted. Additional dimensions can be added to the vertices and quadratics to take various properties of the mesh into consideration, e.g. geometry, normal, color and 2D texture. For our purpose, the quadratics is defined for geometry only for higher computational efficiency. The vertex pairs are stored using a min heap data structure for efficient determination of the pair with the smallest quadratic error. After the contraction, both the quadratic errors of those affected vertex pairs and the min heap are updated. While [7] uses general vertex pair contraction that can merge unconnected regions of the model, we only allow contraction of points connected by an edge, which guarantees that the decimated mesh has the same topology as the original mesh, which is important for medical applications where small structures are of interest. In addition, the evaluation of quadratic error of unconnected vertex pair can be avoided, which increases the speed of mesh decimation.

3.3   Ray-Mesh Intersection

According to Eqn. 3, given a closed mesh of an object with uniform attenuation coefficients, the intensity of mesh-DRR for a given pixel can be generated by shooting a ray from the source to the detector and calculating the distance it travels within the mesh. The calculation of distance requires detection of all the intersections between the ray and the mesh, which is different from standard mesh ray-casting problem where only the closest intersection is of interest and thus detected. In particular, a ray enters and leaves the object alternatively, resulting in an even number of intersections. If all the intersections are detected and sorted by their distance to the source, denoted as $\{q_k\}$, odd and even intersection points then represent the position of the ray entering and leaving the object, respectively. Therefore, the travel distance within the object can be computed as

$$D = \sum_{k=1}^{N} \|q_{2k} - q_{2k-1}\|_2. \tag{5}$$

Calculation of all the intersections of a mesh with a ray is computationally expensive, because unless some sort of culling is performed, each ray must be tested for intersection/non-intersection with all the triangles. A common strategy for intersection culling is space partitioning, which partitions the 3D space into sub-regions, and each sub-region contains a subset of triangles. In this paper, the partitioned sub-region is referred to as a "voxel". During ray-casting, we first perform ray-voxel intersection test to detect the voxels along the path of the ray, and only perform ray-triangle intersection test for triangles in these voxels. In this manner, the intersection tests of a large number of triangles in voxels that are not along the path of the ray can be avoided. There are two popular space partitioning schemes: kd-tree where voxels are of different sizes [8], and constant voxel partitioning [9]. We use constant voxel partitioning because the uniform grid structure makes it straightforward to traverse voxels pierced by the ray in the front-to-back order, which is essential for efficient implementation of mesh-DRR rendering on a Graphic Processing Unit (GPU). The voxel traversal algorithm is shown in Fig. 2, which, for a high efficiency, detects the face through which the ray leaves the current voxel, and tests ray-voxel intersection for only the neighboring voxel in that direction. This process repeats until the ray travels out of the boundary of the volume.

The proposed mesh-DRR rendering algorithm is implemented on GPU for high computational efficiency. In particular, we use ray-based parallelization that lunches one thread for each ray to traverse voxels and compute intersections. The computation of Eqn. 5 requires sorted intersection lists, which are typically achieved by saving all the intersections with their corresponding source-to-intersection distance and performing sorting after traversal. However, saving all intersections is not preferable in GPU implementation because the on-chip shared or per-thread buffer might not be sufficient to store all the intersections for a given ray. Global memory of GPU

Table 1. Pesudo code of the mesh-DRR rendering algorithm

1.	$R \leftarrow$ the ray	17.	$P_{curr} \leftarrow$ intersection point
2.	$N \leftarrow$ current traversed voxel	18.	**end if**
3.	$\lambda_{max} \leftarrow 0$	19.	**end if**
4.	$\lambda_{entry} \leftarrow$ entry distance of R	20.	**end for**
5.	$\lambda_{exit} \leftarrow$ exit distance of R	21.	$\lambda_{max} \leftarrow$ source to P_{curr} distance
6.	$P_{odd} \leftarrow$ nil	22.	**if** P_{curr} is odd intersection (entering mesh)
7.	$P_{curr} \leftarrow$ nil		
8.	$D \leftarrow 0$	23.	$P_{odd} \leftarrow P_{curr}$
		24.	**else**
9.	**while** $\lambda_{entry} < \lambda_{exit}$	25.	$D \leftarrow D + ||P_{curr} - P_{odd}||_2$
10.	**do**	26.	**end if**
11.	$\lambda_{min} \leftarrow$ infinity	27.	**while** $C > 1$
12.	$C \leftarrow 0$	28.	$\lambda_{entry} \leftarrow$ exist distance of the current traversed voxel
13.	**for** all triangles T in N		
14.	**if** R intersects with T in N, and the source to intersection distance $d > \lambda_{max}$	29.	$N \leftarrow$ next neighboring voxel along R
		30.	**end while**
15.	$C \leftarrow C + 1$	31.	**return** D
16.	**if** $d < \lambda_{min}$		

is usually large, but memory access could be very slow when coalesced memory transaction cannot be guaranteed. In addition, as GPU does not allow dynamic memory allocation, designing a data structure to save an arbitrary number of intersections could be problematic.

We propose a triangle traversal algorithm to ensure that all intersections for a given ray are detected in the front-to-back order, so that Eqn. 5 can be updated iteratively during the traversal process with minimum memory consumption. In particular, each thread only needs a buffer for storing one intersection point. When an odd intersection point is detected, it is saved in the buffer, waiting for the following even intersection point. Once the even intersection point is detected, the distance between the two points is calculated and added to D, and the buffer can be used to store the next odd intersection point. Since the front-to-back order of voxel traversal has already been guaranteed by the voxel traversal algorithm [9], we only need to make sure that all the intersections within each voxel are also visited in the front-to-back order. The basic strategy is to traverse all triangles in one voxel multiple times, and only the unprocessed intersection with the smallest distance is processed at a time. This process repeats until there are no more unprocessed intersections in this voxel. The triangle traversal process will then move onto the next voxel until all the voxels are traversed (The pseudo codes are shown in Table 1).

4   Experiments and Results

4.1   Mesh-DRR Rendering and Similarity Profile

We first conducted experiments to evaluate the appearance and speed of the proposed mesh-DRR rendering. The intensity-based similarity profile of mesh-DRR was further

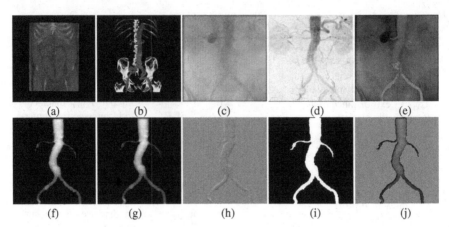

Fig. 3. (a) CT volume. (b) Segmentation meshes for the abdominal aorta. (c) Original fluoroscopic image. (d) Maximum opacity image. (e) Overlay of the 3D model on the fluoroscopic image. (f) CT-DRR. (g) Mesh-DRR. (h) Subtraction image of CT-DRR and mesh-DRR. (i) Binary-DRR as proposed in [3]. (j) Subtraction image of CT-DRR and binary-DRR, showing the significant intensity difference.

computed against volume-DRR for CT (CT-DRR) and clinical X-ray images. The experiment was conducted on clinical datasets from 3 patients undergoing Endovascular Aneurysm Repair (EVAR) procedures, and each patient had a contrast-enhanced pre-operative CT (Fig. 3(a) with vessel segmentations (abdominal aorta, renal arteries and iliac arteries, Fig. 3(b)) and an intra-operative angiographic sequence with contrast injection (Fig. 3(c). Mesh-DRR was generated from the meshes using the proposed method, and CT-DRR was rendered from the pre-operative CT volume with the vessel segmentation mask using conventional volume-DRR rendering. As a comparison, binary mesh rendering as proposed in [2] was also generated and is referred to as binary-DRR. On a modern GPU (Nvida Quadro FX4800), the average runtime for rendering 256×256 mesh-DRR from 3000 triangles is ~3.2 ms, while a CT-DRR rendering using volume ray casting on the same GPU takes ~25 ms for a 256×256×256 CT volume.

Fig. 3 demonstrates the difference between mesh-DRR and CT-DRR. The mesh-DRR rendered from a mesh with 3000 triangles (Fig. 3(g)) has almost no noticeable difference from the CT-DRR (Fig. 3(f)), and their subtraction image is mostly neutral, with a root mean square error (RMSE) of 0.0265 after normalization of the intensities to [0 1] (Fig. 3(h)). In comparison, the subtraction image between binary-DRR and CT-DRR shows a large difference (RMSE of 0.2093), especially at the distal part of the renal and iliac arteries (Fig. 3(j)).

As the main application of mesh-DRR is intensity-based 3D-2D registration, we furthermore analyzed the profile of intensity-based similarity measures on both phantom and real datasets using CT-DRR, mesh-DRR, and binary-DRR. A similarity profile shows the similarity measure of the moving image and the reference image with respect to different offsets from the ground truth position, and is widely used to

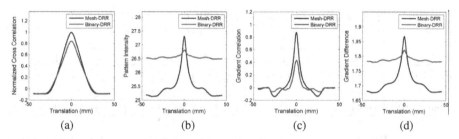

Fig. 4. (a) Normalized Cross Correlation (b) Pattern Intensity (c) Gradient Correlation and (d) Gradient Difference similarity profile for mesh-DRR and binary-DRR on phantom data

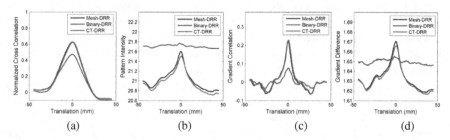

Fig. 5. (a) Normalized Cross Correlation (b) Pattern Intensity (c) Gradient Correlation and (d) Gradient Difference similarity profile for mesh-DRR, binary-DRR, and CT-DRR on real data

evaluate the property of similarity measures. A good similarity measure should have the global maximum at the target position with a wide basin and has few local maximums. We evaluated 4 similarity measures, including Normalized Cross Correlation (NCC), Pattern Intensity (PI), Gradient Correlation (GC) and Gradient Difference (GD). In phantom tests, a CT-DRR rendered from a known pose was used as the reference image with a known ground truth, and the similarity profiles of mesh-DRR and binary-DRR were generated against the CT-DRR (Fig. 4). In tests with real data, the maximum opacity image of the abdominal aorta calculated from the intra-operative angiographic image (Fig. 3(f)) was used as the reference image, and the ground truth pose was manually obtained by an expert. The similarity profiles of CT-DRR, mesh-DRR and binary-DRR were then plotted against the maximum opacity image. Both Fig. 4 and Fig. 5 show that the similarity profile of mesh-DRR has a more dominant peak at the ground truth position and less number of local maxima than that of binary-DRR. Fig. 5 shows that mesh-DRR and CT-DRR have very similar similarity profiles for all similarity measures, indicating that mesh-DRR can be potentially used in intensity-based 3D-2D registration for a wide variety of 3D image modalities other than CT, given the segmentation of the target object.

4.2   Mesh-to-Image Registration Using Mesh-DRR

In this experiment, we further integrated the mesh-DRR renderer into an intensity-based 3D-2D registration framework and evaluated the mesh-to-volume registration accuracy

Table 2. 2D TRE (pixels) using mesh-DRR, CT-DRR and binary-DRR

	NCC			GD		
	Patient 1	Patient 2	Patient 3	Patient 1	Patient 2	Patient 3
Mesh-DRR	2.68±1.22	2.97±1.88	2.29±1.04	1.62±0.92	2.41±1.38	3.11±2.51
CT-DRR	2.14±1.04	3.41±2.35	2.42±1.31	2.24±1.37	2.77±1.51	2.96±2.42
Binary-DRR	16.8±7.48	8.33±4.78	7.19±5.37	14.4±3.47	27.1±14.2	18.7±8.35

on 3 clinical EVAR datasets. We used a two-layer intensity-based 3D-2D registration scheme that performs global search for 3 in-plane parameters (2 translations + 1 rotation), followed by a 6-dimensional rigid-body optimization using Hill-Climbing algorithm. Two similarity measures, NCC and GD, were tested in this experiment. Registration was started from 100 randomly sampled starting poses within a typical offset range for clinical applications (20 mms in translation and 5 degrees in rotation). The registration accuracy is quantitatively measured by the RMSE between the 2D re-projections of pre-defined landmarks (two renal ostia and the bifurcation point of iliac arteries) using the registration pose and the ground truth pose, and is referred to as 2D Target Registration Error (2D TRE). The 2D TRE is measured in pixels, where 1 pixel in the 2D image plane corresponds to ~0.5 mm in the 3D space according to the imaging geometry for these datasets. Table 2 summarizes the registration results, which show that the registration using mesh-DRR achieves similar accuracy as CT-DRR, and significantly outperforms binary-DRR on all the datasets and for both similarity measures. Please note that the registration error using mesh-DRR and CT-DRR are comparable to the inter-observer annotation error, and therefore cannot be compared against each other on their absolute accuracy. In addition, although the similarity profile for NCC using binary-DRR is seemingly close to that using mesh-DRR (Fig. 4(a) and Fig. 5(a)) when translation in only one dimension is concerned, the 3D-2D registration results using binary-DRR and NCC similarity measure are seriously deteriorated compared to that using the proposed mesh-DRR, presumably due to the complication coming from the inter-tangle of all 6 dimensions of a rigid-body transformation model.

4.3   Mesh-DRR from MRI

One of the main advantages of mesh-DRR compared to volume-DRR is its applicability to 3D image modalities other than CT. In this experiment, a head T2-weighted MRI volume was segmented into three categories, air, bones and soft tissues.

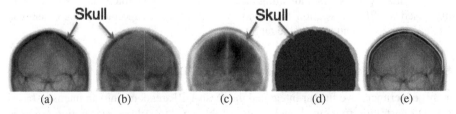

Fig. 6. (a) CT-DRR. (b) Mesh-DRR. (c) MRI-DRR. (d) Alpha-DRR. (e) Registration results using mesh-DRR (yellow) and MRI-DRR (red).

The attenuation coefficient for air is almost zero, and therefore was not used in mesh-DRR rendering. Heuristic attenuation coefficient values were assigned for bones and soft tissues, and a mesh-DRR for the head MRI was rendered following Eqn. 4. For comparison, we also generated a CT-DRR from the CT volume of the same patient, a volume-based DRR rendered directly from MRI (MRI-DRR), and a DRR-like image using alpha blending of two binary images (alpha-DRR) as proposed in [4]. The most dominant feature in X-ray images of the head is the skull, due to its high attenuation coefficient. It can be seen that for both mesh-DRR and CT-DRR, the boundary of the skull is shown as a dark ring (Fig. 6(a)(b)). For MRI-DRR, however, since the bony structure is usually not picked up well by MRI using the standard protocol, the skull is shown as a white ring (pointed by the arrow in Fig. 6(c)). For alpha-DRR, as the thickness of the object is not taken into consideration, it cannot distinguish the boundary of the skull and results in a uniform intensity (Fig. 6(d)).

Intensity-based 3D-2D registration was performed to register the 3D MRI volume using both mesh-DRR and MRI-DRR to the simulated X-ray image using CT-DRR. For the ease of visualization, the boundary of the skull at the registered pose is overlaid onto the CT-DRR in Fig. 6(e). It shows that although there are some details in mesh-DRR that are different from CT-DRR (mainly due to the imperfect segmentation), the quality of the mesh-DRR is sufficient for mesh-to-image registration, which correctly overlays the boundaries of the skull in MRI and CT volumes. In comparison, using MRI-DRR results in an incorrect lower position, which matches the scalp in MRI to the skull in CT.

5   Conclusion

In this paper, we introduced a mesh-based DRR rendering technique that can generate realistic simulated X-ray images from 3D meshes. The proposed mesh-DRR rendering algorithm using ray-casting technique is optimized for GPU architecture to achieve high computation efficiency. We have shown that the proposed mesh-DRR achieves much faster rendering speed than volume-DRR (volume ray-casting), and the resulting rendering can lead to efficient and accurate intensity-based 3D-2D registration for CT volumes and other modalities. Our future work is to quantitatively evaluate the proposed mesh-DRR for 2D-3D registration on a large database and for various 3D image modalities.

Acknowledgement. The authors wish to thank Dr. Wei Hong, Dr. Sajjad Baloch and Dr. Shanhui Sun from Siemens Corporation for their useful comments and advices.

References

1. Liao, R., Zhang, L., Sun, Y., Miao, S., Chefd'hotel, C.: A review of recent advances in registration techniques applied to minimally invasive therapy (2013)
2. Dorgham, O.M., Laycock, S.D., Fisher, M.H.: GPU accelerated generation of digitally reconstructed radiographs for 2-D/3-D image registration. IEEE Transactions on Biomedical Engineering 59(9), 2594–2603 (2012)

3. Thivierge-Gaulin, D., Chou, C.-R., Kiraly, A.P., Chefd'Hotel, C., Strobel, N., Cheriet, F.: 3D-2D registration based on mesh-derived image bisection. In: Dawant, B.M., Christensen, G.E., Fitzpatrick, J.M., Rueckert, D. (eds.) WBIR 2012. LNCS, vol. 7359, pp. 70–78. Springer, Heidelberg (2012)
4. Kaiser, M., John, M., Borsdorf, A., Mountney, P., Ionasec, R., Nottling, A., Kiefer, P., Seeburger, J., Neumuth, T.: Significant acceleration of 2D-3D registration-based fusion of ultrasound and x-ray images by mesh-based drr rendering. In: SPIE Medical Imaging, pp. 867111–867111. International Society for Optics and Photonics (2013)
5. Lorensen, W.E., Cline, H.E.: Marching cubes: A high resolution 3d surface construction algorithm. ACM Siggraph Computer Graphics 21, 163–169 (1987)
6. Whitaker, R.: Reducing aliasing artifacts in iso-surfaces of binary volumes. In: Proceedings of the 2000 IEEE Symposium on Volume Visualization, pp. 23–32 (2000)
7. Garland, M., Heckbert, P.S.: Surface simplification using quadric error metrics. In: Proceedings of the 24th Annual Conference on Computer Graphics and Interactive Techniques, pp. 209–216. ACM Press/Addison-Wesley Publishing Co. (1997)
8. Popov, S., Gunther, J., Seidel, H.-P., Slusallek, P.: Stackless kd-tree traversal for high performance gpu ray tracing. Computer Graphics Forum 26, 415–424 (2007)
9. Amanatides, J., Woo, A., et al.: A fast voxel traversal algorithm for ray tracing. In: Proceedings of EUROGRAPHICS 1987, pp. 3–10 (1987)

Toward Accurate and Robust 2-D/3-D Registration of Implant Models to Single-Plane Fluoroscopy

Shun Miao, Rui Liao, Joseph Lucas, and Christophe Chefd'hotel

Siemens Corporation, Corporate Technology
755 College Rd E, Princeton, NJ, USA

Abstract. A fully automatic and highly accurate 2-D/3-D registration technique with an extended capture range is proposed for registering implant models to single-plane fluoroscopy. The proposed method utilizes library-based registration for pose initialization, followed by an intensity-based iterative registration for pose fine tuning. The algorithm matches the 2-D silhouette of the implant extracted from the fluoroscopy with a pre-computed library of 2-D silhouettes of the implant model to estimate the initial pose. Each library entry represents a combination of out-of-plane rotation parameters. Library matching is performed by computing Shape Context (SC) of the extracted 2-D silhouette and minimizing the Jensen-Shannon Divergence of SCs from the fluoroscopy and the library entry. After pose initialization, iterative optimization is performed to fine tune the registration by maximizing the intensity-based similarity measure between the fluoroscopic image and the simulated X-ray image. In the iterative registration, we use a novel two-layer hierarchical optimization strategy to achieve a high accuracy in depth estimation, to which the projection image is very insensitive. The proposed approach is validated on both computer simulated images and real X-ray images. Validation results show significant improvements over conventional methods in terms of robustness and accuracy.

Keywords: 2-D/3-D registration, robust pose initialization, shape context, implant registration.

1   Introduction

2-D/3-D Image registration is one of the enabling technologies widely used in image-guided therapy and interventional radiology. Among the applications of 2-D/3-D registration techniques, there is a special category where the object to be registered is a metal implant. There are three properties of metal implants that make this particular category different from the general 2-D/3-D registration problems. First, the metal implants are always rigid. Second, the X-ray image of the metal implant is very dark due to its high opacity and hence is relatively easy to segment. Third, the structural model of the implant is usually available as a Computer Assisted Design (CAD) model. By taking advantage of these three properties, an advanced 2-D/3-D registration technique dedicated to metal implants should be able to achieve higher reliability and accuracy than the general 2-D/3-D registration methods.

C.A. Linte et al. (Eds.): MIAR/AE-CAI 2013, LNCS 8090, pp. 97–106, 2013.
© Springer-Verlag Berlin Heidelberg 2013

By far, most 2-D/3-D registration methods in literatures are iterative [1]. These methods iteratively adapt the registration parameters to maximize a matching metric reflecting the quality of registration. The iterative registration algorithms can be further divided into two categories, intensity-based methods [2-5] and feature-based methods [6], depending on the similarity measure to be optimized. Intensity-based methods, which maximize the similarity between the simulated X-ray image produced from the 3-D volume and the real X-ray image, are shown to be very accurate, especially when multiple image planes are employed. However, a constraint of the clinical usage of intensity-based registration methods is their small capture range, and typically manual initialization is required to bring the 3-D model close enough to the target position. On the other hand, feature-based methods, which register landmark and/or salient features that have been manually or semi-automatically extracted from both the 2-D image and the 3-D model, exhibit fast execution time and high robustness in face of large mis-registration. However, it is difficult to achieve fully automatic and accurate landmark/salient feature extraction.

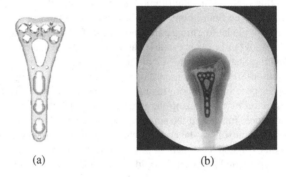

(a)   (b)

Fig. 1. (a) 3-D structural CAD model of the implant. (b) 2-D fluoroscopic image

For the 2-D/3-D registration applications where the 3-D structural CAD model is available, another category called library-based methods has been proposed [7-9]. Library-based methods take advantage of the known 3-D structural model to generate a pre-computed library of expected 2-D projections of the 3-D model, and perform library matching for the given 2-D image to estimate the pose of the 3-D model. However, the library-based methods suffer from a major drawback that the registration accuracy is limited by the density of library entries over the parameter space. To circumvent this burden, Cyr *et al.* [9] borrowed the multi-resolution idea from image registration field and proposed a hierarchical approach, which iteratively narrows down the search range and generates a denser library in the target area. Although this hierarchical approach achieves a higher accuracy, it sacrifices the advantage of offline computation of library generation and feature extraction. Hermans *et a.l* [10] proposed to use the library-based method to provide an initial pose to start the iterative registration algorithm. Our proposed method uses the same workflow as in [10] by concatenating a library-based registration and an iterative optimization of fine-tuning, but with improvements in two aspects: 1. significantly faster library matching using a

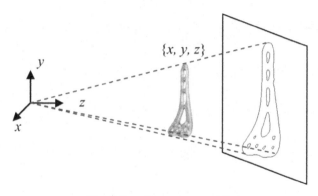

Fig. 2. Imaging system model

more efficient shape encoder and matching metric; 2. higher accuracy in depth position estimation by utilizing a hierarchical optimization strategy.

In our approach, the library consists of 2-D contours extracted from the silhouettes of the implant, and are encoded by Shape Context [11]. We then use Jensen-Shannon Divergence as the matching metric for fast library matching. The proposed library matching scheme achieves a high computational efficiency because it has the Shape Contexts of library entries pre-computed offline, and only leaves the simple Jensen-Shannon Divergence to be computed online. With the initial pose estimated from library matching, a two-layer optimization of intensity-based similarity measure is further performed for the 3-D pose fine tuning.

2   Method

2.1   Overview

The proposed method consists of two steps: (1) The initial pose is estimated by matching the silhouette of the implant in fluoroscopic images to a library of expected 2-D silhouettes of the 3-D model of the same implant from different views. The library matching will provide a pose initialization to bring the 3-D model close to the target position. (2) After pose initialization, the estimated pose is refined by applying a hierarchical optimizer to maximize the similarity between the simulated X-ray image and the fluoroscopic image.

2.2   Camera Setup

The X-ray imaging system is described by the prospective projection model in Fig. 2. The imaging system consists of a point source of X-ray located at the origin and an image detector perpendicular to z axis. X-rays are emitted from the point source, passing through the object and producing images on the image detector. The 3-D pose of the model is described by 6 parameters, $\{x, y, z, \alpha, \beta, \theta\}$, where (x, y, z) is the

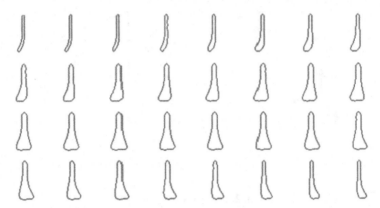

Fig. 3. Examples of library entries

coordinate of the gravity center of the 3-D model, (α, β, θ) are the rotation parameters with respect to x, y, z axis. The iso-center of rotations is at the gravity center.

2.3   Pose Initialization by Library Matching

Since intensity-based 2-D/3-D registration algorithms typically have a very small capture range, an effective 2-D/3-D registration system requires accurate and robust pose initialization. A straight forward approach of pose initialization is global search. However, as the computational complexity of global search grows exponentially with the dimensionality of the searching space, performing global search for transformation parameters with six degrees of freedom (DOF) can be very time consuming and impractical for clinical use. In order to estimate the pose efficiently and accurately, a novel library-based pose initialization method is proposed.

We take advantage of the known 3-D structural model of the implant to generate a library of simulated X-ray images from different views. However, a library that covers the full six DOF for a rigid-body transformation will have a large number of entries. To reduce the size of the library, we utilize the following property of the projection model:

Property 1: Among the six DOF, only the out-of-plane rotation parameters, α and β, significantly affects the geometry of the 2-D projection. The other four DOF only make subtle and negligible impacts on the geometry of the 2-D projection.

In the rest of the paper, the rotation parameter α and β will be referred as geometry-relevant, and the other four DOF as geometry-irrelevant transformation parameters. With the above property, we generate a library to only cover the two geometry-relevant parameters (Fig. 3), and use a shape descriptor that is invariant for 2-D shift, rotation and scaling for library matching. The library matching will provide an initial estimation of α and β. The four parameters for geometry-irrelevant transformations will be further estimated using purely the 2-D shape registration that is described in section 2.C.(2).

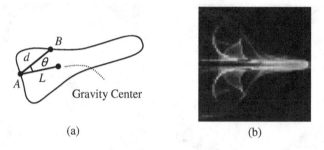

(a)   (b)

Fig. 4. (a) Computation of Shape Context (b) Example of Shape Context

Library Matching --- Estimation of the Geometry-Relevant Transformation
Prior to performing library matching for pose estimation, the implant in the fluoroscopic image is converted to silhouettes by a region growing segmentation method
[12]. The simulated X-ray images are silhouettes by nature in our simplified imaging
system model. However, as shown in Fig.1, for certain implants, nails might be applied and therefore occlude the holes of the implant in fluoroscopic images. To rule
out the impact of nails, we ignore all holes and only use the outline contour of the 2-D
silhouette, which is represented by a sequence of N points P, uniformly sampled on
the contour.

After extracting the contour from the 2-D image, we use Shape Context to encode
the contour. Shape Context is the ideal shape descriptor in our case because it is invariant to translation, rotation and even scaling if the point-to-point distance is normalized to [0, 1].

As shown in Fig. 4, given a fixed point A, all other points can be represented in a
polar coordinate system with pole A and polar axis L connecting A and the gravity
center. Shape Context is defined as a joint histogram of the radius d and the polar
angle θ. In this paper, we use 64 bins for both the radius and the polar angel in the
computation of the joint histogram $H(i,j)$. The library matching metric is then defined as the Jensen-Shannon Divergence (JSD) between the Shape Context of the
fluoroscopic image and a given library entry:

$$JSD = \frac{1}{2}\sum_i H(i,j) \, log\frac{P(i,j)}{Q(i,j)} + \frac{1}{2}\sum_i Q(i,j) \, log\frac{Q(i,j)}{P(i,j)} \tag{1}$$

Where $H(i,j)$ and $Q(i,j)$ are Shape Contexts of target image and library image,
respectively. The library matching selects the library entry that yields the smallest
JSD. Denoting the transformation parameters of the matched library entry as
$\{x_0, y_0, z_0, \alpha_0, \beta_0, \theta_0\}$, the initial estimation of α and β are:

$$\alpha = \alpha_0, \ \beta = \beta_0 \tag{2}$$

It is worthy to point out that the Shape Context of the whole library can be computed offline. The computations that need to be done online include 2-D fluoroscopic
image processing, shape encoding and library matching.

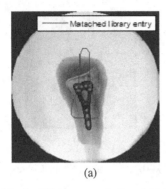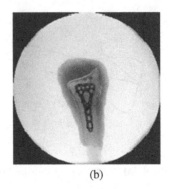

(a)   (b)

Fig. 5. (a) Matched library entry before 2-D shape registration. (b) Matched library entry after 2-D shape registration by SVD.

2-D Shape Registration --- Estimation of Geometry- Irrelevant Transformation.
After the geometry-relevant transformation parameters α and β are estimated by library matching, the remaining four DOF to be estimated are geometry-irrelevant transformation parameters that mainly cause 2-D translation, rotation and scaling. As shown in Fig.5 (a), the contours from the fluoroscopic image and the simulated X-ray image have the same geometry but different 2-D poses. We first register the two contours by 2-D shape registration, and convert the 2-D transformation back to 3-D according to our imaging system model.

As both contours are parameterized by their arc lengths and have the same number of samples, a point-to-point correspondence should exist. To detect this correspondence, for both contours, we plot the profile of the distance from each point to the gravity center of the contour. Then, circular convolution is applied on the two profiles, and the maximum of the convolution indicates the point-to-point correspondence. With the point-to-point correspondence, the 2-D transformation between the two shapes can be directly estimated by Singular Value Decomposition (SVD). An example of 2-D shape registration result is shown in Fig.5 (b).

Given the 2-D transformation parameters of scaling s_{2D}, translation (x_{2D}, y_{2D}) and rotation θ_{2D}, the four geometry-irrelevant transformation parameters in 3-D can be estimated correspondingly. First, the 3-D rotation can be directly inferred because the in-plane rotations are the same in 3-D and 2-D:

$$\theta = \theta_0 + \theta_{2D} \qquad (3)$$

Second, according to the projection model, the depth parameter z is then estimated as:

$$z = \frac{z_0}{s_{2D}} \qquad (4)$$

Last, with the estimated depth position z, translation parameters x and y can be estimated as:

$$x = x_o + \frac{x_{2D}}{SID} \times z, \; y = y_o + \frac{y_{2D}}{SID} \times z \qquad (5)$$

where SID is the source to detector distance, which is assumed to be known in our imaging system model.

2.4   Registration Fine Tuning

The 2-D/3-D registration fine tuning technique is built on the intensity-based iterative registration algorithm proposed by [5]. In particular, we use a simplified Digital Reconstructed Radiograph (DRR) model to render simulated X-ray images. For each pixel, a ray connecting the pixel and the source of X-ray is drawn. If the ray passes through the 3-D CAD model, then the pixel is white, otherwise it is black. The similarity between the simulated X-ray images and the real X-ray image is evaluated using Normalized Cross Correlation (NCC):

$$NCC(I_1, I_2) = \frac{\sum [I_1(x,y) - \bar{I}_1(x,y)][I_2(x,y) - \bar{I}_2(x,y)]}{\sqrt{\sum [I_1(x,y) - \bar{I}_1(x,y)]^2 [I_2(x,y) - \bar{I}_2(x,y)]^2}} \qquad (6)$$

However, the accuracy of depth estimation for mono-plane intensity-based 2-D/3-D registration is relatively poor because a change in depth position only causes small changes in the 2-D silhouette. To achieve a high accuracy of depth estimation, the above similarity measure is optimized by a two-layer hierarchical optimizer. In particular, assuming the starting position is $\{x, y, z, \alpha, \beta, \theta\}$, three hill climbing optimizers are launched independently at three different depth positions of z-10, z and $z+10$, and within a search range of 5 mm in depth. The registration result that yields the largest similarity measure among the three will be selected. After the first layer, the depth position z will be brought closer to the target position, but still has a relative large error because of the large search range. The second layer is very similar to the first layer, but with a much smaller search range and search step. Five optimizers are lunched in the second layer with a 5 mm interval and 2.5 mm search range. The proposed optimization strategy avoids local maxima by dividing the searching space into small bins in the depth direction and performing separate optimization in each bin with a small step size.

3   Experimental Results

In this section, we assess the accuracy and robustness of the proposed method. Many previous 2-D/3-D registration methods reporting high a convergence rate and accuracy only start registration from poses that are very close to the target position. In our experiments, the initial pose will be not provided by the user, and the ability of the proposed method to start registration from arbitrary poses will be demonstrated.

3.1   Synthetic Data

Computer simulation test was conducted to assess the performance of the proposed method. One hundred binary DRRs of the implant were rendered by the perspective

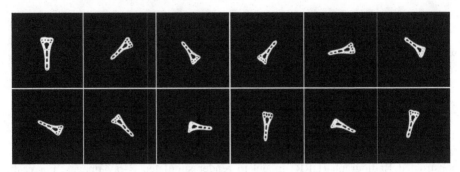

Fig. 6. Examples of artificial X-ray images used in simulation test. The top left image is generated from the reference pose.

projection model with randomly selected poses, and used as artificial X-ray images for simulation test, as shown in Fig. 6. In order to make the pose sampling meaningful, we chose a reference pose according to the typical orientation used clinically. The artificial X-ray image rendered from the reference pose is shown in the top-left image in Fig. 6, which is similar to the real X-ray images shown in Fig. 5. Then, other artificial X-ray images were generated by adding randomly selected offsets to the reference pose, which is within [-100, 100] mm for translation, [-180, 180] degrees for in-plane rotation and [-30, 30] degrees for out-of-plane rotation. The artificial X-ray images and their corresponding poses are then used as ground truth for simulation test. The registration accuracy is quantified by three measurements: 1. The error of the estimated six parameters of rigid-body transformation. 2. The root-mean-square-distance (RMSD) of the 3-D model between the estimated pose and the ground truth pose, referred to as 3D Target Registration Error (3D-TRE). 3. Registration success rate defined by 3D-TRE < 2 mm.

To demonstrate the advantage of the proposed technique in terms of robustness and accuracy, the experimental results of five methods are compared: 1. Library-based initialization only (LM). 2. Library-based initialization followed by hierarchical optimization (prop.) 3. Library-based initialization followed by conventional optimizer (LM+CO) 4. Hierarchical optimization without library-based initialization (HO) 5. The conventional intensity-based iterative method (conv.). For a fair comparison, the same matching metric in Eqn. 6 were used in all the tested methods. It is well recognized that without a good initial pose, iterative 2D-3D registration methods, like method 4 and 5, are very likely to fail due to their small capture range. Therefore, to make the comparison even more challenging for the proposed method, we provided a rough pose initialization for method 4 and 5, which can bring the initial rotation parameters into [-30 30] degrees from the target orientation. The in-plane translation parameters were also initialized by overlaying the projection of the gravity center of the 3-D model and the gravity center of the 2-D silhouette.

The simulation test results are summarized in Table 1. The first three columns show the accuracy of the estimated transformation parameters for 3-D translations and rotations. The average errors of xy position are separated from z position to reflect the accuracy of the algorithm in both in-plane translations and depth direction. The last two columns give the average 3D-TRE and the success rate. It can be seen that due to the small capture range, the conventional intensity-based iterative registration method has large 3D-TRE (32.72 mm) and low success rate (24%). After applying the library matching method for pose initialization, the 3D-TRE is reduced to 2.75 mm and the success rate is increased to 78%. The accuracy of z position is further improved by employing the hierarchical optimization scheme and the final accuracy achieves 1.20 mm in 3D-TRE and 96% in success rate.

Table 1. Experimental results of synthetic data tests

	Average errors				Success rate
	XY difference	Z difference	Angular difference	3D-TRE	
LM	0.237mm	4.56mm	1.42°	4.56mm	50%
Prop.	0.033mm	1.16mm	0.60°	1.20mm	96%
LM+CO	0.043mm	2.65mm	0.98°	2.75mm	78%
HO	5.64mm	9.52mm	28.89°	26.20mm	28%
Conv.	5.34mm	15.49mm	32.23°	32.72mm	24%

3.2   Real Data

Our proposed method (LM+HO) was lastly applied on four real X-ray datasets. For the real X-ray images that do not have the "golden standard" ground truth of the 3-D pose, we are only able to measure the registration accuracy in the 2-D projection. The RMSD between the 2-D contours of the implant's silhouette in the projected image and the fluoroscopic image, referred to as 2D-TRE, is calculated and shown in Table 2. It is shown that for all four real X-ray images, sub-0.1-millimeter 2D-TRE are achieved.

Table 2. 2D-TRE of real data tests

	Image 1	Image 2	Image 3	Image 4
2-D RMSD	0.011mm	0.013mm	0.079mm	0.092mm

4   Conclusion

In this paper, a fully automatic, accurate, and robust 2-D/3-D registration method is proposed for registering metal implants to single-plane fluoroscopic images with an arbitrary pose. The proposed method combines library-based method and intensity-based iterative method to achieve full automation, high accuracy, and a very large capture range. The feasibility of the proposed method is shown using both simulated and real data. In all the simulated datasets, it is shown that the library-based initialization provides a good pose estimation that has RMSD smaller than 10mm. Compared to the conventional optimizer, the proposed hierarchical optimizer shows significant improvements in terms of the accuracy of depth estimation. Future works include clinical testing of the proposed method and investigation of other possible shape encoders that are capable of partial shape matching.

Acknowledgement. We would like to thank Siemens XP for providing the real X-ray images.

References

1. Markelj, P., Tomaževič, D., Likar, B., Pernuš, F.: A review of 3D/2D registration methods for image-guided interventions. Medical Image Analysis 16(3), 642–661 (2012)
2. Yamazaki, T., Watanabe, T., Nakajima, Y., Sugamoto, K., Tomita, T., Yoshikawa, H., Tamura, S.: Improvement of depth position in 2-D/3-D registration of knee implants using single-plane fluoroscopy. IEEE Transactions on Medical Imaging 23(5), 602–612 (2004)
3. Mahfouz, M.R., Hoff, W.A., Komistek, R.D., Dennis, D.A.: A robust method for registration of three-dimensional knee implant models to two-dimensional fluoroscopy images. IEEE Transactions on Medical Imaging 22(12), 1561–1574 (2003)
4. Penney, G.P., Weese, J., Little, J.A., Desmedt, P., Hill, D.L.: A comparison of similarity measures for use in 2-D-3-D medical image registration. IEEE Transactions on Medical Imaging 17(4), 586–595 (1998)
5. Lemieux, L., Jagoe, R., Fish, D.R., Kitchen, N.D., Thomas, D.G.T.: A patient-to-computed-tomography image registration method based on digitally reconstructed radiographs. Medical Physics 21, 1749 (1994)
6. Hipwell, J.H., Penney, G.P., McLaughlin, R.A., Rhode, K., Summers, P., Cox, T.C., Byrne, J.V., Noble, J.A., Hawkes, D.J.: Intensity-based 2-D-3-D registration of cerebral angiograms. IEEE Transactions on Medical Imaging 22(11), 1417–1426 (2003)
7. Hoff, W.A., Komistek, R.D., Dennis, D.A., Walker, S., Northcut, E., Spargo, K.: Pose estimation of artificial knee implants in fluoroscopy images using a template matching technique. In: Proceedings of the 3rd IEEE Workshop on Applications of Computer Vision, WACV 1996, pp. 181–186. IEEE (1996)
8. Banks, S.A., Andrew Hodge, W.: Accurate measurement of three-dimensional knee replacement kinematics using single-plane fluoroscopy. IEEE Transactions on Biomedical Engineering 43(6), 638–649 (1996)
9. Cyr, C.M., Kamal, A.F., Sebastian, T.B., Kimia, B.B.: 2D-3D registration based on shape matching. In: Proceedings of the IEEE Workshop on Mathematical Methods in Biomedical Image Analysis, pp. 198–203. IEEE (2000)
10. Hermans, J., Claes, P., Bellemans, J., Vandermeulen, D., Suetens, P.: Robust initialization for 2D/3D registration of knee implant models to single-plane fluoroscopy. In: Medical Imaging, pp. 651208–651208. International Society for Optics and Photonics (2007)
11. Belongie, S., Malik, J., Puzicha, J.: Shape matching and object recognition using shape contexts. IEEE Transactions on Pattern Analysis and Machine Intelligence 24(4), 509–522 (2002)
12. Adams, R., Bischof, L.: Seeded region growing. IEEE Transactions on Pattern Analysis and Machine Intelligence 16(6), 641–647 (1994)

Ultrasound Image-Guided Mapping of Endoscopic Views on a 3D Placenta Model: A Tracker-Less Approach

Liangjing Yang[1], Junchen Wang[1], Etsuko Kobayashi[1], Hongen Liao[1,2],
Ichiro Sakuma[1], Hiromasa Yamashita[3], and Toshio Chiba[3]

[1] Graduate School of Engineering, The University of Tokyo, Tokyo, Japan
[2] School of Medicine, Tsinghua University, Beijing, China
[3] Clinical Research Center, National Center for Child Health and Development, Tokyo, Japan

Abstract. This work presents a framework for mapping of free-hand endoscopic views onto 3D anatomical model constructed from ultrasound images without the use of external trackers. It is non-disruptive in terms of existing surgical workflow as surgeons do not need to accommodate operational constraints associated with the use of additionally installed motion sensors or tracking systems. A passive fiducial marker is attached to the tip of the endoscope to create a geometric eccentricity that encodes the position and orientation of the camera. The relative position between the endoscope and the anatomical model under the ultrasound image reference frame is used to establish a texture map that overlays endoscopic views onto the surface of the model. This addresses operational challenges including the limited field-of-view (FOV) and the lack of 3D perspective associated with minimally invasive procedure. Experimental results show that average tool position and orientation errors are 1.32 mm and 1.6° respectively. The R.M.S. error of the overall image mapping obtained based on comparison of dimension of landmarks is 3.30 mm with standard deviation of 2.14 mm. The feasibility of the framework is also demonstrated through implementations on a phantom model.

Keywords: surgical navigation, image-guided ultrasound, image mapping.

1 Introduction

1.1 Motivation

Developments in minimally invasive surgical techniques have driven research interests in image-guidance and surgical navigation over the past decades. While the benefits of minimally invasive procedure are now well recognized, such operations are usually associated with challenging visual and dexterous constraints. It is especially demanding in the case of endoscopic fetal surgery where the FOV is extremely small and movement within the surgical site highly delicate. Current practices involve the use endoscopic camera known as fetoscope [1,2] to acquired views inside the womb and ultrasound imaging for a global perspective of the surgical site so as to navigate surgical instruments. Surgeons have to register the two sources of information mentally working with non-intuitive ultrasound images and extremely limited fetoscopic

C.A. Linte et al. (Eds.): MIAR/AE-CAI 2013, LNCS 8090, pp. 107–116, 2013.
© Springer-Verlag Berlin Heidelberg 2013

FOV. Therefore, it is important to equip surgeons with an integrated visualization platform that presents an intuitive 3D navigation perspective of the surgical site together with details and expanded views of the surface anatomy for instance, the placenta vasculature in the case of Twin-to-twin transfusion syndrome [3].

1.2   State-of-the-Art and Existing Limitations

Surgical navigation technology in fetal surgery has been relatively lagging compared to its counterparts in procedures like cardiac or neurosurgery. This is partly due to the unique clinical requirements in fetal surgery which exclude many mainstream imaging modalities that are ionizing in nature. Ultrasound imaging turns out to be one of the best options for image-guidance in fetal surgery. Together with the use of a fetoscope, minimally invasive fetal endoscopic surgery [4, 5] can be performed.

An image stitching approach via feature point correspondence of 2D fetoscopic images for placenta visualization was proposed by Reff *et al.* [6]. While this approach addresses the issue of limited FOV by providing a global 2D map of placenta it does not provide a 3D global perspective and no evaluation of the error due to the use of projective transformation model is presented. Liao *et al.* [7, 8] demonstrated the mapping of 3D fetoscopic view to a prebuilt phantom placenta model based on positional information acquired through a commercial optical tracker. This provides surgeons with an intuitive visualization platform encompassing surface details of the placenta vasculature and the 3D perspective of the operation site. However, it relies on optical tracking system that requires the attachment of markers onto surgical instruments and maintaining line-of-sight throughout the operation workspace [9]. These compromise the usability of the system. Our approach differs in that we construct a visualization platform relying only on the imaging instruments used for the surgery. It obtains the endoscope pose and location using ultrasound image-based localization and constructs a texture map using the endoscopic images.

Ultrasound image-based instrument tracking has been investigated in several applications including visual-servo applications [10] and surgical navigation [11]. A comprehensive analytical study of tracking passive markers in real-time 3D ultrasound is presented by Stoll *et al.* [12]. Mung *et al.* [13] demonstrated sub-mm accuracy with active sensor attached to the tool tip. However, to the best of our knowledge, study that investigates the use of ultrasound image-based localization for mapping of endoscopic views to 3D anatomical model has not yet been presented in existing literature.

1.3   Scope and Organization

The contributions of this work include the application and analytical study of a novel approach that facilitates mapping of endoscopic views to anatomical model constructed from 3D ultrasound without the use of tracking system.

The next section discusses the method for ultrasound image-based localization and texture mapping followed by an explanation of the experimental study. Results are presented and discussed in Section 4. Finally, we conclude the paper by summarizing the important contributions, current limitations, and a brief remark on the future work.

2   Method

2.1   Overview

The novelty of our proposed approach is that it relies only on the imaging devices used in the surgery to facilitate visual guidance. It is non-disruptive in terms of the surgical workflow as attachment of bulky sensors, and the maintenance of line-of-sight is not required. In addition, the relative position between the endoscope and the anatomical model under a common ultrasound image reference frame requires no intermediate registration between multiple sensors. This reduces error due to multiple sensors registration.

The proposed framework consists of an ultrasound initialization phase followed by the mapping of monocular views acquired by a moving free-hand endoscope. Fig. 1 illustrates the workflow of the mapping framework. First, a 3D ultrasound probe is used to scan images of the phantom placenta and the endoscope. The pose and location of the endoscope is encoded by the geometric eccentricity produced by the fiducial marker attached to the endoscope's tip. Ultrasound image-based localization can be used to interpret positional information. Subsequently, registration between the ultrasound and endoscopic images is attained through the ultrasound image-based localization method. As both the position of the phantom placenta and endoscope are defined in the ultrasound image reference frame, their relative position can be obtained. The endoscopic camera is pre-calibrated such that the camera plane's relative position to the fiducial marker is known. With relative positions between the camera plane and the anatomical environment known, 3D-2D projective transformation relationship can be established. This enables the assignment of polygonal patches to the texture map of the endoscopic views which will be discussed in Section 2.3.

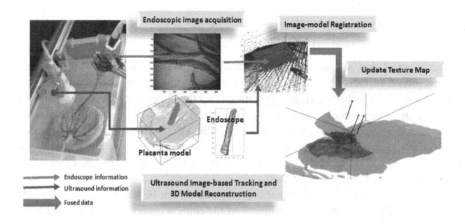

Fig. 1. Texture mapping framework

2.2 Ultrasound Image-Based Localization

Ultrasound image-based localization of the endoscope establishes the relative orientation and position between the endoscope and the relevant anatomical scene. This involves scanning of the 3D anatomy and the endoscope within the same FOV as illustrated in fig. 2(a). Marching Cubes algorithm is used to segment volume data acquired from 3D ultrasound images. This is done by assigning an iso-value to extract the iso-surface. It takes approximately 0.52 s to process a typical volume data constructed from a 440 by 240 image sequence of 60 slices. Geometrical eccentricity adequate to localize the 3 degree-of-freedom in the orthogonal axis of rotation is created by attaching a fiducial marker to the tip of the endoscope as show in fig. 2(b). In fig 2(c), the kinematic configuration of the endoscope which can be represented by a homogenous transformation matrix consisting of its orthogonal rotational axes and position in Cartesian coordinate is computed using Principal Component Analysis (PCA) [14].

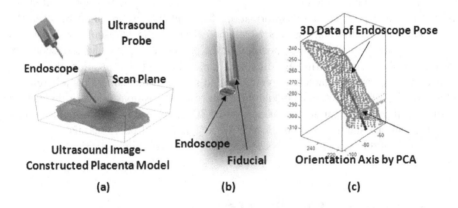

Fig. 2. Ultrasound image-based pose computation

Our method uses an iterative PCA method that is shown to be reasonably robust against image artifacts [15]. A trade-off for this robustness is an increased computational load. Fortunately, tracking information from the ultrasound is not required to be real-time as long as there is sufficient image overlap between images corresponding to the intervals. Updating of every frame of the endoscopic video stream is not necessary for fetoscopic image overlay of the placenta as frame-to-frame image overlap is large. The bidirectional nature of the PCA solution to the respective axis can be resolved using simple logical condition.

The state variables of the kinematic configuration can be define as the roll-pitch-yaw Euler angle and Cartesian coordinates of the camera center position complying to the convention defined in fig. 3. Analytical discussion in Section 4 is referenced to this convention as well.

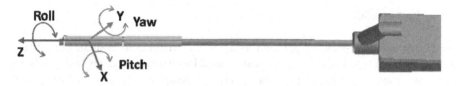

Fig. 3. Convention for defining the endoscope kinematic configuration

2.3   Registration and Texture Mapping

Registration of the endoscopic views and the 3D surface model is based on a projective transformation between the camera plane and the 3D surface. This enables mapping of camera-acquired texture information onto the ultrasound image-constructed surface model. Images from the endoscopic camera are processed as arrays of pixels with pixel values indexed to an RGB color scale as illustrated in fig. 4. Each of the pixel position corresponds to a surface patch on the 3D surface defined by the projective relationship between the camera plane and the face. As subsequent ultrasound image-based tracking data is used to update the endoscope position of the corresponding view and hence the transformation matrix, the updated texture map of the surface is overlaid.

An advantage of this system is that there is no need for intermediate registrations of the surgical image guiding devices with external sensors or tracking systems. Texture mapping can be done directly since the relative position between the surgical instrument and anatomical structure is acquired by a common stationary ultrasound probe used for intraoperative guidance. Therefore, the framework is a self-contained mechanism that performs automatic texture mapping without any disruption to the conventional surgical workflow.

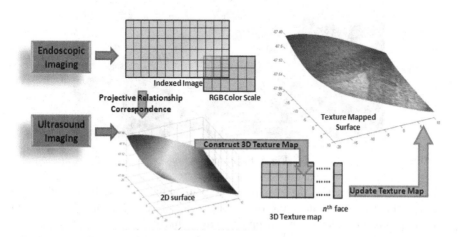

Fig. 4. Texture mapping workflow

3   Experiment

An experiment on a phantom placenta model was carried out to evaluate the efficacy of the system in terms of ultrasound image-based localization accuracy and consistency in image overlay. Fig. 5 depicts the experiment setup with both the endoscope and ultrasound probe imaging a phantom placenta in a water tank environment.

A commercial optical tracking system (POLARIS Spectra, NDI) was used to evaluate the accuracy of positional estimation of a ϕ5.4 mm endoscopic camera (LS501D, Shinko Optical). As shown in fig. 5, a stationary 3D tilt-scanning ultrasound probe was used to acquire ultrasound image sequences at 1 degree angular step and (0.3 x 0.3) mm^2 pixel size through a Prosound α10, Aloka ultrasound imaging system. The ultrasound image-based localization accuracy is therefore benchmarked against the commercial optical tracking system.

To minimize workspace-dependent errors, reference tracking from a proximal marker was performed instead of direct tracking of the endoscope based on the optical tracker's absolute frame. Frame intervals along a camera trajectory constrained to a mechanical pivoting port were tracked by ultrasound image-based method with their corresponding views acquired. The mechanical port constraint is to mimic the condition of minimally invasive procedure. To isolate uncertainties derived from technical issues like ultrasound motion artifacts, we performed localization and pose estimation under a static condition. This is a reasonable operational setting since the updating requirement for the ultrasound image-based localization is not demanding as discussed previously. We are only concerned with the accuracy of the localization.

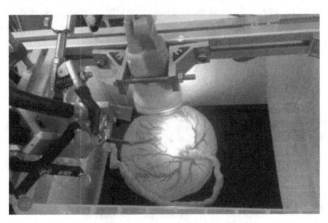

Fig. 5. Experiment setup

To assess the efficacy of the overall texture map on the 3D model, we made use of clearly visible vascular bifurcations on the phantom as physical landmarks. The accuracy and precision of the texture mapping were evaluated by comparing the physical dimension of a 3-point triangular landmark extracted manually across 10 mapped results as illustrated in fig.6 by the screenshot of a particular frame.

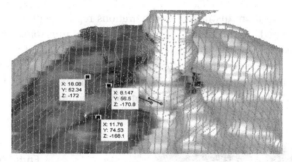

Fig. 6. Selection of vascular bifurcation as evaluation landmarks

4   Results and Discussion

4.1   Evaluation of Ultrasound Image-Based Tracking

The accuracy of the ultrasound image-based tracking based on observation of 10 static intervals along a particular trajectory is presented in Table 1. The mean absolute error was reduced by five times compared to that observed in our previous study [15]. Average angular error also reduced from 2° to current 1.6°. This is done by tuning the gain value of the ultrasound signal to reduce unnecessary image artifacts.

Table 1. Differences between ultrasound image-based tracking and commercial tracker

	mm			*degree*		
	x	*y*	*z*	*roll*	*pitch*	*yaw*
Mean Absolute Error	0.95	0.85	0.35	3.5	0.9	0.3
R.M.S. Error	1.21	1.06	0.45	4.2	1.1	0.4
Standard Deviation	0.99	0.82	0.29	3.8	0.6	0.2

It can be observed that the mean absolute positional errors with Euclidean distance of 1.32 mm are satisfactorily within the dimension of the thickness of a typical blood vessel on the placenta and comparable to the error observed in [11]. While sub-degree pose estimations were achieved in the pitch and yaw direction, significant errors are observed in the roll angle estimation. This can be attributed to the inadequacy in the geometric eccentricity produced by the ultrasound fiducial marker. This is the sole factor responsible for establishing a bias in the symmetry of the endoscope shaft directed along the y-axis (as defined in fig. 3) to be computed based on the iterative PCA. By increasing the gain of the ultrasound signal we can expect better results for roll estimation as reported in our previous work. The trade-off is an increase in ultrasound imaging artifact which affect the overall pose estimation.

While the iterative PCA is designed to be robust even when treating images with severe artifacts, setting extremely high threshold score for outlier rejection is not recommended as it may lead to significant increase in computation time and occasionally failure in converging to a solution if the image is too severely distorted with artifact. A more plausible solution to improve pose estimation accuracy is to redesign the fiducial marker with more distinctive configurations representative of the endoscope pose and better impedance matching to enhance quality of ultrasound images.

Fig. 7 demonstrates the robustness of the iterative PCA method against ultrasound imaging artifact in the water tank texture mapping experiment. Less than three iterations are required in the ultrasound images treated in this experiment. Interested readers may refer to [15] for in-depth discussion of the algorithm.

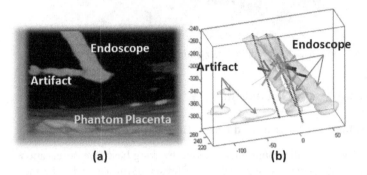

(a)   (b)

Fig. 7. (a) Ultrasound image (b) examples outlier rejection in 3 frames (dotted lines are initial estimation and thickest solid lines represent final estimations of orientation axes)

4.2   Evaluation of Texture Mapping

The error of the texture mapping based on 10 mapped results of the 3-point triangular landmarks has an absolute mean of 2.78 mm and R.M.S. value of 3.30 mm. The standard deviation is 2.14 mm. An example of a 3D ultrasound image constructed placenta model overlaid with free-hand endoscopic views is depicted in Fig. 8. The various poses and locations of the camera are represented by the blue arrows and red spheres respectively.

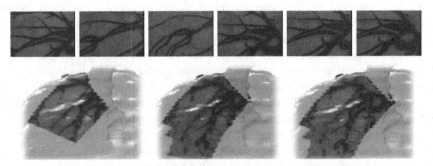

Fig. 8. Endoscopic views (top) overlaid on to 3D placenta model (bottom)

Many factors contributed to the inconsistency of the texture mapping results. Some of these error sources include the inherent uncertainties in ultrasound imaging device, severe image warping due to steep camera-surface angle associated with minimally invasive procedures, internal camera calibration errors and severe lens distortion associated with the wide-angle lens of the endoscope which cannot be adequately rectified even with high order polynomial distortion model. Current mapping region is limited to half of the placenta model due to the vertically positioned probe. Actual procedures do not have this restriction.

As observed in fig. 9, the distortion is prominent at the edges with steep geometries. Although accuracy may be within satisfaction, the overall texture mapping requires further improvement. We are also looking into the combination of other image mapping techniques [16] to address their various individual limitations.

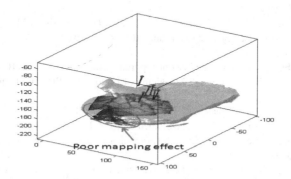

Fig. 9. Deterioration effect at steep geometry remotely situated from camera pivotal point

5   Conclusion

A method for mapping of free-hand endoscopic views onto ultrasound image-constructed 3D anatomical model without the use of tracking system is presented. It contributes to the state-of-the-art by investigating the feasibility of a tracker-less approach in mapping endoscopic views onto a 3D anatomical model. Limitation in FOV and the lack of 3D perspective in minimally invasive procedure are addressed by providing an integrated visualization platform combining endoscopic visual information and ultrasound image-based guidance. Operational constraints disruptive to the surgical workflow are also circumvented using this tracker-less approach.

Current limitations include the need to fix the position of ultrasound probe and the inadequacy in tracking non-static surgical scene. Future work including the investigation of data fusion with endoscopic vision-based techniques to allow effective real-time tracking of the non-static environment will be carried out.

Acknowledgement. This work was supported in part by Grant for Translational Systems Biology and Medicine Initiative (TSBMI) from the Ministry of Education, Culture, Sports, Science and Technology of Japan, and Grant-in-Aid for Scientific Research (Project No. 25350561) of the Japan Society for the Promotion of Science.

References

1. Ville, Y., Hyett, J., Hecher, K., Nicolaides, K.: Preliminary Experience with Endoscopic Laser Surgery for Severe Twin-to-Twin Transfusion Syndrome. N. Engl. J. Med. 332(4), 224–227 (1995)
2. Ville, Y., Hecher, K., Gagnon, A., Sebire, N., Hyett, J., Nicolaides, K.: Endoscopic laser coagulation in the management of severe twin-to-twin transfusion syndrome. BJOG: An International Journal of Obstetrics & Gynaecology 105(4), 446–453 (1998)
3. Bruner, J.P., Anderson, T.L., Rosemond, R.L.: Placental pathophysiology of the twin oligohydramnios-polyhydramnios sequence and the twin-twin transfusion syndrome. Placenta 19(1), 81–86 (1998)
4. Fowler, S.F., Sydorak, R.M., Albanese, C.T., Farmer, D.L., Harrison, M.R., Lee, H.: Fetal endoscopic surgery: Lessons learned and trends reviewed. J. Pediatr Surg. 37(12), 1700–1702 (2002)
5. Rauskolb, R.: Fetoscopy–a new endoscopic approach. Endoscopy 11(2), 107–113 (1979)
6. Reeff, M., Gerhard, F., Szekely, G.: Mosaicing of Endoscopic Placenta Images. GI Jahrestagung (2006)
7. Liao, H., Tsuzuki, M., Kobayashi, E., Sakuma, I.: GPU-based Fast 3D Ultrasound-Endoscope Image Fusion for Complex-Shaped Objects. In: Dossel, O., Schlegel, W. (eds.) World Congress on Medical Physics and Biomedical Engineering, pp. 206–209. Springer, Heidelberg (2009)
8. Liao, H., Tsuzuki, M., Mochizuki, T., Kobayashi, E., Chiba, T., Sakuma, I.: Fast image mapping of endoscopic image mosaics with 3D ultrasound image for intrauterine fetal surgery. Minimally Invasive Therapy & Allied Technologies 18(6), 332–340 (2009)
9. Cleary, K., Peters, T.M.: Image-Guided Interventions Technology Review and Clinical Applications. Annu. Rev. Biomed. Eng. 12, 119–142 (2010)
10. Stoll, J., Novotny, P., Howe, R., Dupont, P.: Real-time 3D ultrasound-based servoing of a surgical instrument. In: IEEE International Conference on Robotics and Automation, pp. 613–618 (2006)
11. Novotny, P.M., Stoll, J., Vasilyev, N.V., del Nido, P.J., Dupont, P.E., Zickler, T.E., Howe, R.D.: GPU based real-time instrument tracking with three-dimensional ultrasound. Med. Image Anal. 11(5), 458–464 (2007)
12. Stoll, J., Ren, H., Dupont, P.: Passive Markers for Tracking Surgical Instruments in Real-Time 3-D Ultrasound Imaging. IEEE T. Med. Imaging 31, 563–575 (2012)
13. Mung, J., Vignon, F., Jain, A.: A Non-disruptive Technology for Robust 3D Tool Tracking for Ultrasound-Guided Interventions. In: Fichtinger, G., Martel, A., Peters, T. (eds.) MICCAI 2011, Part I. LNCS, vol. 6891, pp. 153–160. Springer, Heidelberg (2011)
14. Draper, K.J., Blake, C.C., Gowman, L., Downey, D.B., Fenster, A.: An algorithm for automatic needle localization in ultrasound-guided breast biopsies. Med. Phys. 27, 1971–1979 (2000)
15. Yang, L., Wang, J., Kobayashi, E., Liao, H., Yamashita, H., Sakuma, I., Chiba, T.: Ultrasound Image-based Endoscope Localization for Minimally Invasive Fetoscopic Surgery. In: IEEE International Conference on Engineering in Medicine and Biology Conference, pp. 1411–1413 (2013)
16. Yang, L., Wang, J., Kobayashi, E., Liao, H., Yamashita, H., Sakuma, I., Chiba, T.: An intraoperative framework for mapping of untracked endoscopic vision to 3D ultrasound placenta. Int J. Cars 8(suppl. 1), 152–153 (2013)

An Augmented Reality Approach for Initializing 2D/3D Registration

Ren Hui Gong, Özgür Güler, John Lovejoy, and Ziv Yaniv

The Sheikh Zayed Institute for Pediatric Surgical Innovation, Children's National Medical Center, Washington DC 20010, USA

Abstract. We describe a technique for intraoperative initialization of 2D/3D registration. The technique uses a tracked tool that is already available in the operating room, as part of an image-guided navigation system, to establish the transformation between the preoperative volume and the intraoperative patient. Initialization is performed in two phases: volume-tool pose planning in the virtual world, and patient-tool pose mimicking in the physical world. Depending on the requirements for accuracy and interaction time, the second phase can be done using either instant, coarse, initialization or Augmented Reality (AR) based interactive initialization. The former method is fast and requires no intraoperative modalities, while the latter uses intraoperative x-rays as a guide to continuously refine the initialization. The proposed technique is appropriate for intraoperative 2D/3D initialization as it is contactless, fast, and uses devices already available as part of the navigation system. Evaluation was done using three publicly available reference data sets. The instant, coarse, initialization was able to provide a mean Target Registration Error (mTRE) of 28-40mm, with the majority of the error associated with errors in translation. The AR-based initialization was able to achieve a mTRE on the order of 5-10mm with an average interaction time of 40-60sec.

1 Introduction

The ability to register preoperative 3D images, CT or MR, to the intraoperative setting is a prerequisite of the majority of image-guided navigation systems. Currently, this is primarily performed using fiducials or anatomical landmarks and surfaces which are digitized intraoperatively. An alternative approach is to perform 2D/3D anatomy-based rigid registration, aligning the volumetric data using x-ray images. This subject has been studied extensively resulting in a large number of published algorithms, as surveyed in [1]. These algorithms vary by modality, anatomical structure and algorithmic approach. While the differences are many, all of them have one characteristic in common, they are iterative and require initialization.

In practice, the majority of 2D/3D registration algorithms have not been able to transition from bench to bedside, except in the domain of radiation therapy. The distinguishing feature of this domain as compared to the operating room

C.A. Linte et al. (Eds.): MIAR/AE-CAI 2013, LNCS 8090, pp. 117–126, 2013.

(OR) is that a good initial estimate of the registration parameters is available via accurate patient positioning using other means. In the laboratory setting various approaches to initialization of 2D/3D registration have been used [1,2], including: (1) knowledge of the spatial relationships associated with the clinical setup; (2) coarse paired point registration using skin adhesive fiducials or anatomical landmarks; and (3) manual, keyboard and mouse based, initialization via interactive positioning of the volumetric data using visual comparison between the medical images and the virtual images.

These approaches are often less applicable in a general clinical setting. Knowledge of the clinical setup to estimate an initial transformation is often not sufficiently accurate. Coarse paired-point registration is not always applicable as it either requires placement of fiducials prior to imaging, making the clinical workflow more cumbersome, or requires digitizing anatomical landmarks which may not be accessible. Finally, use of a keyboard and mouse to perform initialization does not fit well in the OR environment due to the requirement for sterility and the fact that the clinical setting is already physically cramped.

We present an Augmented Reality (AR) approach to initializing 2D/3D anatomy-based registration. Our method uses a tracked tool (e.g. a pointer tool) to augment the physical x-ray image with a virtual, volume rendered, image of the anatomy. The user interactively positions and orients the tool so that the virtual and physical images overlap. This approach uses existing hardware found in any navigation system and can be used for all anatomical volumetric imaging modalities. The method was assessed using publicly available reference data sets for evaluation of 2D/3D registration.

2   Method

Our initialization approach is based on the use of a tracked tool to interactively overlay a volume rendering of the anatomy onto the x-ray images. Using multiple AR views, the user manipulates the tool in physical space until the volume rendering of the anatomy overlaps with the corresponding anatomical structures in all x-ray images.

The approach consists of two steps, planning in the *virtual* world, and interaction in the *physical* world. In the planning step the user places a virtual representation of a physical tool next to the volumetric representation of the anatomical structure obtained from CT or MR. In the interaction step, the user mimics the plan in the physical world. That is, they attempt to position the tool in the same pose relative to the anatomy as was done in the virtual world. Figure 1(a) illustrates the concept of this approach.

In Figure 1(b) we present all of the coordinate systems used by our approach. We assume that the transformation from the tool model to its Dynamic Reference Frame (DRF), $T_{toolmodel}^{toolDRF}$, and from the x-ray images to the tracker are known via tool calibration and camera calibration. The transformation from the volume coordinate system to the tool model coordinate system, $T_{volume}^{toolmodel}$, is specified by the user in the planning step, and the patient coordinate system corresponds

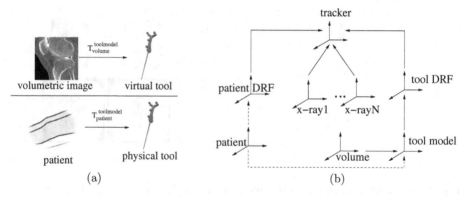

Fig. 1. (a) The user attempts to replicate the pose of the tool defined in the virtual world in the physical world. That is they attempt to position the tool in the physical world such that $T_{volume}^{toolmodel} = T_{patient}^{toolmodel}$. When this happens the volume and patient coordinate systems coincide and we can compute the desired transformation, $T_{patient}^{patientDRF}$. (b) Coordinate systems involved in the registration, solid lines denote known transformations, dashed denote unknown transformations.

to the correct volume pose in the OR, which coincides with the physical location of the patient.

The transformation we seek is given by:

$$T_{patient}^{patientDRF} = (T_{patientDRF}^{tracker})^{-1} T_{toolDRF}^{tracker} T_{toolmodel}^{toolDRF} T_{patient}^{toolmodel}$$

$$\Downarrow$$

$$T_{patient}^{patientDRF} = T_{toolmodel}^{patientDRF} T_{patient}^{toolmodel}$$

If the planned transformation is mimicked accurately in the OR, we have $T_{volume}^{toolmodel} = T_{patient}^{toolmodel}$, which gives us the desired transformation by substitution into the previous equation to yield.

$$T_{patient}^{patientDRF} = T_{toolmodel}^{patientDRF} T_{volume}^{toolmodel} \tag{1}$$

Depending on the accuracy requirements imposed by the subsequent registration algorithm one can use this approach in two ways: instant, coarse, initialization, and interactive AR based initialization. The former is applicable for a variety of intraoperative registration methods as it does not utilize any intraoperative images. The later does require availability of intraoperative images and is thus only applicable to procedures where intraoperative imaging is used.

2.1   Planning

The goal of planning is to define the relative pose between the *tool model* and the *preoperative volume*. This is performed using a graphical user interface (Figure 2(a)), within which the poses of the volume and the tool model can be manipulated individually or concurrently. The tool's pose should match its

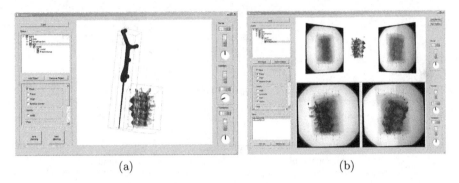

(a)   (b)

Fig. 2. Graphical user interfaces for pose planning in virtual world (a) and pose mimicking in physical world (b)

intended pose in the physical world and it is the user's responsibility to position it in a valid location. This means that the tool cannot overlap with anatomical structures and if using an optical tracking system, its planned position is expected to be visible in the OR.

We use the same approach for registration of CT and MR. Given that in x-ray images the visible structures are primarily bones, we require the user to manipulate the volume rendering transfer function so that these structures are visible to them. This does not imply that the transfer function is optimal, only that for the specific user it yields a visually clear set of anatomical structures.

It should be noted that our approach imposes several requirements on the design of the tracked tool. It must provide six degrees of freedom so that we can manipulate the volume pose in the physical world, and it should not be symmetrical so that the user can visually distinguish between different tool poses. That is, a cylindrical tool such as a needle is best avoided as it defines an infinite number of poses which only differ in rotation about the needle axis. One can design a specific tool based on these requirements, but this is most often not necessary. In our case we utilize a pointer probe which is available as part of the navigation system.

2.2   Instant, Coarse, Initialization

The coarse initialization approach consists of a single step. The planned tool pose is mimicked in the OR by placing the tool besides the patient as planned and initiating the initialization with a foot switch. No further user interaction is required, and $T_{patient}^{patientDRF}$ is estimated instantly. Obviously the accuracy of the result depends on the difference between $T_{volume}^{toolmodel}$, the transformation we use, and $T_{patient}^{toolmodel}$ the correct transformation.

While this method is simple and fast, the initialization accuracy depends on how accurately the planned transformation can be replicated in the OR. By using anatomical landmarks one can plan easy-to-reproduce poses which can provide relatively accurate initializations. As no intraoperative modality is involved, the method can potentially be used to initialize other forms of registration (e.g. point cloud/surface).

2.3 Interactive Augmented Reality Based Initialization

The AR initialization approach is iterative and based on visually guiding the user to the correct pose. We achieve this by real-time direct volume rendering which is overlaid onto the x-ray images. In our case, we perform hardware accelerated volume rendering in parallel for 2-3 images (Figure 2(b)). It should be noted that the camera parameters used to perform the rendering are specific to each x-ray image and are obtained from accurate calibration of the clinical imaging system.

To use the AR based approach, the user starts by performing a coarse initialization as described above. This is required so that there is a reasonable overlap between the rendered image and the x-ray. Then, the user translates and rotates the tracked tool based on the AR views with the goal of maximizing the visual similarity between the overlaid volume rendering and underlying x-ray images. The process continues until a good overall overlay between the x-rays and the corresponding renderings is achieved. The maximal overlap is obtained when $T_{volume}^{toolmodel} = T_{patient}^{toolmodel}$, and the desired transformation is computed as described above. Again, the accuracy of the result depends on the difference between these two transformations.

3 Experiments

3.1 Data

We evaluate our initialization approach using three publicly available reference data sets for 2D/3D registration. The first data set [3] is from the Image Science Institute (ISI), Netherlands, and consists of images from a spine phantom containing three vertebra. The second data set [4] is from the University of Ljubljana, from a phantom consisting of five lumbar vertebra. The third data set [5] is from the Medical University of Vienna, and consists of a cadaver animal head. Unlike the previous two data sets, this data set contains a significant amount of soft tissue which is visible in the x-ray images.

For each of the data sets, we selected two x-ray images, one CT, one MR, and the reference transformations for the CT and MR. The reference transformations position the volumes in the "tracker", common, coordinate frame to match the corresponding x-ray images. Figure 3 shows the x-ray images from all reference data sets.

3.2 Evaluation Scheme

In the reference data sets, only reference transformations with respect to their own "trackers", common coordinate frame, were provided. We need to link these

ISI   U. Ljubljana   Med. U. Vienna

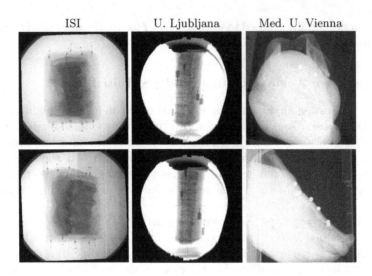

Fig. 3. X-ray images of the reference data sets. First row: AP view. Second row: lateral view.

"tracker" coordinate frames to our physical setup and tracking system. Figure 4(a) illustrates how the reference transformation is established, and how the error transformation is computed. $T_{patient}^{tracker'}$, $T_{xray\_ap}^{tracker'}$ and $T_{xray\_lat}^{tracker'}$ were provided as part of the reference data. The transformation we are interested in, $T_{patient}^{patientDRF}$, is unknown as we do not have the physical phantoms from which the reference data sets were created. We thus need to make an arbitrary choice, relating a physical, tracked, reference frame to the phantom. Once this

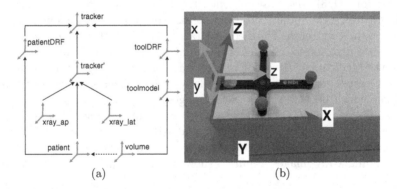

(a)   (b)

Fig. 4. (a) Transformations involved in the validation of the initialization approach. The *tracker'* coordinate system is the common/world coordinate system used by the reference data set. (b) Definition of reference transformation. The patient and DRF coordinate frames are shown in red and green colors, respectively, and the transformation between the two was used as the reference of our experiments.

transformation is established we can compute the transformation $T_{tracker'}^{tracker}$ accordingly to obtain the reference transformations with respect to our tracker. Then the error transformation between the estimated and ground-truth pose is computed as

$$T_{volume}^{patient} = (T_{patientDRF}^{tracker} T_{patient}^{patientDRF})^{-1} T_{toolDRF}^{tracker} T_{toolmodel}^{toolDRF} T_{volume}^{toolmodel} \quad (2)$$

Note that when the user is able to exactly mimic the planned tool position in the physical world we have $T_{volume}^{patient} = I$.

In our experiments, $T_{patient}^{patientDRF}$ was chosen based on the bounding box of the volume. First, a cardboard box, Figure 4(b), was used to represent the physical patient. The box roughly matches the volume's bounding box in size, and its coordinate frame is aligned with the volume's coordinate frame. Then the patient DRF was placed at the lower-left corner of the xz-surface of the box. Finally, we obtained the coordinates of three known points on the box in the DRF's coordinate system. Thus we have the coordinates of the same points in the patient coordinate system and in the DRF coordinate system. From this setup, $T_{patient}^{patientDRF}$ is readily available via paired point rigid registration [6].

We used the Polaris Vicra optical tracking system from Northern Digital Inc. (Waterloo, ON, Canada) to evaluate our approach. Initialization accuracy is evaluated using the mean Target Registration Error (mTRE):

$$mTRE(e; S) = \frac{1}{N} \sum_{i=1}^{N} \| T_{volume}^{patient} p_i \|, \quad (3)$$

where $T_{volume}^{patient}$ is the error transformation with parameters e, computed as Eq. 2, p_i is a point on our target bone surface S, and N is the total number of surface points.

For each data set, combination of x-ray/MR and x-ray/CT, we created ten plans. We thus had 60 planned tool poses in the virtual world. For each of the sixty plans we had two users perform initialization using the coarse and AR based approaches. For the AR-based initialization approach we also recorded the interaction time.

3.3   Results

Table 1 summarizes the results for the coarse initialization. This method resulted in a relatively high mTRE (28-40mm). However it should be noted that the rotational errors are relatively low, while the translational errors are high. This fact can benefit registration algorithms as correcting rotation errors is more challenging than correcting translation errors. We observed that for each data set the rotational errors are more dominant along one axis. Not surprisingly this axis corresponds to the long axis of our tool. As we noted in section 2.1, the uncertainty in orientation when using a cylindrical like tool is higher around its main axis. This theoretical observation is reflected in practice by our results. We also note that the translational errors have large standard deviations. This is

Table 1. Experimental results for coarse initialization (summary of all 120 initialization trials)

	ISI	U. Ljubljana	Med. U. Vienna
mTRE (mm)	28.1 ± 15.4	29.8 ± 14.0	39.9 ± 19.9
θ_x (°)	0.8 ± 3.6	-0.9 ± 1.7	4.4 ± 8.2
θ_y (°)	-6.3 ± 6.6	-0.3 ± 1.3	2.0 ± 1.9
θ_z (°)	2.0 ± 2.5	-5.1 ± 5.0	-0.5 ± 2.8
t_x (mm)	-10.3 ± 13.3	-25.4 ± 17.8	-8.1 ± 12.5
t_y (mm)	7.3 ± 10.1	7.5 ± 15.2	2.6 ± 17.7
t_z (mm)	-10.4 ± 16.3	8.4 ± 11.8	11.7 ± 6.7

primarily due to the variations in pose planning. In our current implementation we did not provide quantitative feedback (i.e. distances between the tool and anatomy), thus the user visually judges the distance in the virtual world and attempts to mimic it in the physical world. This variability can potentially be minimized by allowing the user to measure distances in the virtual world, which they can then mimic more accurately in the physical world.

Figure 5 summarizes the results for the AR-based interactive initialization. With an average interaction time of 40-60 seconds, an average mTRE of 5-10mm can be achieved. These numbers satisfy the requirements of most 2D/3D registration applications.

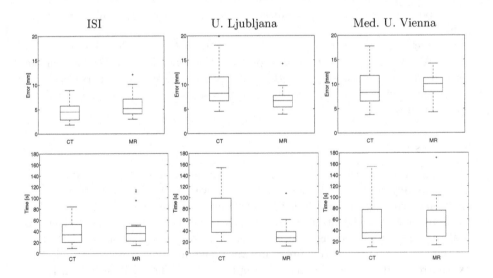

Fig. 5. Experimental results for AR-based interactive initialization. Results from the two users were combined: (top row) mTRE, and (bottom row) interaction time.

3.4   Discussion

The subject of 2D/3D rigid registration is often considered a solved problem. One would assume this is the case given the large number of solutions presented in the literature. Unfortunately, the majority of these methods assume reasonably accurate initialization, mTRE < 10mm, is available, yet they do not specify how it is obtained. While there are specific clinical settings where such an initialization is available, this is not the case in general. As a consequence 2D/3D registration has not been able to transition from bench to bedside.

We propose an AR based solution to initialization which is applicable for image-guided navigation when x-ray images are available. Our method was inspired by an observation made in [7] in the context of segmentation which is equally relevant for registration: Humans are highly adept at determining the presence and rough location of an object of interest in an image. In the context of registration, we provide an intuitive interaction approach which allows us to take advantage of the operators recognition abilities. As a result, the initialization is quick and robust to occlusions in the x-ray image.

To evaluate our approach we used three publicly available reference data sets. On the one hand, this enables a fair comparison between our approach and other methods, all evaluated on the same data sets. On the other hand, these reference data sets do not fully reflect the complexity of the clinical setting. This is primarily visible in the spine data sets which have much less soft tissue than their clinical counterparts. We do not expect this to significantly effect the accuracy of our approach as the operator will implicitly compensate for these differences while interactively setting the volume transfer function during the planning phase. An additional difference between our setting and the OR is that the anatomy of interest may not be visible due to sterile drapes. This can potentially have a significant effect on the results of the coarse registration phase as it solely relies on visually positioning the tool relative to the anatomy without acquiring any intraoperative images. We do not expect this to have a significant effect on our overall results. Our only requirement from the coarse initialization is that the resulting transformation enables us to augment the x-ray images. That is, the volume rendering should have some overlap with the x-ray images which is the case even when the transformation we use is far from the correct one. The user then manipulates the tracked tool based on the AR view which is not effected by the draping. As a consequence we expect similar accuracy in the OR to that obtained in our phantom studies.

4   Conclusion

We described an AR-based approach for initializing 2D/3D registration as part of an image-guided navigation system. The approach does not require any additional equipment and uses a tracked tool which is already part of the navigation system. As our approach is interactive it is equally applicable to registration of CT or MR. In addition, our initialization is based on visual alignment of anatomical structures which simplifies the clinical workflow as there is no requirement for placement of fiducials prior to imaging.

Acknowledgement. We would like to thank E. Wilson for his help creating the mesh model of the tracked tool.

References

1. Markelj, P., Tomaževič, D., Likar, B., Pernuš, F.: A review of 3D/2D registration methods for image-guided interventions. Medical Image Analysis 16(3), 642–661 (2012)
2. Yaniv, Z.: Rigid registration. In: Peters, T., Cleary, K. (eds.) Image-Guided Interventions: Technology and Applications. Springer (May 2008)
3. van de Kraats, E.B., Penney, G.P., Tomaževič, D., van Walsum, T., Niessen, W.J.: Standardized evaluation methodology for 2-D-3-D registration. IEEE Trans. Med. Imag. 24(9), 1177–1189 (2005)
4. Tomaževič, D., Likar, B., Pernuš, F.: Gold standard data for evaluation and comparison of 3D/2D registration methods. Computer Aided Surgery 9(4), 137–144 (2004)
5. Pawiro, S., Markelj, P., Pernus, F., Gendrin, C., Figl, M., Weber, C., Kainberger, F., Nöbauer-Huhmann, I., Bergmeister, H., Stock, M., Georg, D., Bergmann, H., Birkfellner, W.: Validation for 2D/3D registration I: A new gold standard data set. Med. Phys. 38(3), 1481–1490 (2011)
6. Horn, B.K.P.: Closed-form solution of absolute orientation using unit quaternions. Journal of the Optical Society of America A 4(4), 629–642 (1987)
7. Udupa, J.K., et al.: A framework for evaluating image segmentation algorithms. Comput. Med. Imaging Graph. 30(2), 75–87 (2006)

Surface Reconstruction from Tracked Endoscopic Video Using the Structure from Motion Approach

Deyu Sun[1,2], Jiquan Liu[1,*], Cristian A. Linte[2], Huilong Duan[1], and Richard A. Robb[2]

[1] College of Biomedical Engineering & Instrument Science,
Zhejiang University, Hangzhou, China
[2] Biomedical Imaging Resource, Mayo Clinic, Rochester, MN, USA

Abstract. The lack of 3D vision and proper depth perception associated with traditional endoscopy significantly limits the quality of the diagnostic examinations and therapy delivery. To address this challenge, we propose a technique to reconstruct a 3D model of the visualized scene from a sequence of spatially-encoded endoscopic video frames. The method is based on the structure from motion approach adopted from computer vision, and uses both the intrinsic camera parameters, as well as the tracking transforms associated with each acquired video frame to calculate the global coordinates of the features in the video, and generate a true size 3D model of the imaged scene. We conducted a series of phantom experiments to evaluate the robustness of the proposed method and the accuracy of a generated 3D scene, which yielded 1.7 ± 0.9 mm reconstruction error. We also demonstrated the application of the proposed method using patient-specific endoscopic video image samples acquired during an *in vivo* gastroscopy procedure.

Keywords: reconstruction, endoscopy, motion tracking device, structure from motion, hand-eye calibration.

1   Introduction

Endoscopy is the gold standard imaging modality for screening many types of cancers in soft cavities, such as gastric and colorectal cancer. However, the limitations of endoscopic video, including lack of 3D vision and depth perception, as well as radial image distortions, present challenges to clinicians as far as hand-eye coordination and operating field localization, which, in turn, impact the quality of the endoscopic exam. As an example, during endoscopy procedures, the digestive tract is examined segment by segment, but it is difficult to keep track of any segments that might have been left unexamined. In fact, ~13% of examinations are incomplete, leading to a high "miss rate" for pathological conditions [1, 2].

A visualization approach that conveys the 3D relationship between the imaged structures would greatly improve this technique. However, 3D scene reconstruction from video images of soft cavity organs remains a difficult problem. Due to the deformability of soft cavity organs, conventional modeling methods of reconstruction

---

* Corresponding author.

C.A. Linte et al. (Eds.): MIAR/AE-CAI 2013, LNCS 8090, pp. 127–135, 2013.
© Springer-Verlag Berlin Heidelberg 2013

from pre-operative imaging data have limited success. In recent years, computer vision based algorithms have attracted great attention, for their potential to provide *in vivo*, intraoperative reconstructions of the soft cavity organs using endoscopes. Stoyanov *et al.* used a stereo vision algorithm to create a 3D model of a laparoscopic video scene [3]. Nevertheless, given the limited baseline length (on the order of the endoscope diameter), the stereo vision algorithm cannot precisely reconstruct 3D scenes at a relatively large distance. To overcome this shortcoming, some researchers even proposed to change the position of optical cameras to the lateral side of the endoscope [4]. Another attempt was led by Fuchs *et al.* [5], who replaced the traditional endoscopic camera with a structured light projector and scanner to provide an augmented reality visualization of the soft tissue. Although adequate, this approach requires additional surgery to acquire the 3D structure. In addition, both stereo reconstruction and reconstruction based on structured light cannot make use of typical monocular endoscope.

We propose a novel 3D reconstruction method based on a well-known computer vision algorithm - the structure from motion (SFM), which enables 3D structure reconstruction from a single moving camera. Hartley *et al.* have shown that the SFM method can only reconstruct a true size 3D model from an un-calibrated camera, if the positions of several reference points in the imaged scene are known [6]. To compensate for the inability to annotate reference points on the patient's organ during endoscopic procedures, our method uses a motion tracking device (i.e., tracking sensor) attached to the endoscope to estimate the position and pose of endoscope in real time. For robotic applications, this approach is known as hand-eye calibration [7] and several groups have proposed various approaches to perform the calibration, by imposing special requirements on the endoscope positions and poses during image acquisition. Unfortunately, such requirements are difficult to meet in a clinical setting, as humans do not possess the same precision as robots, and the optimal tracking volume associated with the employed magnetic tracking system is also a limiting factor (a small cuboid of 31cm x 46cm x 30 cm).

Here, we propose a new approach to solve hand-eye calibration problem. By tracking the position and orientation of the endoscope in real time, the true coordinates of the imaged scene can be identified, and a 3D surface model of the viewed scene can be generated. Comparing with existing reconstruction algorithms, the advantage of our method is that it applies to typical monocular endoscopes. The method is implemented and validated using a traditional gastroscope (GIF-QX240, Olympus Corp., CA, USA).

2   Materials and Methods

2.1   Outline of the Method

Given the homologous pixel coordinates $x_i \leftrightarrow x_i'$ of a 3D point X_i imaged in two different frames, according to the SFM theory, the global 3D coordinates of X_i can be computed by solving the following linear equations:

$$\begin{cases} x_i = PX_i \\ x_i' = P'X_i \end{cases}$$

(1)

where P and P' are projection matrices of the endoscope at two positions. The projection matrix is defined by the intrinsic parameters and extrinsic parameters of the endoscope.

$$P = \begin{bmatrix} f_x & 0 & c_x \\ 0 & f_y & c_y \\ 0 & 0 & 1 \end{bmatrix} \begin{bmatrix} 1 & 0 & 0 & 0 \\ 0 & 1 & 0 & 0 \\ 0 & 0 & 1 & 0 \end{bmatrix} \begin{bmatrix} R & t \\ 0^T & 1 \end{bmatrix}$$

(2)

where f_x, f_y are dependent on the endoscope focal length and physical size; and c_x, c_y represent the intersection of endoscope optical axis and imaging plane.

These four parameters describe the optical properties of the endoscope, referred to as intrinsic parameters, while R and t describe the transform between the world coordinate system and the camera coordinate system, referred to extrinsic parameters. Based on the description above, our method can be divided into six steps (Fig. 1). In the paper, we only focused on hand-eye calibration and briefly introduced other steps.

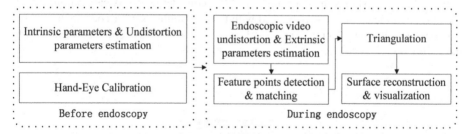

Fig. 1. Flow-chart of the reconstruction method

The lens of endoscope is similar to a fish-eye lens and the acquired images appear distorted. To correct for these distortions, the intrinsic parameters of the endoscope can be determined before endoscopy using the widely-accepted method proposed by Zhang's et al. [8], and used to un-distort the images.

Then the extrinsic parameters of the endoscope was estimated by the hand-eye calibration method which was detailed in section 2.2.

To obtain the corresponding points $x_i \leftrightarrow x_i'$ in the two frames, we chose to use the Features from Accelerated Segment Test (FAST) detector [9] , as it is a scale and rotation invariant and features faster performance and a higher detection rate than other commonly used detectors, such as the Scale-Invariant Feature Transform (SIFT) and Speeded Up Robust Features (SURF) detectors. After detection, a multi-dimensional vector was then extracted to describe each feature, followed by matching of homologoues features from the two frames using the k-nearest neighbor algorithm.

Triangulation is the process of computing the 3D coordinate from two different views using the linear equations in (1). Since there might be errors in the detected corresponding points $x_i \leftrightarrow x_i'$, the 3D coordinates solved from (1) are only an approximation of real point. To obtain a robust and meaningful solution, the geometric error cost function was used to solve the optimization problem, the solution of which is the closest point on the epipolar line [6].

Based on the 3D coordinates determined from equation (1), the triangle patches were generated to form a surface model, which was visualized using a surface rendering method.

2.2   Hand-Eye Calibration and Estimation of Extrinsic Parameters

The endoscope was instrumented by attaching an Ascension magnetic tracking sensor (Ascension, Northern Digital Inc. Waterloo, Canada) (Fig. 2(c)), enabling real-time identification of the endoscope position and pose within the magnetic field generated by the transmitter (Fig. 2(a)). Currently, the tracking sensor and its cable were attached to the endoscope by surgical tape; before endoscopy, the endoscope as well as the attached sensor were sterilized. In future, we considered to incorporate tracking sensor into endoscope directly, e.g. attached the tracking sensor through the endoscope tube in a way similar to how biopsy forceps and endoscopic ultrasonography is utilized. Fig. 2(d) shows the coordinate systems considered in this calibration: world (global) coordinate system – associated with the transmitter; sensor coordinate system – associated with the tracking sensor; and camera coordinate system – associated with the acquired images.

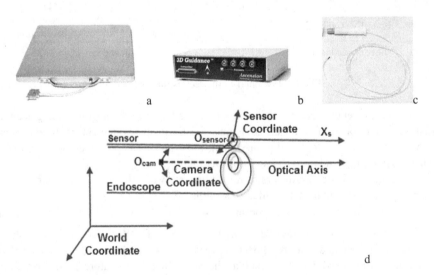

Fig. 2. (a-c): 6DOF magnetic tracking system, including a flat transmitter (a), power unit (b), and tracking sensor (c). (d): coordinate systems considered in this application.

The extrinsic parameters represent the transform between the world and camera coordinates. Since the transform between the sensor and world coordinates is provided by the tracking system, the key to compute the extrinsic parameters is to determine the transform between the sensor and camera coordinate, (i.e. the hand-eye calibration transform) determined using the method illustrated below Fig. 3.

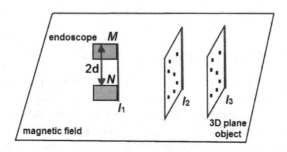

Fig. 3. Determination of the hand-eye calibration transform: A checker-board pattern is imaged from two different endoscope positions, while maintaining the optical axes parallel

To determine this transform, we imaged a checker-board pattern from two different endoscope positions precisely marked to ensure that the endoscope optical axis is maintained parallel between the two different acquisitions. The endoscope was first places at position M, and image M-l_2 of the checker-board patterns in position l_2 was acquired, containing K features (corners). The pattern was then shifted to position (l_3) 10 mm away and maintained, and image M-l_3 was acquired. This protocol was repeated with the endoscope at position N, keeping the optical axes at the two positions parallel, and images N-l_2 and N-l_3 were acquired. With the images M-l_2 and N-l_2, we can calculate the 3D coordinates of the first K points at the position of l_2 by using the stereo vision triangulation theory:

$$Z_i = \frac{2f_x d}{x_{i,M} - x_{i,N}}, \, X_{i,M} = \frac{Z_i}{f_x}\left(x_{i,M} - c_x\right), Y_{i,M} = \frac{Z_i}{f_y}\left(y_{i,M} - c_y\right) \qquad (3)$$

where f_x, f_y, c_x, c_y are endoscope intrinsic parameters, $(x_{i,M}, y_{i,M})$ are the pixel coordinate of feature point i in the imaging plane with the endoscope positioned at M, $(X_{i,M}, Y_{i,M}, Z_i)$ are the 3D camera coordinates with the endoscope positioned at M, and $x_{i,M} - x_{i,N}$ is referred to as the disparity. The second set of K features at the position of l_3 can be obtained in a similar fashion. The world coordinate of the two sets of K features were measured by selecting them with the tracked stilus. After defining the world-to-camera coordinate transform ($R_{c->w}, t_{c->w}$) using the two sets of K homologous features, the transform from the camera to sensor coordinate ($R_{c->s}, t_{c->s}$) can be calculated:

$$R_{c->s} = R_{s->w}^{-1} R_{c->w}, \, t_{c->s} = R_{s->w}^{-1}\left(t_{c->w} - t_{s->w}\right) \qquad (4)$$

Following hand-eye calibration, the extrinsic parameters of the endoscope at any position can be calculated by equation (5), and all imaged features can be transposed from the image coordinate frame into the world coordinate frame.

$$R_{w->c} = \left(R_{s->w} R_{c->s}\right)^{-1}, t_{w->c} = -R_{c->s}^{-1} R_{s->w}^{-1} \left(R_{s->w} t_{c->s} + t_{s->w}\right) \tag{5}$$

3   Results

3.1   Validation of Hand-Eye Calibration Method

To evaluate the precision of our hand-eye calibration method, we computed the sensor-to-camera transform at three different positions in the magnetic field. Ideally the transform should be reproducible, however, due to the measurement and computational uncertainty, slight differences were observed (Table 1).

The error associated with the translation vector is measured by calculating the Euclidean distance from each measured vector $t_{c->s,i}$ to their mean. To determine the error associated with the rotation matrix, we computed the difference between the mapping of a unit vector under the mean transform, and each of the three transforms, and used the maximum angle between the resulting vectors as a measure of error:

$$Error \leq \sqrt{\max\left(eig\left(\left(R_{c->s,i} - \overline{R}_{c->s}\right)^T \left(R_{c->s,i} - \overline{R}_{c->s}\right)\right)\right)} \tag{6}$$

where $R_{c->s,i}$ is the rotation matrix measure at position i and $\overline{R}_{c->s}$ is their mean.

Table 1. Results of Hand-Eye Calibration

Position	$t_{c->s}$ (mm)	Rotation angle around X, Y, Z axes (degree)	Error of $t_{c->s}$ (mm)	Error of $R_{c->s}$ (radian)
1	(-1.96, -8.55, -3.76)	(89.87, -4.51, 84.97)	0.14	0.0028
2	(-1.96, -8.71, -3.19)	(89.66, -4.62, 85.05)	0.05	0.0029
3	(-2.03, -8.65, -3.26)	(89.93, -4.76, 85.17)	0.02	0.0035
Average	(-1.98, -8.64, -3.40)	(89.82, -4.63, 85.06)	/	/

3.2   Estimation of Reconstruction Error

To evaluate the error associated with the reconstruction of the 3D scene, we designed a phantom experiment using a gastric model with 28 markers attached on its inner wall (Fig. 4 (a)). The model was imaged from two different positions using a gastroscope (Fig 4.b&c) and Fig. 4(d) shows the reconstructed 3D surface model of the imaged scene. The reconstruction error was determined as the Euclidean distance between the reconstructed and true marker coordinates (identified by discretization with a tracked stylus) and which resulted in 1.7±0.9 mm, equivalent to a root mean square (RMS) error of 1.9 mm.

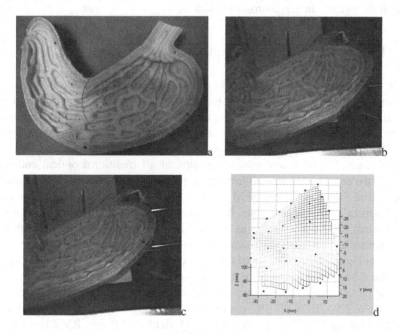

Fig. 4. 3D reconstruction of the gastric model containing 28 markers (a) imaged from two different views (b) and (c), and reconstructed as a 3D rendered surface (d)

3.3   Reconstruction from an *in vivo* Gastroscopy Procedure

To demonstrate the value of the proposed method in the context of an intended clinical application, Fig. 5(a & b) shows a pair of video images acquired during an *in vivo* gastroscopy procedure, from which features of interest were detected and matched. The black hole in the image is pylorus.

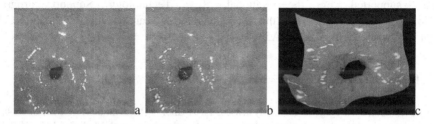

Fig. 5. (a) & (b) *In vivo* demonstration of feature detection and matching from two (a) & (b) clinical gastroscopy images, with the 3D reconstructed scene in (c) displayed as a rendered surface. The arrow direction and length represent the direction and strength of the feature vector, respectively. The features with same direction and strength represent the matched features.

Fig. 5 (c) is the surface reconstructed from the frames pairs in Fig. 5(a) & (b). In the reconstructed model we can also see the pylorus, the black hole in the center, and the region around the pylorus is slightly convex, which just accords with the shape of the pylorus in the gastroscopic videos.

4   Discussion and Conclusion

In this paper, we proposed an fast and efficient surface reconstruction approach for soft cavity organs based on typical monocular endoscopic video frames acquired while the position and orientation of the endoscope is tracked using magnetic tracking system. To determine the intrinsic parameters of the endoscopic camera, we used the method proposed by Zhang *et al.*, which assumes an invariant endoscope focal length the procedure. This is a common assumption of all traditional optical endoscopes, requiring the determination of all intrinsic parameters only once, prior to a procedure. Compared to the conventional SFM method, our method is more accurate in estimation of camera's position and pose. According to Velez et al [10], the translation error of traditional SFM was as large as 27.7122 mm while ours was no more than 0.14 mm. Another advantage featured by our method is the computation of the extrinsic parameters simply by several matrix computations, without the need for any complex algorithms. Moreover, by employing high-speed feature detectors and using GPU acceleration to un-distort the acquired video frames, our method performs in less than 30 ms on a 2.5 GHz CPU PC running 64-bit Windows 7 with 4G RAM and an NVIDIA Quadro FX 570 graphics card, and yields a 1.9 mm RMS reconstruction error. Compared to the stereo reconstruction method proposed by Stoyanov et al [11], our method has a lower reconstruction error (1.9 mm compared to 2~10 mm).

To date, the method had been used in an image-guided biopsy marking system for gastroscopy [12]. Future efforts will be channeled to improve computer-aided endoscopy, as a means to provide better real-time visualization for superior clinical evaluation and examination quality.

Acknowledgement. We thank Dr. Si Jianmin and Dr. Hu Weiling from Sir Run Run Shaw Hospital, Hangzhou for their help to improve the algorithm. The project was supported by the National Key Technology Support Program (No. 2011BAI12B01) and the Fundamental Research Funds for the Central Universities (No. 2013QNA5018).

References

1. Pickhardt, P.J., Nugent, P.A., Mysliwiec, P.A., Choi, J.R., Schindler, W.R.: Location of adenomas missed by optical colonoscopy. Annals of Internal Medicine 141, 352–359 (2004)
2. Shah, H.A., Paszat, L.F., Saskin, R., Stukel, T.A., Rabeneck, L.: Factors associated with incomplete colonscopy: A population-based study. Gastroenterology 132, 2297–2303 (2007)

3. Stoyanov, D., Scarzanella, M.V., Pratt, P., Yang, G.-Z.: Real-time stereo reconstruction in robotically assisted minimally invasive surgery. In: Jiang, T., Navab, N., Pluim, J.P.W., Viergever, M.A. (eds.) MICCAI 2010, Part I. LNCS, vol. 6361, pp. 275–282. Springer, Heidelberg (2010)
4. Czamek, R., Kolff, J.: Stereo laparoscope with discrete working distance. US patent 6767321 (2004)
5. Fuchs, H., et al.: Augmented reality visualization for laparoscopic surgery. In: Wells, W.M., Colchester, A.C.F., Delp, S.L. (eds.) MICCAI 1998. LNCS, vol. 1496, pp. 934–943. Springer, Heidelberg (1998)
6. Hartley, R., Zisserman, A.: Multiple View Geometry in Computer Vision. Cambridge University Press, New York (2001)
7. Tsai, R.Y., Lenz, R.K.: A new technique for fully autonomous and efficient 3D robotics hand/eye calibration. In: International Conference on Robotics and Automation, vol. 1, pp. 554–561 (1988)
8. Zhang, Z.: A flexible new technique for camera calibration. IEEE Transactions on Pattern Analysis and Machine Intelligence 22(11), 1330–1334 (2000)
9. Rosten, E., Drummond, T.: Machine learning for high-speed corner detection. In: Leonardis, A., Bischof, H., Pinz, A. (eds.) ECCV 2006, Part I. LNCS, vol. 3951, pp. 430–443. Springer, Heidelberg (2006)
10. Vélez, A.F.M., Marcinczak, J.M., Grigat, R.-R.: Structure from motion based approaches to 3D reconstruction in minimal invasive laparoscopy. In: Campilho, A., Kamel, M. (eds.) ICIAR 2012, Part II. LNCS, vol. 7325, pp. 296–303. Springer, Heidelberg (2012)
11. Stoyanov, D., Mylonas, G.P., Deligianni, F., Darzi, A., Yang, G.Z.: Soft-tissue motion tracking and structure estimation for robotic assisted MIS procedures. In: Duncan, J.S., Gerig, G. (eds.) MICCAI 2005. LNCS, vol. 3750, pp. 139–146. Springer, Heidelberg (2005)
12. Sun, D., Hu, W., Wu, W., Liu, J., Duan, H., Si, J.: Design of the image-guided biopsy marking system for gastroscopy. Journal of Medical Systems 36(5), 2909–2920 (2012)

Towards CT Enhanced Ultrasound Guidance for Off-pump Beating Heart Mitral Valve Repair

Feng P. Li[1,2], Martin Rajchl[1,2], James A. White[1,3], Aashish Goela[4], and Terry M. Peters[1,2]

[1] Imaging Research Laboratories, Robarts Research Institute, London, ON
[2] Biomedical Engineering Graduate Program, Western University, London, ON
[3] Division of Cardiology, Department of Medicine, Western University, London, ON
[4] Department of Medical Imaging, Western University, London, ON

Abstract. Off-pump beating heart interventions require a good guidance system to show both cardiac anatomy and motion. Over the years, echocardiography has become a popular solution for such a purpose because of its real-time imaging capability, flexibility, non-invasiveness, and low cost. However, it can be difficult for surgeons to appreciate the position and orientation of 2D images and to keep surgical tools and targets both shown in the image plane with only ultrasound guidance. In this paper, we propose to use CT images as high-quality 3D context to enhance ultrasound images through image registration to provide a better guidance system with very few changes to standard workflow. We have also developed a method to generate synthetic 4D CT images through non-rigid registration, when dynamic pre-operative CT images are not available. The validation of synthetic CT images was performed by comparing them to real dynamic CT images and the validation of CT-ultrasound registration was performed with static, dynamic, and synthetic CT images.

Keywords: image-guidance, beating-heart interventions, synthetic CT, CT-enhanced ultrasound guidance.

1 Introduction

Mitral valve prolapse (MVP) is a common valvular abnormality that can cause severe non-ischaemic mitral regurgitation[3]. The cause of MVP can be histological abnormalities of valvular tissue, geometric disparities between the left ventricle and mitral valve (MV), or various connective tissue disorders[4]. Implantation of artificial chordae tendineae is a widely used technique for correction of both posterior and anterior leaflet prolapse[2]. The conventional surgical approach for mitral valve repair usually requires a full or partial sternotomy and the use of a heart-lung machine, also referred as the "pump". Recent developments in cardiac surgery, however, have made it possible to perform the repair in a minimally-invasive manner on a beating heart ("off-pump")[1]. However, these

C.A. Linte et al. (Eds.): MIAR/AE-CAI 2013, LNCS 8090, pp. 136–143, 2013.

minimally invasive approaches are often limited by the lack of a direct view of surgical targets and/or tools, a challenge that is compounded by potential movement of the target during the cardiac cycle. For this reason, sophisticated image-guided navigation systems are required to assist in procedural efficiency and therapeutic success.

Guidance systems for off-pump beating heart interventions must show both cardiac anatomy and tissue motion. Echocardiography (ultrasound), because of its real-time imaging capability, flexibility, non-invasiveness, and low cost, is frequently employed in cardiac surgery as both a monitoring and imaging modality. However, safety concerns exist since it can be difficult for surgeons to appreciate the position and orientation of 2D images relative to a surgical tool, and to keep the tool tip and target in the image plane simultaneously. As alternatives, fluoroscopy can only provide real-time 2D projection images , while poorly demonstrating the target anatomical structures; intra-operative MRI has the capability of displaying cardiac anatomy and motion dynamically during interventions[7], but is very expensive, requires developments of novel, non-ferromagnetic tools and devices, and is unavailable in most institutions. To overcome these limitations, Moore et al.[9] described a navigation system for off-pump beating heart mitral valve repair, in which the bi-plane transesophageal echocardiogram (TEE) images were augmented by a virtual presentation of selected anatomical models, i.e. mitral valve annulus (MVA) and aortic valve annulus (AVA), which were defined by manually identified feature points on the TEE images right before the surgery started. Animal studies showed that the augmented virtuality guidance that they employed significantly improved the efficiency, accuracy, and safety of the procedure that involved guiding the surgical tool from the entry point at the cardiac apex to the target area, compared to TEE-only guidance. However, the virtual anatomical model were not dynamically updated and could be centimeters away from the actual position due to physical movement of the target during the surgery.

In this paper, we propose a guidance system that improves on Moore's work by employing CT-enhanced ultrasound images for guiding such procedures. Both CT and ultrasound are commonly used in the standard clinical workflow for cardiac interventions, so the proposed approach requires very few changes in the image acquisition workflow. In this guidance system, intra-operative TEE images display the real-time cardiac anatomy and motion, while the pre-operatively acquired high spatial resolution CT images are dynamically fused with the TEE images to provide a high quality 4D context. We also developed a method to generate patient-specific synthetic 4D CT image sequences based on a static CT image and 4D ultrasound images to avoid the need to acquire high-dose retrospectively-gated CT scans[5]. We validated and compared the accuracy and efficiency of different registration approaches with both real and synthetic CT images, with respect to the mitral valve annulus, the target for procedures that aim to repair the mitral valve.

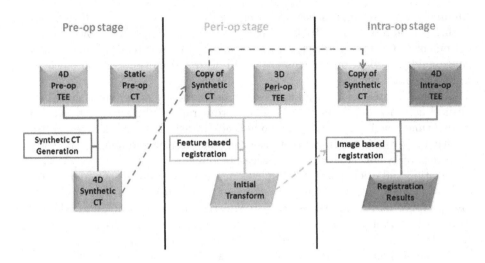

Fig. 1. The suggested clinical workflow of how to use CT-enhanced ultrasound guidance for off-pump beating heart interventions

2   Methods

2.1   Suggested Clinical Workflow

The suggested clinical workflow for using CT-enhanced ultrasound guidance is illustrated below (Fig. 1). In the pre-operative stage, 4D CT images are either acquired by performing a retrospectively gated CT scan or generated based on a static CT and 4D ultrasound images from the same patient using the proposed synthetic CT generation method. The 4D CT images are transferred to the guidance system and brought to the operation room prior to surgery.

In the peri-operative stage, an initial registration is performed between a peri-operatively required 3D ultrasound volume and a CT image at the same or closest cardiac phase using feature based registration. Features, such as the inner walls of the left ventricles, are semi-automatically segmented using an approach described in [11]. The resulting registration transform is then saved and used as an initialization for the intra-operative CT to ultrasound registration.

In the intra-operative stage, CT images are registered to the intra-operatively acquired TEE images using rapid GPU-based algorithm. The registered images can be visualized in different formats according to surgeon's preference, such as directly overlaying TEE images onto CT, displaying the volume rendering CT images within the visualization environment, or simply extracting critical features from these images and displaying them fused the CT or TEE volumes. In this way, visual linkage can be provided between the intra-operative images, pre-operative image, anatomical models, and surgical tools within the same guidance framework.

2.2   Generation of 4D Synthetic CT

The generation of the synthetic dynamic CT images is performed through non-rigid registrations between ultrasound images [12] over a single cardiac cycle to obtain patient specific heart motion maps, in the form of deformation fields, and to apply these vector maps to CT images to provide synthetic animation. In this approach, at least one sequence of 3D TEE images, representing at least one complete cardiac cycle, and one single frame cardiac CT images must be acquired pre-operatively.

The procedure begins with the selection of a single 3D TEE image, acquired at a cardiac phase close to the static CT image as a reference and rigidly registering it to the static CT image. The rigid registration is performed by semi-automatically segmenting the inner wall of the left ventricles from both the reference TEE image and the static CT image, aligning the segmented ventricles with the Iterative Closest Point (ICP) method, and refining the alignment with a mutual information based registration [6] . All the other TEE images in the 4D sequence are then rigidly registered to the reference image as initialization for the later non-rigid transform.

After the initial rigid registration step, non-rigid registrations are performed amongst the ultrasound images in the 4D sequence. To obtain the deformations fields that relate the reference image to all the other images in the sequence, we can either perform registration directly between the reference image and each member of the sequece, between temporally adjacent images, or in a group-wise manner [13]. The deformation fields are then employed as cardiac motion maps and applied to the static CT image to generate a synthetic dynamic CT sequence. By performing this approach for each frame, we can generate an entire sequence of synthetic dynamic CT images with the same temporal resolution as the 4D TEE images. The non-rigid registration method we employed is the mult-resolution fast free-from (F3D) deformation registration method described by Modat et al. [8], because of its capability of handling the morphological deformation due to cardiac motion and providing relatively smooth deformation fields.

2.3   GPU-Based Real-Time Registration

During the intra-operative stage, real-time image registration is performed between intra-operative and pre-operative images. Dynamic CT images obtained from retrospectively gated scans, synthetic CT images generated by our method, and pre-operative 4D TEE images, can potentially fulfill the role of pre-operative images in the proposed system. CT images can be registered to the intra-operative TEE images in two different ways. The first is to perform online registration directly between the CT images and intra-operative TEE images, using a multi-modality registration method. The second is to perform the registration between CT images and pre-operative TEE images prior to the surgery, perform online registration between intra-operative and pre-operative TEE images during the surgery, and then combine the two transforms to achieve registration between CT and intra-operative TEE images. The potential benefit of the second method is that the off-line registration can be verified by clinicians prior to the procedure to ensure optimized results, and the online registration is between images of a single modality (i.e. ultrasound), which can potentially be performed more efficiently and reliably. We used mutual information (MI) as the similarity metric for CT to TEE registration, while employing sum of squared differences (SSD) for TEE to TEE registration. Validation of these methods is presented below.

In this project we perform rigid registration between intra- and pre-operative images at corresponding cardiac phases. To accelerate this process, bringing it close to real-time, the registration algorithms are parallelized on graphic processing units (GPUs). The registration pipeline contains three components: image transform, linear interpolation, and similarity metric computation. In this case, image transform and interpolation can be completely parallelized and very efficiently implemented on a GPU, since the operation on each voxel is identical and independent. However, the similarity metric computation, either MI or SSD, cannot be perfectly parallelized due to potential race conditions [10], that is caused by access to a shared memory address by multiple processing threads without proper synchronization which can lead to unexpected results. We therefore use a recursive method, that divides the entire volume into small blocks first and then iteratively sums up the intermediate results, to achieve partial parallelization for this computation.

3   Experiments and Results

3.1   Validation of Synthetic CT

The validation of the quality of synthetic CT images is perform by comparing the synthetic images to real dynamic CT volumes. We performed the validation the data from five patient. For each patient we acquired a dynamic CT sequence representing one cardiac cycle and a 4D TEE sequece representing several cardiac cycles. The first images in the dynamic CT sequence was used as a static CT image from which synthetic CT images were generated. Then, we manually segmented the left ventricles from both dynamic and synthetic CT images and compared them at corresponding cardiac phases with respect to the Dice Similarity Coefficient(DSC) and root mean square errors (RMSe). The results are shown in Table 1.

Table 1 demonstrates that the left ventricles in the synthetic CT images were quite similar as the ones in the dynamic CT images with a mean DSC of 0.82 and mean RMS of 2.96mm. However, the comparison results at diastolic frames, such as frame 2 and 10, are better than the results at systole (frame 4 and 5). One possible reason for this phenomenon is that patients were under general anesthesia when taking TEE scans, while they were awake when taking dynamic CT scans.

Table 1. Comparison of left ventricles between synthetic and dynamic CT images over one cardiac cycle of five patients

# of frame	2	3	4	5	6	7	8	9	10
DSC(mean)	0.86	0.81	0.77	0.77	0.80	0.83	0.83	0.85	0.87
DSC(σ)	0.03	0.02	0.05	0.05	0.03	0.04	0.05	0.04	0.03
RMS(mean)	2.48	3.11	3.67	3.63	3.28	2.74	2.71	2.59	2.42
RMS(σ)	0.60	0.46	0.88	0.58	0.77	0.84	0.43	0.21	0.27

*RMS measurements in mm

3.2 Validation of CT-TEE Registration

In order to examine the impact of introducing dynamic and synthetic CT images to the guidance system, we performed CT-TEE registration using static, dynamic, and synthetic CT images. The static CT images used in this experiment were acquired at end-diastole. We manually segmented the mitral valve annulus (MVA), which indicates the target area in the mitral valve repair procedure, and used it for the target registration error (TRE) tests. Two registration approaches were used. The first directly performs multi-modality registration between pre-operative CT and intra-operative TEE images, while the second separates the registration into two stages, CT-TEE registration at pre-operative stage and TEE-TEE registration at intra-operative stage. The first approach uses mutual information as a similarity metric, while the second uses SSD. The validation was performed on five patients' data and for each patient we used image sequences representing two cardiac cycles. The result is shown in Table 2.

Table 2. Comparison of TRE w.r.t. MVA with static, dynamic, and synthetic CT images (mm)

CT-TEE Registration						
CT type	Static		Dynamic		Synthetic	
Cardiac phase of TEE	ES	ED	ES	ED	ES	ED
RMS (mean)	9.00	4.90	3.94	4.94	4.59	4.12
RMS (σ)	2.51	0.95	1.37	0.74	1.22	0.41

CT-TEE + TEE-TEE Registration						
CT type	Static		Dynamic		Synthetic	
Cardiac phase of TEE	ES	ED	ES	ED	ES	ED
RMS (mean)	10.37	5.56	4.59	5.23	5.91	4.29
RMS (σ)	1.36	2.25	0.33	1.52	2.08	1.03

*ES: end-systole, ED:end-diastole

Table 2 shows that, with both registration approaches, using only a static CT image for registration can result in large TRE errors when the TEE image was acquired at a different cardiac phase. However, this error can be reduced by using dynamic or synthetic CT images. The result showed that using the synthetic CT images generated by our method led to results similar to those obtained from

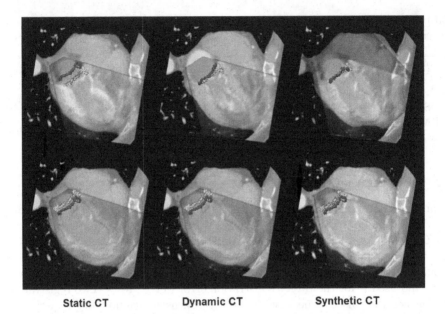

Static CT   **Dynamic CT**   **Synthetic CT**

Fig. 2. An example of registration results. First row: results at end systole; Second row: results at end diastole; Left column: registration using static CT; Middle column: registration using dynamic CT; Right column: registration using synthetic CT. TEE images are shown in yellow, while CT images are shown in grey. The yellow curves represent MVA from TEE, while the red curves represent MVA from CT.

actual dynamic CT images. However, using synthetic CT can greatly reduce the radiation dose applied to patients.

Comparing the two registration approaches, it can be observed that the result of directly CT-TEE approach was slightly better than the two-stage approach. A possible reason for this is that the two-stage method introduced registration errors in both of the stages and these errors were accumulated. However, the two-stage approach showed better efficiency at the intra-operative stage, requiring 227 ± 63ms to perform a TEE-TEE registration using SSD, while the direct approach required 430 ± 182ms to perform a CT-TEE registration using mutual information.

4   Discussion and Conclusion

We proposed a CT-enhanced ultrasound guidance system in which pre-operative CT images and intra-operative TEE images are fused to provide both real-time cardiac motion and high quality 3D anatomy context. The proposed solution can provide a linkage between pre-operative and intra-opertive images and flexibility in visualization formats. It is cost-effective and requires very few changes to the current standard workflow. We have also developed a method to generate synthetic 4D CT images to be used in the guidance system. The validation showed that by introducing synthetic CT images to the system, we can achieve better results than using a static CT image and similar results to the use of actual dynamic images, without applying high radiation dose to the patient.

References

[1] Bajona, P., Katz, W.E., Daly, R.C., Zehr, K.J., Speziali, G.: Beating-heart, off-pump mitral valve repair by implantation of artificial chordae tendineae: an acute in vivo animal study. The Journal of Thoracic and Cardiovascular Surgery 137(1), 188–193 (2009)

[2] David, T.E., Ivanov, J., Armstrong, S., Christie, D., Rakowski, H.: A comparison of outcomes of mitral valve repair for degenerative disease with posterior, anterior, and bileaflet prolapse. The Journal of Thoracic and Cardiovascular Surgery 130(5), 1242–1249 (2005)

[3] Freed, L., Levy, D., Levine, R., Larson, M., Evans, J., Fuller, D., Lehman, B., Benjamin, E.: Prevelence and Clinical Outcome of Mitral Valve Porlapse. The New England Journal of Medicine 341(1), 1–7 (1999)

[4] Hayek, E., Gring, C.N., Griffin, B.P.: Mitral valve prolapse. Lancet 365(9458), 507–518 (2005)

[5] Hirai, N., Horiguchi, J., Fujioka, C., Kiguchi, M., Yamamoto, H., Matsuura, N., Kitagawa, T., Teragawa, H., Kohno, N., Ito, K.: Prospective versus Retrospective ECG-gated 64-Detector Coronary CT Angiography: Assessment of Image Quality, Stenosis, and Radiation Dose. Radiology 248(2), 424–430 (2008)

[6] Maes, F., Collignon, A., Vandermeulen, D., Marchal, G., Suetens, P.: Multimodality image registration by maximization of mutual information. IEEE Transactions on Medical Imaging 16(2), 187–198 (1997)

[7] Mcveigh, E.R., Guttman, M.A., Kellman, P., Raval, A.N., Lederman, R.J., Cardiology Branch A N R.: Real-time, Interactive MRI for Cardiovascular Interventions. Acad. Radiol. 12(9), 1121–1127 (2005)

[8] Modat, M., Ridgway, G.R., Taylor, Z.A., Lehmann, M., Barnes, J., Hawkes, D.J., Fox, N.C., Ourselin, S.: Fast free-form deformation using graphics processing units. Computer Methods and Programs in Biomedicine 98(3), 278–284 (2010)

[9] Moore, J., Wedlake, C., Bainbridge, D., Guiraudon, G., Chu, M., Kiaii, B., Lang, P., Rajchl, M., Peters, T.: A navigation platform for guidance of beating heart transapical mitral valve repair. IEEE Transactions on Biomedical Engineering (2012)

[10] Netzer, R.H.B., Miller, B.P.: What Are Race Conditions? Some Issues and Formalization of Wisconsin. Journal ACM Letters on Programming Languages and Systems 1(1), 74–88 (1992)

[11] Rajchl, M., Yuan, J., White, J.A., Nambakhsh, C.M.S., Ukwatta, E., Li, F., Stirrat, J., Peters, T.M.: A fast convex optimization approach to segmenting 3D scar tissue from delayed-enhancement cardiac MR images. In: Ayache, N., Delingette, H., Golland, P., Mori, K. (eds.) MICCAI 2012, Part I. LNCS, vol. 7510, pp. 659–666. Springer, Heidelberg (2012)

[12] Wierzbicki, M., Drangova, M., Guiraudon, G., Peters, T.: Validation of dynamic heart models obtained using non-linear registration for virtual reality training, planning, and guidance of minimally invasive cardiac surgeries. Medical Image Analysis 8(3), 387–401 (2004)

[13] Wu, G., Yap, P.-T., Wang, Q., Shen, D.: Groupwise Registration from Exemplar to Group Mean: Extending Hammer to Groupwise Registration. In: Proceedings of the Conference on Information Processing in Medical Imaging, pp. 396–399 (2010)

A Bayesian Approach for Construction of Sparse Statistical Shape Models Using Dirichlet Distribution

Ali Gooya[1,2,*], Elaheh Mousavi[1], Christos Davatzikos[2], and Hongen Liao[3,4]

[1] Tarbiat Modares University, Tehran, Iran
[2] Department of Radiology, The University of Pennsylvania, US
[3] School of Medicine, Tsinghua University, China
[4] Graduate School of Engineering, The University of Tokyo, Japan
a.gooya@modares.ac.ir,
christos.davatzikos@uphs.upenn.edu,
liao@bmpe.t.u-tokyo.jp

Abstract. Statistical shape models (SSMs) made using point sets are important tools to capture the variations within shape populations. One popular method for construction of SSMs is based on the Expectation-Maximization (EM) algorithm which establishes probabilistic matches between the model and training points. In this paper, we propose a novel Bayesian framework to automatically determine the optimal number of the model points. We use a Dirichlet distribution as a prior to enforce sparsity on the mixture weights of Gaussians. Insignificant model points are determined and pruned out using a quadratic programming technique. We apply our method to learn a sparse SSM from 15 manually segmented caudate nuclei data sets. The generalization ability of the proposed model compares favorably to a traditional EM based model.

1 Introduction

Statistical shape models, originally invented by Cootes *et. al.* in [1], have a long history in aiding automatic segmentation of anatomical structures using prior shape based information [2][3]. Learning a shape prior from training data can be in general described as the problem of density estimation in pattern analysis. Parametric modeling of statistics from training data is a popular method mainly due to its compactness and computational efficiency. However using these methods, an optimal model complexity must be chosen. This is an important issue because it affects the generalization efficiency of the trained model. For SSMs with no exact point correspondences, the model complexity can refer to the number of the points representing the mean shape, which is usually selected prior to construction of the model [4][5].

One of the traditional approaches for determining an optimal model during the training phase is to enforce sparsity on an initially maximal model. To the

---

* Corresponding author.

C.A. Linte et al. (Eds.): MIAR/AE-CAI 2013, LNCS 8090, pp. 144–152, 2013.

best of our knowledge, no prior such work has been published in the context of SSMs to address the problem of selecting the number of points on the mean model. Zhang *et.al.* proposed a method for sparse shape representation in [6]. However, their method needs all the training set to be saved in a large shape repository. Durrelman *et.al.* [7] proposed a L1-type prior to enforce sparsity on the deformation fields, which encode the shape variations. Hence, their method is different from ours in the respect that they do not enforce sparsity on the number of the points of the mean model.

In this chapter, we propose a novel Bayesian framework to learn a sparse SSM from point cloud training sets. The major novelty of the method is our formulation which allows us to use quadratic programming as a tool for determining the optimal number of mean shape points during the alignment procedure. We formulate the problem as estimation of mixture weights of Gaussians. To enforce sparsity, we impose a symmetric Dirichlet distribution as a prior on the weights of the mixture and estimate the unknown parameters using EM algorithm [12]. The hyper-parameter controlling the sparsity level is determined using cross validation. As an example application, we apply our method to learn variations of caudate nuclei within a set of manually segmented data sets [9]. We show the importance of selecting optimal number for model points and compare our method to a state-of-the-art model proposed in [4]. This chapter is organized as following: we introduce our formulation in Section 2, and present the results in Section 3 which is followed by a conclusion in Section 4.

2   Methods

Let $\mathcal{X} = \{X_k \in (\mathbb{R}^D)^{N_k}\}, 1 \leq k \leq K$ denote the set of K observed D dimensional point sets, and $\mathcal{M} = \{m_j \in \mathbb{R}^D\}, 1 \leq j \leq N_M$ be a model point set. In addition, let $\mathcal{T} = \{T_k = (s_k, R_k, b_k)\}$ be the set of K rigid transformations where each T_k globally transforms the model points $m_j \in \mathcal{M}$ onto the space of X_k, i.e. $T_k \star m_j = s_k R_k m_j + b_k$. We consider $\mathrm{x}_{ki} \in X_k$ to be a noisy observation vector sampled from a Gaussian distribution centred at $T_k \star m_j$ such that: $p(\mathrm{x}_{ki}|T_k, m_j) = \mathcal{N}(\mathrm{x}_{ki}|T_k \star m_j, \Sigma)$, where $\Sigma = diag(\sigma_1^2, \cdots, \sigma_D^2)$ is a diagonal covariance matrix. Since N_M points exist on $\mathcal{M}$, the conditional pdf of x_{ki} can be given as a mixture of Gaussians: $p(\mathrm{x}_{ki}|T_k, \mathcal{M}, \pi) = \sum_{j=1}^{N_M} \pi_j p(\mathrm{x}_{ki}|T_k, m_j)$ where $\pi = (\pi_1, \cdots, \pi_{Nm})^T$.

Now, assuming that all N_k observed points on X_k are independent, the probability of X_k can be written as: $p(X_k|T_k, \mathcal{M}, \pi) = \prod_{i=1}^{N_k} p(\mathrm{x}_{ki}|T_k, \mathcal{M}, \pi)$. Finally, to model the pdf of the total observation $\mathcal{X}$, we further assume the given K points sets are jointly independent and identically distributed (*i.i.d.*) such that:

$$p(\mathcal{X}|\mathcal{T}, \mathcal{M}, \pi) = \prod_{k=1}^{K} p(X_k|T_k, \mathcal{M}, \pi). \tag{1}$$

Next, we formulate the problem of estimating the set of parameters in a Bayesian framework and maximize the following posterior probability:

$$\hat{\mathcal{T}}, \hat{\mathcal{M}}, \hat{\pi} = \underset{\mathcal{T}, \mathcal{M}, \pi}{\mathrm{argmax}} \, log[p(\mathcal{T}, \mathcal{M}, \pi|\mathcal{X})] = \underset{\mathcal{T}, \mathcal{M}, \pi}{\mathrm{argmax}} \, [log\, p(\mathcal{X}|\mathcal{T}, \mathcal{M}, \pi) + log\, p(\pi)] \tag{2}$$

2.1   Dirichlet Prior on the Mixture Coefficients

In this section we propose a prior pdf for the set of mixture coefficients π defined in previous section, which leads to sparse estimation of the model points. To enforce sparsity, we let π be drawn from a symmetric Dirichlet distribution function [11] which is given by:

$$p(\pi) = \frac{\Gamma(N_M(N(\alpha - 1) + 1))}{\Gamma(N(\alpha - 1) + 1)^{N_M}} \prod_{j=1}^{N_M} \pi_j^{N(\alpha-1)} \qquad (3)$$

in which N denotes the total number of the observed points ($N = \sum_{k=1}^{K} N_k$), Γ is the Gamma function and α is the *concentration* parameter. This form is slightly different from standard symmetric Dirichlet distribution in the way that we have replaced $\alpha - 1$ by $N(\alpha - 1)$ to effectively enforce the sparsity. Also, the gamma functions are also modified so that that the integral of (3) over π results in one. For $\alpha = 1$, this distribution reduces to a uniform distribution. For values of $\alpha > 1$, all π_i coefficients will be close to $1/N_M$. However, for $\alpha < 1$ the distribution prefers sparsity on the mixture coefficients, *i.e.* , some π_i will be close zero.

2.2   Optimization Using EM

Direct solution of the problem in (2) does not have a closed form thus we use the EM algorithm [12] to find a tractable solution. Having an estimate of the parameters $\Theta = \{\mathcal{T}, \mathcal{M}, \Sigma, \pi\}$ at the current iteration (n), EM maximizes a lower bound on the right hand of (2) which has the following form:

$$Q(\Theta|\Theta^{(n)}){=}\sum_{k=1}^{K}\sum_{i=1}^{N_k}\sum_{j=1}^{N_M}\{E_{kij}^{(n)}[log(\pi_j){+}log(\mathcal{N}(\mathrm{x}_{ki}|T_k \star m_j, \Sigma))]\}{+}log(p(\Pi))\,(4)$$

The EM algorithm consists of two iterative steps. In the **E-Step**, the posterior probabilities $E_{kij}^{(n)}$ are updated using current estimates of parameters:

$$E_{kij}^{(n)} = \frac{\pi_j^{(n)}\mathcal{N}(\mathrm{x}_{ki}|T_k^{(n)} \star m_j^{(n)}, \Sigma^{(n)})}{\sum_{l=1}^{N_M} \pi_l^{(n)}\mathcal{N}(\mathrm{x}_{ki}|T_k^{(n)} \star m_j^{(n)}, \Sigma^{(n)})} \qquad (5)$$

In the **M-Step**, the value of (4) is maximized w.r.t. the unknown parameters. We have followed the same principle outlined in [13] in order to derive update equations of the parameters $\mathcal{T}, \mathcal{M}, \Sigma$. The obtained equations are the same as those in [13] and omitted here due to the limitation of space. In this paper, we give our emphasis to derive the update equations for the vector π which results in sparsity of the estimated model $\mathcal{M}$.

We replace (3) in (4) and keep the relevant terms to π. Next, we apply the constraint that $\sum_{j=1}^{N_M} \pi_j = 1$ by a Lagrangian parameter λ, and we arrive at following expression which should be maximized for each π_j, $1 \leq j \leq N_M$:

$$Q(\Theta|\Theta^{(n)}){=}\sum_{k=1}^{K}\sum_{i=1}^{N_k}\sum_{j=1}^{N_M}\{[E_{kij}^{(n)} + (\alpha - 1)]log(\pi_j)\} + \lambda(\sum_{j=1}^{N_M} \pi_j - 1) + O.T. \,(6)$$

Taking derivative w.r.t. π_j and eliminating λ we obtain:

$$\pi_j^\star = \frac{\gamma_j^{(n)} + \alpha - 1}{N_M(\alpha - 1) + 1} \tag{7}$$

where N denotes the total number of the observed points ($N = \sum_{k=1}^K N_k$) and $\gamma_j^{(n)} = 1/N \sum_{k=1}^K \sum_{i=1}^{N_k} E_{kij}^{(n)}$. This value can be regarded as the *total responsibility* which the model point m_j admits. For $\alpha = 1$, (7) reduces to classic maximum likelihood based estimation of mixture weights where no sparsity is imposed.

It is important to note that the mixture weights which are computed using (7) may take negative values, because no positivity constraint is considered in (6). In fact, it is easy to see that for $1 - 1/N_M \leq \alpha$, if $\gamma_j^{(n)} < 1 - \alpha$ then $\pi_j^\star < 0$. In other words, if the total responsibility of the model point m_j drops beyond the value of $1 - \alpha$, its corresponding mixture weight will be negative. However, since this is not a plausible value, for such model points we set $\pi_j = 0$ using a quadratic programming scheme explained below. Note that sparsity can increase when α is very close to $1 - 1/N_M$. Hence, we define an auxiliary variable as $z \in (0, 1)$ to specify α using: $\alpha = (1 - 1/N_M)z + (1 - z)$. With this definition, sparsity will be proportional to z. Having estimated all values of $\pi_j^\star$, we update the mixture weights by solving the following convex optimization problem using the generalized sequential minimal optimizer proposed in [8]:

$$\pi_1^{(n)}, \cdots, \pi_{N_M}^{(n)} = \underset{\pi_1, \cdots, \pi_{N_M}}{\operatorname{argmin}} \sum_{j=1}^{N_M} (\pi_j^\star - \pi_j)^2, \; s.t : \sum_{j=1}^{N_M} \pi_j = 1 \; \wedge \; 0 \leq \pi_j, \forall j \tag{8}$$

The method breaks this problem into a series of small sub-problems by identifying those mixture weights that violate the constraints. We have observed that even for a large number of model points ($N_M \simeq 1e4$), the convergence rate is typically less than a second. At the end of the M-Step, we identify and prune out those model points whose corresponding mixture weights are zero. Next, we update N_M by counting the remaining *alive* points. The algorithm iteratively alters between E and M steps until convergence.

2.3   Construction of Statistical Shape Model

A popular method for construction of a shape model is using Principal Component Analysis [1]. The method requires one-to-one point correspondences between the training data set aligned with the mean shape. To identify such relations, we use the idea of "virtual correspondence" proposed in [4] which resolves the problem as follows: For any model point m_j a virtually correspondent point, denoted by $\breve{x}_{kj}$, is induced by the training sample X_k according to:

$$\breve{x}_{kj} = \sum_{i=1}^{N_s} \frac{E_{kij}}{\sum_l E_{klj}} T_k^{-1} \star x_{ki} \tag{9}$$

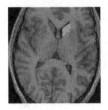 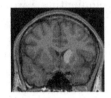 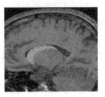

Fig. 1. Manually segmented caudate nuclei in axial, coronal and sagital slices

We compute these correspondences for all training samples and obtain $K + 1$ virtually aligned shapes (including the mean shape). Next, we convert each shape into a vector by a column-wise concatenation and apply the PCA to the co-variance matrix of these vectors. As a result we obtain the average vector $\bar{X} \in \mathbb{R}^{DN_M}$ and the matrix of eigenmodes $P \in \mathbb{R}^{DN_M \times n}$, where $n \leq K$ is the number of the principal components considered. Having defined these components, any unseen sample vector X can be considered as: $X = \bar{X} + Pb$, where b is the coefficients vector. To eliminate the noise from X, each coefficient is constrained by: $|b_i| \leq 3\sqrt{\lambda_i}$ where λ_i is the ith eigenvalue of the co-variance matrix of training vectors [1].

3   Results

In this section we first describe our available data sets of caudate nuclei and provide details of the training point sets. Finally, we present the results of the proposed method and compare its generalization ability with [4].

3.1   Specifications of Data and Point Sets

The caudate data consists of 15 data sets acquired from subjects with Schizoptypal Personality Disorder [9]. Each caudate nucleus was manually segmented by an expert (see Fig.1). In this paper, we use a mixed type of coordinates-levelset values as a feature vector at each point to facilitate representation of the surfaces using implicit definition. Let ϕ_k denote the signed distance function from the surface of the kth segmented training set. The points specifying X_k, are defined as $\mathbf{x}_{ki} = [x_{ki}, y_{ki}, z_{ki}, \phi_k(x_{ki}, y_{ki}, z_{ki})]^T$. We only consider the points in a narrow band surrounding the surface of the segmented structures. For the thickness of 2.0 mm, approximately 4000 points are obtained per a single nucleus. Next, each point set is individually decimated to around 400 points by setting $z = 0.9$ and estimating no transformation. The resulting point sets are then used to construct the shape models in the subsequent steps. Fig.2 shows a few samples of these point sets prior to registration in (a) and after it in (b).

3.2   Experiments

In the first part of our experiments we aimed at determining an optimal value for z (hence an optimal model) by measuring generalization efficiency of the

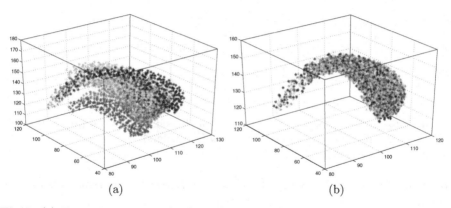

Fig. 2. (a) Ten training point clouds represented by the points in a narrow band of thickness 2.0, (b) The same point sets registered by our proposed method

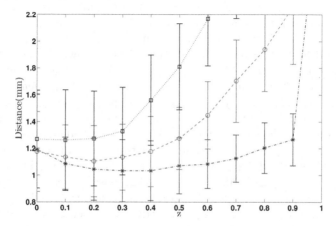

Fig. 3. Estimated generalization error (see Section 3.2) for different numbers of training versus test samples: 10 vs. 5 (*blue*), 5 vs. 10 (*red*), and 3 vs. 12 (*black*)

estimated SSMs. With 15 point sets generated as explained in Section 3.1, we performed three sets of cross-validations by using 10, 5 and only 3 point sets as training data and leaving the rest as the test sets. To evaluate the generalization, PCA analysis was first performed using the co-registered training sets (see Section 2.3). Next, each test point set was first aligned with the trained model and subsequently projected to its PCA space. The number of eigenmodes used in this projection was equal to the number of training sets. Then, the average distance between the surfaces of the original and the projected test set was measured. To reconstruct surfaces from point sets, the level set values on the points were interpolated using radial basis functions [10] and then the zero level set was extracted. For each evaluation, we increased the sparsity by varying z from 0 to 1 in increments of 0.1. The number of model points N_M was initially set to the

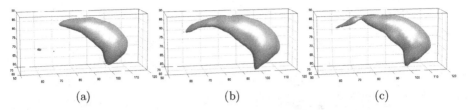

(a)   (b)   (c)

Fig. 4. Estimated mean shape from 10 segmented caudate nuclei at:(a)$z = 0$ (3601 points), (b)$z = 0.3$ (630 points) and (c)$z = 0.9$ (186 points)

total number of available points (typically $N - K$ to avoid extreme over-fitting) and later reduced by the imposed sparsity.

Fig.3 shows the results of these experiments applied on a single caudate nucleus. As seen, for each number of training data sets, there is an optimal sparsity level which is implied by z. For instance, using 10 training data sets, the minimum average generalization error of $1.03 \pm 0.23\,mm$ occurs at $z = 0.3$ (sparsity level of 82.7%). Models with more points suffer from over-fitting, and models with decreased number of points lose details. This is shown in Fig.4. The presence of small apart pieces in Fig.4-(a) can be explained as follows: due the large number of points (3601) the estimated variance of the components, *i.e.* Σ, is rather small. Consequently, the registration of the training point sets hasn't been accurate enough and the zero level of these points sets do not coincide as good as the other models in (b) and (c), where we have had a better registration performance. Furthermore, as the number of training data sets decreases, the generalization ability reduces and less sparsity levels are preferred by the model.

We compared our sparse SSM with an EM-ICP based model by closely following the principle outlined in [4] and performing 3 fold cross validation scheme (10 training data set). The parameters needed to be set in this method were as follows: $N_m = 400$ (equal to a typical number of points on a single training set), variance reduction factor of 0.85 and 20 number of EM iterations. A t-test showed the attained errors of $1.10 \pm 0.22\,mm$ were significantly higher than those attained using our sparse model (p-value: 0.0043). Fig.5 shows the mean model and variations along the first and second principal components for both caudate nuclei. These are estimated using all $K = 15$ data sets and $z = 0.3$ which led to a model with 1181 points decimated from 7875 training points. As seen, the variation along the first component changes the length of the tails in (a), whereas the variation along the second component displaces the tail position.

4   Conclusion

In this paper we approached the problem of model selection in the context of statistical shape models. Our method is a Bayesian estimation framework which imposes sparsity on the number of mixture components using a Dirichlet distribution. The method is able to automatically identify an optimal number of mean

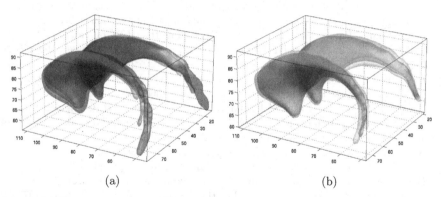

(a)   (b)

Fig. 5. (a) First principal and (b) second principal modes of variation are shown. In both figures the mean shape ($\bar{X}$) is specified in red and other colors specify the positive and negative variations along with the principle modes $\bar{X} \pm \lambda_i P_i$.

shape points. We successfully applied our method to learn the variations within the segmented caudate data sets and showed that it favorably compares with a classic EM-ICP method. The proposed algorithm can generate highly sparse (over 80%) yet reasonable models. The trained model can be used for shape based segmentations and classifications. In the current framework, we determine the concentration parameter using cross-validation. In future, we will estimate this hyper-parameter by its explicit optimization in the training phase.

References

1. Cootes, T.F., Taylor, C.J.: Active Shape Models-Their Training and Application. Computer Vision and Image Understanding 61, 38–59 (1995)
2. Heimann, T., Meinzer, H.: Statistical shape models for 3D medical image segmentation: A review. Medical Image Analysis 13(4), 543–563 (2009)
3. Leventon, M.E., Grimson, W.E.L., Faugeras, D.O.: Statistical Shape Influence in Geodesic Active Contours. In: CVPR, pp. 1316–1323 (2000)
4. Hufnagel, H., Pennec, X., Ehrhardt, J., Ayache, N., Handels, H.: Generation of a Statistical Shape Model with Probabilistic Point Correspondences and EM-ICP. International Journal for Computer Assisted Radiology and Surgery 5, 265–273 (2008)
5. Granger, S., Pennec, X.: Multi-scale EM-ICP: A Fast and Robust Approach for Surface Registration. In: Heyden, A., Sparr, G., Nielsen, M., Johansen, P. (eds.) ECCV 2002, Part IV. LNCS, vol. 2353, pp. 418–432. Springer, Heidelberg (2002)
6. Zhang, S., Zhan, Y., Dewan, M., Huang, J., Metaxas, D.N., Zhou, X.S.: Deformable Segmentation via Sparse Shape Representation. In: Fichtinger, G., Martel, A., Peters, T. (eds.) MICCAI 2011, Part II. LNCS, vol. 6892, pp. 451–458. Springer, Heidelberg (2011)

7. Durrleman, S., Prastawa, M., Korenberg, J.R., Joshi, S., Trouvé, A., Gerig, G.: Topology Preserving Atlas Construction from Shape Data without Correspondence Using Sparse Parameters. In: Ayache, N., Delingette, H., Golland, P., Mori, K. (eds.) MICCAI 2012, Part III. LNCS, vol. 7512, pp. 223–230. Springer, Heidelberg (2012)

8. Keerthi, S.S., Gilbert, E.G.: Convergence of a Generalized SMO Algorithm for SVM Classifier Design. Machine Learning 46, 351–360 (2002)

9. Levitt, J., et al.: MRI study of caudate nucleus volume and its cognitive correlates in neuroleptic-naive patients with schizotypal personality disorder. American Journal of Psychiatry 159(7), 1190–1197 (2002)

10. Bochkanov, S., Bystritsky, V.: ALGLIB, http://www.alglib.net

11. Bishop, C.: Pattern Recognition and Machine Learning. Springer (2006)

12. Dempster, A.P., Laird, N.M., Rubin, D.B.: Maximum Likelihood from Incomplete Data via the EM Algorithm. Journal of the Royal Stat. Soc. 39(1), 1–38 (1977)

13. Myronenko, A., Xubo, S.: Point Set Registration: Coherent Point Drift. IEEE Tran. on Pat. Anal. and Mach. Intel. 32(12), 2262–2275 (2010)

Brain-Cloud: A Generalized and Flexible Registration Framework for Brain MR Images

Minjeong Kim[1], Guorong Wu[1], Qian Wang[2], and Dinggang Shen[1]

[1] Department of Radiology and BRIC, University of North Carolina at Chapel Hill
[2] Department of Computer Science, University of North Carolina at Chapel Hill

Abstract. Image registration, which aligns a pair of fixed and moving images, is often tackled by the large shape and intensity variation between the images. As a remedy, we present a generalized registration framework that is capable to predict the initial deformation field between the fixed and moving images, even though their appearances are very different. For the prediction, we learn the prior knowledge on deformation from pre-observed images. Especially, our method is significantly differentiated from previous methods that are usually confined to a specific fixed image, to be flexible for handling arbitrary fixed and moving images. Specifically, our idea is to encapsulate many pre-observed images into a hierarchical infrastructure, termed as *cloud*, which is able to efficiently compute the deformation pathways between the pre-observed images. After anchoring the fixed and moving images to their respective *port* images (similar images in terms of intensity appearance) in the cloud, we predict the initial deformation between the fixed and moving images by the deformation pathway between the two *port* images. Thus, the remaining small deformation can be efficiently refined via most existing deformable registration methods. With the cloud, we have obtained promising registration results on both adult and infant brain images, demonstrating the advantage of the proposed registration framework in improving the registration performance.

1   Introduction

Deformable registration of brain MR images is a key step in neuroscience and clinical studies. Although many algorithms have been proposed during past decades, most of them aim to directly estimate the deformation field that deforms a moving image to a fixed image. Ignoring the potentially high variation between the two images might undermine the registration quality, as it is well known that the registration of two images with different appearance is much more challenging than the registration of two images with similar appearance. Specifically, the registration would be extremely vulnerable to structural ambiguities in detecting anatomical correspondences between the two very different images, and also suffer from high computational cost.

One of effective remedies to overcome the inter-image variation in registration is to predict the deformation pathway based on prior knowledge. Thus, by providing the predicted deformation as a good initialization to existing registration methods, the complete deformation between two images can be easily estimated via efficient

C.A. Linte et al. (Eds.): MIAR/AE-CAI 2013, LNCS 8090, pp. 153–161, 2013.
© Springer-Verlag Berlin Heidelberg 2013

deformation refinement [1-4]. In the existing methods, the correlation between appearance and deformation statistics of moving images with respect to a fixed image is often established in the training stage. Then, given a new moving image, its deformation field (or coefficients) can be predicted to initialize the registration from the learned correlation model. However, learning of the appearance-deformation correlation is generally confined to a *specific fixed image*, which limits the flexibility of the framework since the fixed image may change in different applications.

In this work, we present a generalized registration framework that provides on-demand access to any arbitrary fixed and moving images, even though the shape and intensity variation between the two images might be large. Specifically, we create an infrastructure, in which a large number of pre-observed brain images are carefully organized and the deformation field between each pair of them can be easily calculated. Thus, every image in the infrastructure may serve as the port image, to which a to-be-registered image can be anchored if they are similar. After anchoring the fixed and moving images to their respective ports, we assert that the desired deformation between the two images can be well approximated by the deformation between the two ports. The deformation pathway determined by our infrastructure can be regarded as a well-performing initialization and further refined efficiently by existing registration methods. We further term the infrastructure of brain images as the *cloud*, resembling the popular cloud computing, due to its capability in providing registration services that are transparent to varying fixed and moving images. That is, the cloud is adaptive to any input fixed and moving images, and can predict satisfactory deformation field as the initialization to the existing registration methods for further refinement, even though the variation between the images is large.

It is clear that the key of our registration framework is to construct the cloud and use it for guiding image registration. A straightforward solution is to build the cloud with a simple graph, where (1) nodes representing similar images are directly linked by edges; (2) all pairs of nodes/images in the cloud are essentially (directly or indirectly) connected. Meanwhile, we calculate the deformation field associated with each (connected) graph edge. Then, given a new pair of fixed and moving images, the shortest route between their respective ports can be identified in the cloud. After that, the deformation between two port images can thus be computed by integrating all deformations on the graph edges along the shortest route. The solution by the simple graph, however, may suffer from the large number of pre-observed images included in the cloud, which is often required to well understand the distribution of the high-dimensional images. Specifically, the critical issue is that the route between the fixed and moving images may travel along too many nodes in the graph, thus resulting in accumulated errors when integrating deformation fields along individual edges.

A hierarchical design of the cloud, which potentially reduces the length of the identified route between the fixed and moving images, obviously can better predict the initial deformation to register the two images. Bearing this point, we automatically partition all pre-observed images into several groups, with each group consisting of only similar images in terms of their intensity appearances. After building the simple graph to describe the image distribution in each group, we introduce inter-group links that connect each pair of groups and finally acquire the hierarchical infrastructure as the cloud. Taking advantages of this hyper-graph, the fixed and moving images can thus be better registered by following the shortest route inside the cloud.

We have evaluated our cloud registration framework integrated with one of the state-of-the-art registration methods [5]. Promising experimental results on both real and simulated brain images demonstrated that our cloud registration method is able to substantially improve the registration results, indicating its potential to be applied to the challenging registration problems, e.g., infant and elderly brain images.

2   Methods

2.1   Cloud with Simple Graph

Given the fixed image F and moving image M, the goal of image registration is to estimate the deformation pathway φ that deforms M to the space of F. The conventional registration methods usually estimate the deformation pathway φ between F and M directly. However, the optimization of φ could be very difficult and vulnerable to local minima, when the appearance difference between F and M is large. In order to alleviate this concern, we utilize a simple graph of pre-observed images to provide good initialization for registration.

Simple Graph Construction: Here, we consider all pre-observed images $I = \{I_i | i = 1, ..., N\}$ sitting in a high-dimension manifold. Thus, two images with similar appearances are close to each other on the manifold. We then introduce a graph to approximate the manifold, as only similar images are connected in the graph. Two criteria are applied to build the graph: (1) each pair of nodes (images) should be linked (directly or indirectly); (2) the number of edges should be as less as possible. Given a well-defined graph, we only calculate the deformation fields for the images directly connected in the graph, thus avoiding the challenge of registering two faraway images.

To acquire the desired graph, we first calculate the distance matrix $D = [d_{ij}]_{N \times N}$, where each entry $d_{ij} = d(I_i, I_j)$ encodes the distance between the image I_i ($i = 1, \cdots, N$) and the image I_j ($j = 1, \cdots, N$). The sum of squared difference (SSD) of intensity is used for measuring image distance due to its simplicity. To meet the two criteria above, we use a line-search-based method to determine the optimal threshold h upon image distances. Specifically, we set the search range with the low bound $b_L = 0$ and the upper bound $b_H = \max_{i,j} d_{ij}$. Then, the threshold h is updated following $h = b_L + \lambda(b_H - b_L)$, where the scalar $\lambda \in (0,1)$ specifies the step size in line search. If the constructed graph satisfies criterion (1), b_H will be decreased to h; otherwise, b_L will be increased to h. We repeat these steps until b_L meets with b_H. After obtaining the optimal threshold h, we can determine the edges by following

$$e_{ij} = \begin{cases} 1 & d(I_i, I_j) < h \\ 0 & otherwise \end{cases}. \tag{1}$$

Here, $e_{ij} = 1$ represents that there is an edge between I_i and I_j, while $e_{ij} = 0$ indicates no direct link between I_i and I_j.

Next, we deploy deformable image registration to estimate the deformation pathway φ_{ij} for the connected nodes (images) I_i and I_j (φ_{ji} is used to deform I_j to I_i, vice versa). Note, to locate the shortest route from the node I_i to the indirectly connected node I_j, we apply the classic Dijkstra's algorithm, as the edges in the graph are weighted by the distances between their end nodes (images). In the final, we define the cloud **B** as:

$$B = \left(I, \{e_{ij}\}, \{d_{ij}\}, \{\varphi_{ij}\}\right), \ i, j = 1, \dots, N. \tag{2}$$

Registration with Cloud: The registration with the simple graph cloud is demonstrated in **Fig. 1**. To register the moving image M (red box in **Fig. 1**) with the fixed image F (red circle in **Fig. 1**), we first find the closest node I_f in the graph with respect to the fixed image, where $f = \arg\min_{f=1,\dots,N} d\left(F, I_f\right)$. Similarly, we can obtain the closest node I_m with respect to the moving image M. We name the nodes I_f and I_m as the *port* images to which F and M are anchored in terms of the cloud **B** (depicted by the solid arrows in **Fig. 1**), respectively. Then, we use Dijkstra's algorithm to establish the shortest route $Y_{f \to m}$ (red dashed arrows in **Fig. 1**) from I_f to I_m within the cloud **B** by considering the distance d_{ij} between I_i and I_j as the traveling cost. Finally, we can obtain the deformation pathway $\varphi_{f \to m}$ by sequentially composing the deformations of all edges along the route $Y_{f \to m}$.

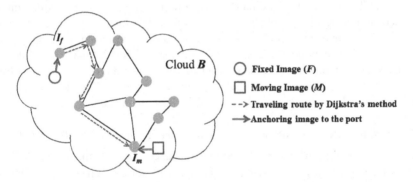

Fig. 1. Demonstration of proposed framework with the cloud constructed by simple graph

Since we assume both F and M can find the similar port images in the cloud **B**, it is reasonable to presume that the deformation from F to M and deformation from I_f to I_m are highly alike. Thus, the deformation pathway $\varphi_{f \to m}$ can be used as the good initialization for existing registration methods to refine and finally acquire the complete deformation. To validate this assumption, we need to include as many images as possible to construct the cloud **B**. However, it raises the critical concern that a single simple graph is unable to well describe the distribution of large population dataset. Thus, we extend our cloud construction method from the simple graph to the scenario of the hyper-graph in Section 2.2.

2.2   Cloud with Hyper-Graph

Given a large number of pre-observed images, we propose to construct the cloud that describes the image distribution in a hierarchical manner. *First*, we use affinity propagation (AP) [6] to cluster all images into several groups based on the distance matrix D. For each clustered group, we build a simple graph to represent the interior image distribution following Section 2.1. In the example of **Fig. 2**, the entire population of pre-observed images is partitioned into three groups. *Then*, for any two groups, we exhaustively calculate the distance d_{ij} between each node I_i in the first group and the node I_j in the second group. The K pairs of images that yield K smallest distances are selected, such that edges between the K pairs of nodes are added to bridge the graphs for the two groups. Thus, the inter-group edge $e_{ij}^{inter} = 1$ (shown by the black double lines in **Fig. 2**) if the distance between I_i and I_j (I_i and I_j belonging to different groups) is among the K smallest. Otherwise, $e_{ij}^{inter} = 0$.

In the framework of our cloud registration, the fixed image F and the moving image M might anchor to the different groups, as demonstrated in **Fig. 2**. Since any pair of groups are essentially connected via inter-group edges, it is straightforward to apply Dijkstra's algorithm to determine the route $\Upsilon_{f \to m}$ across individual groups and obtain the initial deformation pathway $\varphi_{f \to m}$ by concatenating the deformations of all edges along $\Upsilon_{f \to m}$.

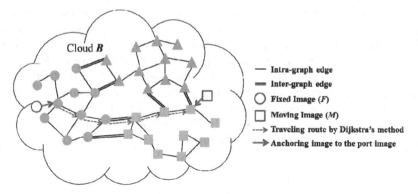

Fig. 2. Demonstration of proposed framework with the cloud constructed by hyper-graph

3   Experiments

We here use one of the state-of-the-art intensity-based registration algorithms [5] as a baseline registration method in our cloud registration framework. Note that other deformable registration methods can also be used for improving the performance via our proposed framework. The evaluation of registration performance was conducted by comparison with the original registration method (1) without deformation initialization, (2) with initial deformation estimated by support vector regression (SVR) [1], and (3) with initial deformation estimated by tree hierarchy [2].

In our experiments, we follow the method in [1] to simulate MR brains images from the learned statistical model on image appearance and deformation fields in order to have enough number of images to build the cloud. Since the simulation method needs to specify a template image, we simulate the image in each group by regarding the exemplar image in affinity propagation (AP) as the center node. Specifically, for each group in the cloud, we first align all nodes with the center node. Then we apply PCA to these deformation fields for obtaining eigenvectors to represent the characteristic of the statistical deformation fields. Finally, to simulate brain images in this graph, we randomly perturb each eigenvector within the statistically valid range for generating the new deformation fields, which are used to deform the exemplar images to simulate the new brain images in the cloud.

3.1 Simulated Dataset

For quantitatively evaluating the registration performance of our proposed framework, we conducted the deformation simulation algorithm proposed in [7]. We simulated 60 images, based on the deformation statistics on an elderly brain database by the simulator, and then divided them into 3 groups (i.e., # of groups in the cloud = 3) by AP method. The images in each group are used for building the hyper-graph in the cloud.

Fifty pairs of fixed and moving images, along with their ground-truth deformation fields, are also generated using the simulator. By predicting the initial deformation followed by estimating the residual deformations between 50 pairs of fixed and moving images, we compare their complete deformation fields by the original registration method without deformation prediction, as well as three deformation initialization based registration methods, with the ground-truth deformations. As the result, the averaged magnitude of residual deformations by the four registration methods for 50 pairs of data, compared to the ground-truth deformations, are 0.58, 0.49, 0.47 and 0.38 mm (ours), respectively. This indicates that our cloud registration method is the best in predicting initial deformations for further registration.

3.2 Infant Brain Dataset

Longitudinal brains of seven infant subjects are used in this experiment, with each subject having the serial images acquired at 6 time points (0, 3, 6, 9, 12, and 18 months old). Due to the lack of enough images (totally 42 images), our experiments with this dataset were performed in a leave-two-out (LTO) fashion by randomly choosing two images as fixed and moving images from the dataset. For each LTO case, the rest 40 images are divided into 2 groups by the AP method.

To qualitatively evaluate the performance of deformation prediction, we display the warped moving images w.r.t. a selective fixed image by three deformation initialization methods in **Fig. 4**. The visual inspection on the similarity between the warped moving images (**Fig. 4**c-e) w.r.t. the fixed image (**Fig. 4**b) indicates our cloud registration method can provide the best initialization for infant brain images. Especially, the aggressive warping in the warped moving images (depicted by red arrows in **Fig. 4**) by tree-based and SVR-based methods is not shown in the result by our cloud registration method. This aggressive warping is mainly caused by the accumulated deformation error when forcing the deformation pathway to go through the fixed template in other two methods.

Due to lack of label information in this dataset, we classified all voxels into three tissue categories, white matter (WM), gray matter (GM) and ventricular CSF (VN), by using a publicly available software (http://www.nitrc.org/projects/ibeat/). The averaged Dice overlap ratios achieved by four registration methods (the original registration method + three deformation initialization based registration methods) are shown in Table 1, demonstrating the best registration accuracy by our cloud registration method. The outperformance of all three deformation initialization based registration methods over the original registration method is apparent, indicating the importance of using good deformation initialization to help register infant brain images with large anatomical and dynamic intensity changes.

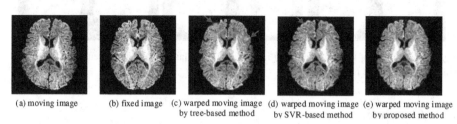

(a) moving image   (b) fixed image   (c) warped moving image   (d) warped moving image   (e) warped moving image
                                        by tree-based method   by SVR-based method   by proposed method

Fig. 3. Demonstration of three warped versions of a moving image (a) w.r.t. a fixed image (b) by tree-based method (c), SVR-based method (d), and our cloud-based method (e)

Table 1. Averaged Dice overlap ratios of WM, GM and VN tissue maps on the registered images, by the original registration method and three initialization based registration methods

	Original registration	Tree-based method	SVR-based method	Proposed method
WM	71.3	73.3	73.5	**74.7**
GM	71.1	72.9	73.4	**74.5**
VN	69.3	71.2	71.6	**73.1**

3.3   IXI Dataset

The 30 images in IXI dataset (http://brain-development.org/), each with 83 manually labeled ROIs, were used in this experiment. Similar to the experiment in Section 3.2, in each LTO case, two images are selected as the fixed and moving images and the rest 28 images are divided into 2 groups by AP method. We repeated this cross-validation for 50 times (IXI-1). For quantitatively evaluating the registration performance, we measure the registration accuracy based on the averaged Dice overlap scores of 83 ROIs from all 50 LTO cross-validation cases. The averaged Dice overlap scores are 78.9%, 79.1% and **79.8%** by tree-based method, SVR-based method, and **our proposed method**, respectively, and 78.3% by the original registration method.

We further selected 5 pairs of fixed and moving images (IXI-2) from above 50 LTO cross-validation cases, which are difficult to register due to their large shape and intensity differences. **Fig. 4** shows 3 of those 5 pairs of fixed and moving images. The averaged Dice overlap scores on these 5 pairs are 63.8%, 66.2%, 66.7%, and **70.3%** by the original registration method, tree-based method, SVR-based method, and **our proposed method**, respectively. For both IXI-1 and IXI-2 datasets tested above, our cloud registration method consistently outperforms all other registration algorithms. Especially, our method significantly improves the registration performance for the difficult cases (IXI-2), even compared to other two deformation initialization based registration methods.

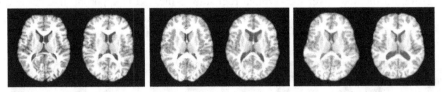

Fig. 4. Three pairs of fixed and moving images that have large shape and intensity differences, which challenges the registration

4   Conclusions

In this paper, we present a novel registration framework to anchor any pair of fixed and moving images to the cloud of images, for immediately providing the initial deformation between the two images. Especially, our cloud is built on the hyper-graph to organize image distribution hierarchically. Therefore, it is not restricted for new to-be-registered images to follow the fixed template, thus enabling adaptive and immediate establishment of the deformation pathway between the two images. Since our proposed framework is general enough to use any other deformable registration algorithm (with reasonable performance) to build the cloud, we will test other registration methods, e.g., diffeomorphic demons algorithm, in our framework. Moreover, we will apply the proposed method to huge datasets, e.g., Alzheimer's Disease Neuroimaging Initiative (ADNI), to better show the usefulness the hyper-graph in our framework.

References

1. Kim, M., et al.: A General Fast Registration Framework by Learning Deformation-Appearance Correlation. IEEE Transactions on Image Processing 21(4), 1823–1833 (2012)
2. Jia, H., Yap, P.-T., Shen, D.: Iterative multi-atlas-based multi-image segmentation with tree-based registration. Neuroimage 59(1), 422–430 (2012)
3. Tang, S., et al.: RABBIT: rapid alignment of brains by building intermediate templates. Neuroimage 47(4), 1277–1287 (2009)

4. Loeckx, D., Maes, F., Vandermeulen, D., Suetens, P.: Non-rigid image registration using a statistical spline deformation model. In: Taylor, C.J., Noble, J.A. (eds.) IPMI 2003. LNCS, vol. 2732, pp. 463–474. Springer, Heidelberg (2003)
5. Shen, D.: Fast image registration by hierarchical soft correspondence detection. Pattern Recognition 42(5), 954–961 (2009)
6. Frey, B.J., Dueck, D.: Clustering by Passing Messages Between Data Points. Science 315(5814), 972–976 (2007)
7. Xue, Z., et al.: Simulating deformations of MR brain images for validation of atlas-based segmentation and registration algorithms. Neuroimage 33(3), 855–866 (2006)

Realtime Wide-Baseline Registration of the Uterus in Laparoscopic Videos Using Multiple Texture Maps

Toby Collins, Daniel Pizarro, Adrien Bartoli, Michel Canis, and Nicolas Bourdel

ISIT UMR 6284 CNRS/UdA, Clermont-Ferrand, France

Abstract. We present a way to register the uterus in monocular laparoscopy in realtime using a novel two-phase approach. This differs significantly to SLAM, which is currently the leading approach for registration in MIS when scenes are approximately rigid. In the first phase we construct a 3D model of the uterus using dense SfM. This involves a method for semi-automatically masking the uterus from background structures in a set of reference frames, which we call Mask Bootstrapping from Motion (MBM). In the second phase the 3D model is registered to the live laparoscopic video using a novel wide-baseline approach that uses many texture maps to capture the real changes in appearance of the uterus. Capturing these changes means that registration can be performed reliably without needing temporal priors, which are needed in SLAM. This simplifies registration and leads to far fewer tuning parameters. We show that our approach significantly outperforms SLAM on an *in vivo* dataset comprising three human uteri.

1 Introduction

One of the main current goals of computer assisted intervention in Minimal Invasive Surgery (MIS) is to enrich the surgeon's video data using Augmented Reality (AR). Examples of this include being able to visualise sub-surface structures [16], enlarge the surgical field of view [18] and overlay information from other imaging modalities [14]. AR in MIS involves solving a fundamental open problem, namely registration. Depending on the application this may involve registering optical images to one another, or to register them to another modality. A challenging problem is how to achieve registration accurately, reliably and in realtime. In this paper we focus on the problem of registering laparoscopic images of the uterus. Solving this problem would open up several important clinical applications, including AR-assisted resection of lesions such as uterine fibroids and endometriosis.

The uterus is a flexible organ that can exhibit strong deformation when manipulated with laparoscopic tools [12]. However when observing the uterus during intervention prior to resection it remains quite rigid and does not deform significantly due to respiration. Optical registration in laparoscopy has

C.A. Linte et al. (Eds.): MIAR/AE-CAI 2013, LNCS 8090, pp. 162–171, 2013.

been studied previously for other organs using the assumption of rigid, or approximately rigid motion. This has been developed with monocular [4,6,7] and stereo [13,18] laparoscopes. These solve the problem using a general paradigm called visual Simultaneous Localisation and Mapping (SLAM). Visual SLAM relies only on raw optical data, and does not need other hardware such as magnetic [14] or optical [16] tracking devices. SLAM involves building a 3D representation of the environment, known as the *map*, and determining the rigid transform which positions the map in the camera's coordinate frame. The core challenge in SLAM is how to achieve *data association*. SLAM requires data association in two respects. The first is for *map building*. The second is for *localisation*, which is to determine where the map's points are located in a new input image. SLAM offers a fast solution to these problems and has found considerable success in man-made environments. However SLAM in MIS is still proving challenging. This is due to the repeated nature of tissue texture, rapid camera motion and photo-constancy violations caused by blood or mucous.

SLAM also has considerable difficulty when the scene is not globally rigid. When the scene is made up of independently moving structures SLAM can make errors by merging features from different structures into one map. For laparoscopic procedures involving the uterus a typical scene will comprise the uterus, ovaries, peritoneum, small intestine and bladder. In most procedures a cannula is inserted into the uterus through the vagina and is operated externally by an assistant. The assistant's hand movement causes the uterus to move independently of the surrounding structures. As we will show, one cannot apply off-the-shelf monocular SLAM in these conditions. One problem is to ensure the map comprises features from the uterus and not background structures. We therefore have in conjunction with registration a segmentation problem. This amounts to computing binary *masks* which label pixels as either being on the uterus body or not. However achieving this automatically is difficult and has not been studied in the literature.

The focus of this work is to solve registration using a minimal amount of manual segmentation. A naive way to proceed would be to mask the uterus manually in one or more frames and enforce that SLAM uses features found only within the masks. However, there is no guarantee that SLAM will not eventually use features from surrounding organs, thus leading to mapping and localisation errors. By contrast it is infeasible to mask frames manually for every frame.

Proposed Approach and Registration Pipeline. Our solution is to step away from the SLAM paradigm and solve the mapping problem with dense multi-view Structure-from-Motion (SfM) [8]. We use SfM to *explicitly decouple* the map building process from localisation. Using SfM has the advantage that data association is done without requiring input images come from a video. Rather, it works using a collection of unorganised images, and unlike SLAM assumes nothing about temporal continuity. We propose a SfM-based method for registering the uterus in two distinct phases. We illustrate this in Figure 1. Phase 1 involves estimating a dense 3D model of the uterus from a set of *reference frames*. These are recorded whilst the surgeon views the uterus from a range of different viewpoints. This involves a novel process that we call *Mask*

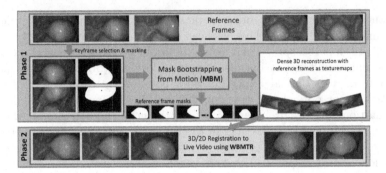

Fig. 1. Proposed approach pipeline divided into two phases. Phase 1 uses a reference video to construct a dense 3D surface model of the uterus. Phase 2 registers the model to new video frames in realtime.

Bootstrapping from Motion (MBM). The idea behind MBM is to use a small number of manually-segmented masks to bootstrap computing the masks in all reference frames. First a small number of reference frames are selected, called *keyframes*, which are masked manually. An initial dense 3D uterus model is computed using SfM with only these masked keyframes. The model is then registered to all other reference frames, and their masks are predicted using the model's projected silhouette. We then can use *all* reference frames and masks to compute a more accurate 3D model. Importantly, the masks do not need to be particularly accurate, because modern SfM algorithms are inherently robust. Rather the mask's job is to prevent confusion during SfM by background structures transforming according to different motion models.

Phase 2 involves using the 3D model from Phase 1 to register the uterus in realtime. In contrast to SLAM, we present a way to achieve this that does not rely on a prediction using the registration in previous frames. Rather each frame can be registered independently. This is achievable due to the rich appearance data provided by the model's many reference frames. We call this Wide-Baseline Multi-Texturemap Registration (WBMTR).

Materials. Data has been acquired with a standard Karl Stortz 10mm zero-degree HD laparoscope, capturing videos at 25fps at 1920×1080 pixels. The laparoscope was calibrated using standard methods immediately before intervention using OpenCV's calibration library. Algorithms have been implemented in a combination of C++ and CUDA, and run on a standard Intel i7 desktop PC with an NVidia GTX 660 CUDA-enabled graphics card.

2   Phase 1: Dense 3D Reconstruction Using MBM

2.1   Creating the Exploratory Video and Frame Pre-processing

The exploratory video begins at the point during intervention after abdominal inflation, instrument and camera insertion and once the uterus has been localised by the surgeon. The goal of this video is two-fold. The first is to provide sufficient data so that the uterus body can be reconstructed with SfM. The second is to provide sufficiently different views of the uterus in order to capture how its appearance changes as it is viewed from different viewpoints. This second point is crucial for achieving reliable registration in Phase 2. To achieve these goals we capture the exploratory video in somewhat controlled conditions with a simple protocol. By contrast in Phase 2 the surgeon can view the uterus as they wish.

The protocol is as follows. The uterus is centred in the video so that the uterus fundus is fully visible to the camera (Figure 1, top keyframe). At this point video capture begins. The uterus is then tilted by manipulating the cannula to reveal the posterior side of its body (Figure 1, bottom keyframe). It is then moved in a rotary fashion to reveal lateral and anterior views. Once completed video capture stops. We denote the length in seconds of the exploratory video with T. In practice $T \simeq 30$ seconds. From the capture we select a subset of 60 reference frames. We do this automatically by partitioning the video into 60 even time intervals: $\{t_1, t_2, ...t_{60}\}$. At each time t_k we create a local window comprising the frames at $t_k \pm \frac{T}{60 \times 2}$. From this window we select the sharpest frame. We do this by computing the response of a 5×5 smooth Laplacian filter and measuring a robust maximum (specifically at the 90th percentile). The frame with the highest robust maximum in the kth interval is chosen to be the kth reference frame. From the reference frames we select a subset of 8 uniformly-spaced *keyframes*. For each keyframe we create a mask by manually outlining the uterus body with an interactive polygon. This process is quick because the masks do *not* need to be particularly accurate, and takes approximately 1-2 minutes to perform.

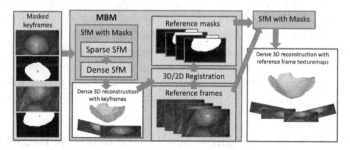

Fig. 2. Mask Bootstrapping from Motion (MBM) applied to the uterus

2.2   Mask Bootstrapping from Motion (MBM)

In Fig. 2 we have expanded out the MBM component in Fig. 1. MBM takes as inputs the set of keyframes and their respective masks. The first step of MBM is to perform dense SfM using the masked keyframes. Modern dense SfM works in two stages. The first stage is to perform sparse SfM using local features extracted from the images. The well established method for this is to estimate the camera poses from feature correspondences, and then refine them with bundle adjustment [8]. The second stage involves reconstructing a dense surface using multi-view stereo [17]. The masks come into play in both stages. In the first stage features are only used that lie within the masks. In the second stage only pixel information within the masks is used to constrain dense reconstruction. There exist several mature libraries for performing dense SfM. We have found good success for both the sparse and dense stages using Agisoft's Photoscan [1]. For reconstructing the uterus we did not need to change Photoscan's default parameters for mesh smoothness and resolution. With a set of 8 keyframes Sparse SfM takes about 15 seconds on our hardware and Dense SfM takes about 1 minute, returning a 3D model in the order of 20,000 vertices.

The next stage of MBM is to take this 3D model and perform registration using WBMTR for the remaining reference frames. We postpone details of WBMTR to §3, as it is the same algorithm used for live registration. For each reference frame WBMTR either gives us the model's 3D pose, or it returns a failure to register. For all frames with 3D pose estimates, we render the model with OpenGL and compute the model's silhouette. We then morphologically dilate the silhouette to grow its area to allow the next run of SfM to be able to discover more of the uterus surface. Empirically we have found a dilation of amount 15% area to be effective. There is a compromise here, as we do not want significant background regions being included in the masks. We then pass the reference images and their masks back to dense SfM, which returns a second 3D surface model, and the 3D poses of the model with respect to the reference frames. Sometimes it may fail to estimate pose. The reasons for this are the same as the reason why WBMTR may fail, chiefly if there is excessive motion blur. We call the set of reference images for which pose *was* estimated the *texturemap images*. We use this term because these images allow us to texturemap the model. However unlike traditional texturemapping where the images are combined to form a *single* aggregated texturemap, we keep *all* texturemap images. By doing so we capture the real changes of appearance of the uterus as it is viewed from different viewpoints. This is important because state-of-the-art feature detectors and descriptors can still have difficulty in handling viewpoint changes due to the complex interaction between tissue reflectance, illumination angle and surface orientation. When we use many texturemap images, we are reducing the requirement for features to be invariant to these changes.

3   Phase 2: Wide-Baseline Multi-texturemap Registration

In this section we describe WBMTR for registering the 3D model in realtime. WBMTR is a feature-based method. That is, registration is achieved by determining feature correspondences between the 3D model's texture maps and a given input image. Unlike SLAM, WBMTR requires no initial pose estimate.

3.1   Preparing the Model for Registration

For each texturemap image, we render the 3D model with OpenGL and store the corresponding 3D position of all pixels that lie within the model's silhouette. Using this we can immediately determine the 3D positions of any 2D image features located within the model's silhouette. Note that without computing a dense 3D model this is not possible in general. For each texturemap image we extract a large set of image features. Specifically we use GPU-SURF features [2] because they can be computed very quickly and, as shown in the evaluation section, work well for the uterus. Similar or better accuracy would be expected with SIFT [11], however these are far slower to compute. We use OpenCV's GPU-SURF implementation with default settings, giving descriptors of length $d = 128$ bytes. For a typical 1920×1080 images of the uterus, between 70-500 features are usually found, taking less than 10ms with our hardware. We use the average of the green and blue channels to compute features, rather than the standard approach of using average intensity. The reason is that green and blue light penetrates human tissue superficially and do not exhibit as much sub-surface scattering as with red light. The difference is very prominent with the uterus [3]. To mitigate tracking specularities we detect saturated pixels as those with intensity greater than 250, and any feature that lies within 5 pixels to a saturated pixel is discarded. We concatenate the features from all texturemap images into a single list, represented by $\mathcal{F} = \{(\mathbf{x}_m, I_m, \mathbf{d}_m)\}$, where $\mathbf{x}_m$ denotes the mth feature's 3D position in the model coordinate frame, I_m denotes the index of the texturemap from which it was detected and $\mathbf{d}_m$ denotes its descriptor.

3.2   Registration

For a given input image we compute its GPU-SURF features using the average of its green and blue channels. We denote this with the set $\mathcal{G} = \{(\mathbf{y}_i, \tilde{\mathbf{d}}_i)\}$. $\mathbf{y}_i$ denotes the ith feature's image position and $\tilde{\mathbf{d}}_i$ denotes its descriptor. WBMTR follows a RANSAC-based hypothesis and test framework [5]. Specifically this splits registration into three components. The first involves computing a set of candidate matches between $\mathcal{F}$ and $\mathcal{G}$. The second involves searching for a pose hypothesis that can best explain these matches. The third involves taking the best hypothesis and refining with efficient gradient-based optimisation [10].

Computing candidate matches. Candidate matches are found between $\mathcal{F}$ and $\mathcal{G}$ as those pairs with *(i)* strong descriptor agreement and *(ii)* have a low likelihood of being false. *(ii)* can be achieved with Lowe's Ratio Test (LRT) [11]. For each member of $\mathcal{F}$ we compute the member in $\mathcal{G}$ with the nearest descriptor. If this descriptor distance is less than τ times the distance to the second nearest descriptor in $\mathcal{G}$, it is deemed a candidate match. The LRT is very standard in feature-based pose estimation and we use a default value of $\tau = 0.8$. A novelty of using *multiple* texture maps is that we can also exploit match *coherence*. What we mean by coherence is that correct matches are likely to be those which come from similar texturemap images. Enforcing coherence can reduce false matches because it prevents matches occurring from wildly different texture maps. We enforce coherence with a winner-takes-all strategy. We first find the index I^* of the texturemap with the most amount of candidate matches after applying LRT. This indicates the texturemap image which is 'closest' to the input image. Because SURF is invariant to scale changes and image rotation, close means a texturemap image which views the uterus from a similar viewpoint, up to a change in depth and a rotation of the laparoscope about its optical axis. We then recompute the candidate matches with LRT, but using *only* features from I^*. Performing these processes is very quick. This is because $\mathcal{F}$ is completely pre-computed, and evaluating descriptor distances can be distributed trivially on the GPU.

Computing 3D Pose. Given the set of candidate matches, we perform RANSAC to find the most compatible rigid 3D pose. This involves sampling many match subsets of size 4, and for each sample creating a pose hypothesis using PnP [10]. Each hypothesis is tested for support by measuring how many of the other matches are predicted well by the hypothesis. Sampling and hypotheses testing is very parallelisable, and we use OpenCV's existing implementation for this. There are two free parameters which govern performance. The first is the deviation τ_r (in pixels) below which a match is considered to support a hypothesis. The second is the minimum number of matches n_c which must support a hypothesis. We have found good default values to be $\tau_r = 12$ pixels and $n_c = 15$, and terminate RANSAC if more than 500 hypotheses have been sampled. If no pose has been found with more than n_c supported matches, then we say the uterus' pose cannot be estimated for that image. Because registration is achieved independently for each frame there may be some registration jitter between frames which is undesirable for AR. This can be handled easily by applying some temporal smoothing. Currently we output a weighted average the pose estimates over a short time interval comprising the previous $m = 5$ frames, using the weighting scheme $w_t = (m - t)/m + 1$.

4   Experimental Results

In this section we evaluate WBMTR using real *in vivo* data from three different human uteri captured before hysterectomy. We name these U_1, U_2 and U_3. The video data for each uterus is divided into two sections. The first is the exploratory section. The second is a *free-hand* section, where the surgical team observed the uterus but were free to move the laparoscope and cannula as they wished. The free section lasted approximately one minute and started immediately after the exploratory section.

Marker-Based Ground Truth Evaluation. Before starting the exploratory section, artificial markers were introduced on the uterus to give us accurate pose estimates that could be used for Ground-Truth (GT) evaluation. The surgeon marked the uterus with a coagulation instrument at 12-15 locations spread over the uterus body. This gave a set of small regions approximately 3mm in diameter which could be tracked. We show snapshots of these markers in Figure 3, middle-left column. We performed marker tracking using correlation-based tracking. The markers were tracked using a small patch surrounding each marker, and fitted using a 2D affine transform that was optimised with gradient descent. We manually verified the tracks, and manually initialised if the tracks became lost. We then ran bundle adjustment [8] to compute the markers' positions in

3D, and the 3D poses of the uterus in each frame. If fewer than four markers were visible in a frame we said GT pose could not be estimated for that frame. Care was taken to avoid WBMTR exploiting the additional texture introduced by the markers. This was done by masking out the markers in each frame, thus preventing SURF from finding features on the markers.

Method Comparison. We compared our method against the most recent SLAM system applied to laparoscopic images [7], which is based on EKF. The public code accompanying [7] uses FAST features [15]. We have found FAST to perform very poorly with the uterus because it comprises few corner-like features, and [7] could perform better using SURF features. We use this as the baseline method which we refer to as SLAM+SURF. We also tested the performance of PTAM [9]. However PTAM also uses FAST, and to work requires a good initialisation. This is done by tracking points in the first ten or so frames and performing stereo. For each uterus very few PTAM tracks could be found, despite the motion being smooth, and were insufficient to successfully initialise the maps.

We summarise the results of WBMTR against SLAM+SURF in Figure 4. The three rows correspond to results for the three uteri. We plot error with respect to position (in mm) in the first column, and error with respect to rotation (in degrees) in the second column. The vertical black line corresponds to the point in time when the exploratory section stopped, and the free-hand section started. WBMTR and SLAM+SURF give translation up to a global scale factor. This is a property of *all* visual SLAM and SfM methods. To give translation estimates in mm, it must be rescaled by a scale factor given by GT. For both methods, this was done by computing the least-squares scale factor which minimised the translation error with respect to GT. We can see from Figure 4 that WBMTR significantly outperformed SLAM+SURF, with respect to rotation and translation, and across both the exploratory and free-hand sections. As time increases the translation error of SLAM+SURF steadily increases, indicating that it suffers significant pose estimation drift. By contrast WBMTR suffers no such drift, and the translation error is usually below 2mm. There are some error spikes in WBMTR, particularly in the free-hand sections. This occurs when the uterus is only partially visible to the camera. In these cases only features on a fraction of the surface can be estimated, and hence we have fewer features with which to constrain pose. There are some gaps in the graphs for which error could not be computed. These occur when fewer than four markers were visible in a frame. In the third column of Figure 4 we show the 3D trajectories of the camera estimated by WBMTR and SLAM+SURF. GT is shown as blue dots. Here the performance improvement of WBMTR over SLAM+SURF is very clear. In the third and fourth columns of Figure 3 we show snapshots of the registered 3D model overlaid in two frames. One can see WBMTR handles cases when the surface is partially visible and occluded by tools. Note that the boundary of the reconstructed 3D model should not necessarily align to the occluding contour of the uterus in the image. This is because the 3D models are only partially reconstructed by SfM. The boundary does not correspond to anything physical, but rather the region on the uterus for which SfM could reconstruct shape.

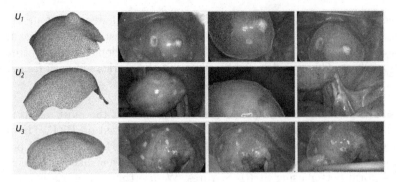

Fig. 3. Column 1: the dense 3D models built in Phase 1. Column 2: the coagulation markers. Columns 3&4: the registered models using WBMTR.

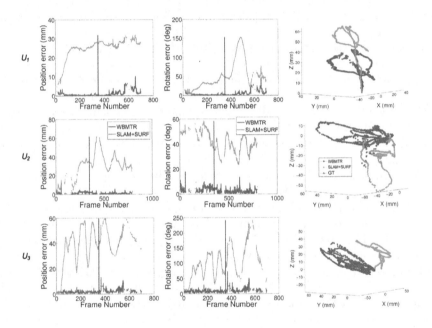

Fig. 4. In vivo evaluation of pose estimation accuracy for three uterus datasets

5   Conclusion and Future Work

We have presented a reliable and fast way to register the uterus in monocular laparoscopy using a novel two-phase approach. The approach differs to SLAM by decoupling 3D mapping and segmentation (done in Phase 1) from live registration (done in Phase 2). Phase 2 is achieved in realtime at approximately 26fps using standard hardware, and does not depend on successful registration in previous frames. It is thus simpler than EKF-SLAM and PTAM because it does not require switching between tracking and re-localisation. We have shown that our approach significantly outperforms EKF-SLAM for this problem. In the future we aim to enlarge our evaluation dataset and to explore the new opportunities that our method opens up for AR-assisted resection planning in uterine laparosurgery.

References

1. Agisoft: Photoscan, http://www.agisoft.ru/products/photoscan
2. Bay, H., Ess, A., Tuytelaars, T., Van Gool, L.: Speeded-up robust features (SURF). Comput. Vis. Image Underst. 110(3) (June 2008)
3. Collins, T., Bartoli, A.: Towards live monocular 3D laparoscopy using shading and specularity information. In: Abolmaesumi, P., Joskowicz, L., Navab, N., Jannin, P. (eds.) IPCAI 2012. LNCS, vol. 7330, pp. 11–21. Springer, Heidelberg (2012)
4. Davison, A.J., Reid, I.D., Molton, N.D., Stasse, O.: MonoSLAM: Real-time single camera SLAM. PAMI 29(6), 1052–1067 (2007)
5. Fischler, M.A., Bolles, R.C.: Random sample consensus. Commun. ACM (1981)
6. Grasa, O.G., Civera, J., Guemes, A., Muñoz, V., Montiel, J.M.M.: EKF monocular SLAM 3D modeling, measuring and augmented reality from endoscope image sequences. In: AEMI-ARCAI (2009)
7. Grasa, O.G., Civera, J., Montiel, J.M.M.: EKF monocular SLAM with relocalization for laparoscopic sequences. In: ICRA (2011)
8. Hartley, R.I., Zisserman, A.: Multiple View Geometry in Computer Vision. Cambridge University Press (2004) ISBN: 0521540518
9. Klein, G., Murray, D.: Parallel tracking and mapping for small AR workspaces. In: ISMAR, Nara, Japan (November 2007)
10. Lepetit, V., Moreno-Noguer, F., Fua, P.: EPnP: An accurate O(n) solution to the PnP problem. IJCV (2009)
11. Lowe, D.G.: Distinctive image features from scale-invariant keypoints. IJCV (2004)
12. Malti, A., Bartoli, A., Collins, T.: Template-based conformal shape-from-motion-and-shading for laparoscopy. In: Abolmaesumi, P., Joskowicz, L., Navab, N., Jannin, P. (eds.) IPCAI 2012. LNCS, vol. 7330, pp. 1–10. Springer, Heidelberg (2012)
13. Mountney, P., Stoyanov, D., Davison, A.J., Yang, G.Z.: Simultaneous stereoscope localization and soft-tissue mapping for minimal invasive surgery. In: Larsen, R., Nielsen, M., Sporring, J. (eds.) MICCAI 2006. LNCS, vol. 4190, pp. 347–354. Springer, Heidelberg (2006)
14. Nakamoto, M., Nakada, K., Sato, Y., Konishi, K., Hashizume, M., Tamura, S.: Intraoperative magnetic tracker calibration using a magneto-optic hybrid tracker for 3-d ultrasound-based navigation in laparoscopic surgery. TMI (2008)
15. Rosten, E., Drummond, T.: Machine learning for high-speed corner detection. In: Leonardis, A., Bischof, H., Pinz, A. (eds.) ECCV 2006, Part I. LNCS, vol. 3951, pp. 430–443. Springer, Heidelberg (2006)
16. Simpfendörfer, T., Baumhauer, M., Müller, M., Gutt, C., Meinzer, H., Rassweiler, J., Guven, S., Teber, D.: Augmented reality visualization during laparoscopic radical prostatectomy. Endourology (2011)
17. Strecha, C., von Hansen, W., Gool, L.J.V., Fua, P., Thoennessen, U.: On benchmarking camera calibration and multi-view stereo for high resolution imagery. In: CVPR (2008)
18. Totz, J., Mountney, P., Stoyanov, D., Yang, G.-Z.: Dense surface reconstruction for enhanced navigation in MIS. In: Fichtinger, G., Martel, A., Peters, T. (eds.) MICCAI 2011, Part I. LNCS, vol. 6891, pp. 89–96. Springer, Heidelberg (2011)

3D Robotic Catheter Shape Reconstruction and Localisation Using Appearance Priors and Adaptive C-Arm Positioning

Alessandro Vandini, Stamatia Giannarou, Su-Lin Lee, and Guang-Zhong Yang

The Hamlyn Centre for Robotic Surgery
Imperial College London, UK
{a.vandini12,g.z.yang}@imperial.ac.uk

Abstract. Accurate catheter navigation is necessary in endovascular interventions to avoid endothelial injury and subsequent complications. Although the use of robotic assistance has facilitated the navigation of catheters through complex anatomies, ambiguity in the catheter shape due to the 2D visualization provided by fluoroscopy can result in catheter and arterial wall collisions. The need for accurate shape reconstruction and localisation of the catheter has motivated the development of a range of 3D sensing techniques and augmented intraoperative imaging. The purpose of this paper is to present a 3D vision-based catheter shape reconstruction and localisation technique without the need for additional hardware. It is based on adaptive C-arm positioning under spatial constraints by incorporating appearance priors. On-line estimations of the 3D catheter shape can be achieved from the fluoroscopic images alone and are used to define the C-arm rotation that is optimal to reconstruct and localise the 3D catheter shape. The method is fully automatic and carried out without the burden of additional radiation and nephrotoxic risk to the patient. Detailed validation has been performed to demonstrate the potential clinical value of the technique.

1 Introduction

Catheter-based endovascular interventions have been increasingly used due to its minimal trauma to the patient. However they are associated with increased complexity as manipulation of the guidewire and catheter is difficult. Moreover there is a loss of direct access to the anatomy and poor visualisation of the surgical site. Endovascular robotic systems have been introduced in order to improve navigation through complex anatomies, enhancing the control and stability of the catheter [1]. However, clinically, the current imaging for intraoperative guidance is still limited to X-ray fluoroscopy which is a 2D projection of the 3D scene generated by an interventional X-ray (C-arm) system. Although the use of ultrasound, real-time MRI and additional 3D tracking devices attached to the catheter is gaining momentum, these solutions are not fully integrated into the clinical workflow yet. In parallel, the underlying technologies for interventional X-ray are also steadily improving owing to the development of accurate C-arm

C.A. Linte et al. (Eds.): MIAR/AE-CAI 2013, LNCS 8090, pp. 172–181, 2013.

movements, robot actuation (e.g. Artis zeego by Siemens and Discovery IGS by GE), hardware and software for enhancing the image quality, and incorporation of CT-like reconstruction capabilities. In order to minimise radiation exposure, nephrotoxic risk (due to excessive use of contrast agent) and endothelial damage (caused by unwanted collisions of the catheter with the vessel walls), it is necessary to maximise the information content of the available intraoperative imaging with technological solutions that are easy to integrate into the existing clinical workflow. Therefore, the reconstruction and localisation in 3D space of the catheter using fluoroscopy is necessary in order to minimize the aforementioned factors and ensure safe navigation through the endovascular system. Moreover, the reconstruction and localisation of the entire 3D shape of the catheter is particularly important for tendon driven robotic catheters with multiple bending segments (such as the Hansen Sensei system) as cross-talk is inevitable. It is not only the catheter tip that can collide with the artery walls; endothelial damage can be caused by any point along the catheter length. This 3D shape information can aid the clinician when performing robotic catheterisation, providing safe guidance through complex anatomy by identification of critical locations.

3D shape reconstruction of the catheter can be achieved with biplane C-arm systems using triangulation [2] or 3D/2D registration [3]. Although these approaches are well developed, biplane C-arm systems are not always available due to their high cost or operation workspace constraints during endovascular interventions. To achieve 3D localisation with monoplane C-arm systems, additional information is required. These include the use of preoperative data of the vessel morphology combined with back projection [4] and other patient specific anatomical priors. For these approaches, achieving an accurate registration of the preoperative model and handling anatomy deformations remains a challenge. To partially overcome these limitations a 3D probability distribution of the current plausible positions of the catheter, which was calculated using a particle filter and was based on fluoroscopic images and 3DRA, has been introduced [5]. Several non-rigid 3D/2D registration methods have also been proposed to estimate the position of deforming vascular structures [6,7]. However, these alone are difficult to apply to catheter shape reconstruction as a 3D model of the object is required in advance and the projection of a catheter shape is less informative than a projection of a vessel structure in order to recover its shape from projections images. Catheter localisation using limited C-arm rotation has also been investigated using non-rigid structure from motion combined with a kinematic model of the catheter [8]. However, the kinematic model cannot deal with catheter deformation caused by collisions with the surrounding environment.

The purpose of this research is to propose a 3D catheter reconstruction and localisation scheme based on a monoplane C-arm system with adaptive positioning in order to ensure safe and accurate online navigation. The optimal C-arm position used for reconstructing and localising the catheter is calculated using an initial 3D catheter shape estimated via appearance priors. To this end, we will use the Hansen Artisan robotic catheter as the exemplar to illustrate the overall concept and theoretical background of the system. The robotic catheter part

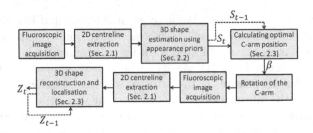

Fig. 1. The 3D catheter shape reconstruction and localisation workflow. The dashed lines represent inputs used at time t but estimated at time $t - 1$.

modelled in this work was the leader (shown in Figure 4(a)). With the proposed method, the rotation of the C-arm is limited to small angles to ensure speed, safety and minimal disturbance to the operation workspace during endovascular intervention. Although a complex navigation path might require several limited rotations, the achieved 3D catheter localisation can decrease the overall procedure time which is affected by the challenge in 2D navigation. Detailed validation of the method is performed to illustrate its potential clinical value.

2   Methods

The proposed online catheter reconstruction and localisation consists of the following steps: 2D catheter centreline extraction, 3D catheter shape estimation using appearance priors, optimal C-arm positioning and 3D shape reconstruction and localisation. The workflow of the method is shown in Figure 1.

2.1   Learning and Filter-Based Methods for Centreline Extraction

To automatically detect the catheter centreline in the fluoroscopic sequences, a learning-based technique combined with a filter-based method was used. The catheter is first detected using a cascade of boosted classifiers with Haar-like features [9]. Instead of training the classifiers to detect the whole catheter as a single object, small segments are detected first by treating the catheter as a set of connected small rigid segments. The entire projected shape is then estimated connecting the detected segments. The cascade was trained using data different to that used for validation. Catheter segments were manually annotated in fluoroscopic images and used as positive samples while fluoroscopic images with no catheter were used to generate negative samples for the training phase. The cascade had 20 stages. After initial detection false positives were filtered out taking into account the density of the detections, namely the overlap between bounding boxes (detected regions). In this study, the minimum number of overlapping detections that an accepted detected patch has to present is five, which was empirically estimated.

While the result of the learning-based approach provides an approximate automatic segmentation of the catheter, the positions of the bounding boxes is not accurate enough for a precise centreline localisation. A filter based on the Hessian matrix [10] was applied on the detected regions in order to have a precise segmentation of the catheter. The eigenvalue of the Hessian matrix encapsulates information regarding the presence of line-like objects in the filter area. The Hessian matrix is calculated as: $H = \begin{pmatrix} L_{xx} & L_{xy} \\ L_{xy} & L_{yy} \end{pmatrix}$ where L_{xy} is the result of the convolution of a scaled Gaussian derivative. Thus, the eigenvalues are estimated as: $\lambda_{1,2} = \frac{1}{2} \left(L_{xx} + L_{yy} \pm \sqrt{(L_{xx} - L_{yy})^2 + 4L_{xy}^2} \right)$. Finally, for each bounding box, the centre of mass of the cloud of pixels that respond positively to the filter was calculated. This resulted in a line of points along the centreline of the catheter. A cubic spline was then fitted to the point cloud to form a smooth and continuous 2D catheter centreline.

2.2 3D Catheter Shape Estimation Using Appearance Priors

To estimate the 3D shape of the catheter S using appearance priors, the 2D centreline extracted was first divided into n small segments defined as $c_z, z = 1 \ldots n$. For each of these 2D segments their 3D orientation in the image plane (θ) was estimated considering the orientation of the segment in the image, as shown in Figure 2(a). Their 3D orientation out of the image plane (ϕ) was estimated using a database of visual appearance priors at different degrees of bending angle, as shown in Figure 2(b). The database of visual appearance priors was generated offline and was composed by fluoroscopic projections of segments of the catheter recorded at different C-arm positions, simulating controlled and known rotations of the catheter out of the image plane. Rotations modelled in the database ranged between 0° to 50° around the Z axis (defined along the length of the imaging bed). The cardinality of the database used was six (one template every 10°, as shown in Figure 2(b)) as it was observed that no significant visual changes occurred on the catheter segment for shorter angle intervals. As the projection of each segment cannot differentiate positive or negative angles, i.e., the catheter bending into or out of the projection plane, this ambiguity is resolved by incorporating a smoothness constraint of the catheter. Each segment c_z had the length of the templates used in the database of visual appearance priors.

The estimated catheter shape S was modelled using a graph representation, where each 3D edge corresponds to the centreline of each 3D segment of the catheter and the nodes their connections. Spherical coordinates were adopted to define the edge connecting two consecutive nodes x_i and x_j. The 3D coordinates of the root of the graphs were x_1 and were initialised to the origin of the coordinate system of the shape. Hence, as shown in [6], the 3D position of a generic k^{th} node can be calculated as:

$$x_k = x_1 + \sum_{i,j \in A_k} \begin{bmatrix} r \cos \theta_{ij} \sin \phi_{ij} \\ r \sin \theta_{ij} \sin \phi_{ij} \\ r \cos \phi_{ij} \end{bmatrix}, \tag{1}$$

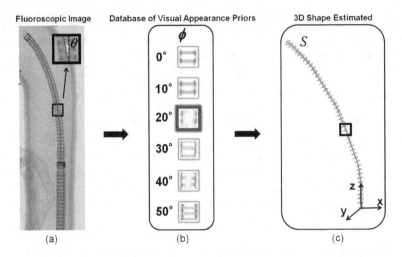

Fig. 2. The estimated catheter shape S (c) is calculated using the appearance priors. In order to calculate the 3D orientation of each catheter segment (one catheter segment is highlighted in the fluoroscopic image) their 3D orientation in the image plane (θ) was estimated considering the orientation of the segment in the image (a) while their 3D orientation out of the image plane (ϕ) was estimated using a database of visual appearance priors at different degrees of bending angle (b).

where r is the length of the edge that links the ith and j^{th} nodes respectively, ϕ_{ij} and θ_{ij} are the two angles of the polar notation and A_k is the set of ancestors of the kth node. This gave a recursive definition of the catheter shape.

In this study, r was calculated by dividing the length of the catheter (in mm) by n. Therefore, to define S starting from the root node, every edge has to be defined by estimating ϕ_{ij} and θ_{ij}. θ_{ij} is the slope of c_i (highlighted in yellow in Figure 2(a)) and was calculated by approximating c_i with a line that passes through its first and last point. ϕ_{ij} is the slope of the ith 3D segment along the projection plane and is estimated using the database of appearance priors. Based on this database, a similarity measurement was calculated using normalised cross-correlation between each template of the database and the projection of the ith 3D segment. The template with the highest similarity indicated the value of ϕ_{ij}. During template matching, each template was rotated by θ_{ij} to match the orientation of the ith 3D segment projected in the image plane.

Once all nodes were defined, a Catmull-Rom spline was used to interpolate between them to generate a smooth and continuous 3D catheter centreline. The 3D centreline was discretised into m equidistant nodes which represent the estimated catheter shape S. m was empirically chosen to be 20 in this study in order to best represent the shape without increasing the complexity of the model. S is defined in the coordinate system of the shape and it is different than the C-arm coordinate system where the catheter has to be localised. Therefore S encapsulates approximated 3D shape and orientation information of the catheter with respect to the C-arm but does not provide the absolute position of the shape.

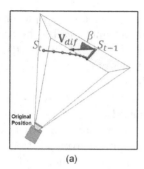 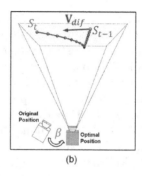

(a)   (b)

Fig. 3. (a) shows the estimated catheter shapes S_{t-1} and S_t at the original C-arm position. This position is not optimal for the 3D reconstruction and localisation of the catheter at time t as the deformation described by $\mathbf{V}_{dif}$ lies outside the image plane creating the angle β. In (b) the C-arm has been rotated by β in order to reach the optimal position where $\mathbf{V}_{dif}$ lies on the image plane.

2.3 Optimal C-Arm Positioning and 3D Catheter Shape Reconstruction and Localisation

We define S_{t-1} and S_t (at two time points $t-1$ and t) to be two estimated catheter shapes found. S_{t-1} and S_t are used to calculate the optimal C-arm position for the catheter shape reconstruction and localisation at time t. An estimation of the deformation between S_{t-1} and S_t was found as $S_{(t-1,t)} = S_t - S_{t-1}$. It can be appreciated that large reconstruction errors due to ambiguities of the single view would occur when the catheter deformation $S_{(t-1,t)}$ is out of the image plane (Figure 3(a)). To minimise this error, it is necessary to acquire a different view, optimised with due consideration of $S_{(t-1,t)}$ and the limitations of the C-arm rotation. Therefore, an online optimal small-angle reprojection method is proposed.

The optimal C-arm position is calculated using the optimal orientation vector defined as $\mathbf{V}_{dif} = \overrightarrow{S_{t-1}^{tip}B}$, where S_{t-1}^{tip} is a 3D point that describes the position of the tip of S_{t-1}, $B = S_{t-1}^{tip} + \bar{S}_{(t-1,t)}$ and $\bar{S}_{(t-1,t)}$ is the mean of $S_{(t-1,t)}$. Although $\mathbf{V}_{dif}$ is a 3D vector and coarsely approximates the deformation between the two catheter shapes, it encapsulates information of the main deformations regarding their relative displacement and orientation with respect to the C-arm view. The C-arm should be oriented in such a way that $\mathbf{V}_{dif}$ is aligned to the detector (the deformation lies on the image plane, as shown in Figure 3(b)) and therefore the deformation can be recovered without any ambiguities due to the single view used. The optimal rotation of the C-arm β is calculated as $\beta = \arctan(\mathbf{V}_{dif_y}/\mathbf{V}_{dif_x})$ where $\mathbf{V}_{dif_y}$ and $\mathbf{V}_{dif_x}$ are the y and x components of $\mathbf{V}_{dif}$ respectively. This constrains the rotation of the C-arm around the Z axis.

The shape Z_t is the 3D catheter shape that is reconstructed and localised in the C-arm coordinate system. It is composed by q equidistant 3D nodes, where $q = 20$. Z_t is found from the optimal C-arm view (rotating the C-arm by β, as shown in Figure 3(b)) using Z_{t-1} as prior knowledge of the shape and the 2D catheter centreline extracted on the fluoroscopic image acquired at the optimal C-arm position. To reconstruct and localise this catheter shape in the C-arm coordinate system, the energy function $\mathbf{E}(\mathbf{u}) = \mathbf{D}(\mathbf{u}) + \alpha S_l(\mathbf{u}) + \gamma S_{\mathbf{D}}(\mathbf{u})$ was minimized. $\mathbf{u}$ are the displacements of the nodes of Z_{t-1} to minimize the function and localise the current catheter shape Z_t, which is estimated as $Z_t = Z_{t-1} + \mathbf{u}$. S_l is the length preserving term and $S_{\mathbf{D}}$ is the smoothness term as described in [7]. $\mathbf{D}$ is the image-based difference measure between the projections of Z_{t-1} displaced of $\mathbf{u}$ and the 2D catheter centreline extracted from the fluoroscopic image acquired at the optimal C-arm position. It is defined as: $\mathbf{D} = \frac{1}{q} \sum_{i=1}^{q} \mathbf{M}^2(\mathbf{d}(\mathbf{y_i}))$ where q is the number of nodes of Z_{t-1}, $\mathbf{y_i}$ is the projection in the image plane of the ith node of Z_{t-1} after a displacement $\mathbf{u_i}$ and $\mathbf{M}$ is the distance map calculated using the 2D centreline. Since a 2D to 3D correspondence between the 2D centreline and Z_{t-1} is known, the distances of the projections of the displaced endpoints of Z_{t-1} used to find $\mathbf{D}$ were calculated considering the endpoints of the 2D centreline instead of $\mathbf{M}$. The coefficients α and γ were empirically chosen to be 120 and 4.5, respectively.

2.4   Experiment Design and Validation

To validate the achievable accuracy of the proposed method, detailed experiments were performed with a silicone phantom of the aortic arch (Elastrat Sarl, Geneva, Switzerland) and a Hansen Artisan robotic catheter (Hansen Medical, Mountain View, CA, USA). A GE Innova 4100 for interventional radiology (GE Medical Systems, Buc, France) was used to acquire the fluoroscopic images and the CT scans for validation. The experimental setup is shown in Figure 4. The calibration of the C-arm was performed using a customised grid phantom. To obtain the ground truth data, the catheter was manually segmented from the CT volumes and a 3D centreline was extracted from the segmented meshes [11].

For this study, two comprehensive data sets were collected. For the first set, the robotic catheter was scanned at a fully extended (straight) shape as well as at two different bending shapes. For each shape, fluoroscopy images were acquired with projection planes from 0° to +40° RAO (Right Anterior Oblique), with image acquisition every 2°. 3D CT scans of the catheter were also acquired for validation. The second set of data consisted of two sequences of the catheter in the silicone phantom: a pullback along the aortic arch from the aortic root and one cannulating the left subclavian artery starting from the descending aorta. The procedure was divided into five steps for the cannulation of a left subclavian artery and four steps for the aortic arch. At each step, fluoroscopy images were acquired with projection planes from 0° to +40° RAO, with image acquisition every 2°. 3D CT scans of the catheter were also acquired for validation. The catheter was moved 10 to 15 mm at each step.

For the first dataset, the fully extended shape was used as initialisation Z_{t-1} in order to reconstruct the two curved shapes. For each C-arm position (every 10° from 0° to 40°) the curved shapes were reconstructed and localised from that X-ray projection and at the optimal C-arm position found for that particular position. The mean errors were calculated as the mean of the distances between

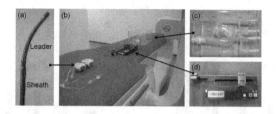

Fig. 4. The experimental setup (b): Hansen Artisan robotic catheter (a), a silicone phantom of the aortic arch (c) and an automatic pullback device (d)

each point along the calculated 3D catheter centreline to the closest point on the ground truth centreline and the distances between each point along the ground truth centreline to the closest point on the 3D calculated catheter centreline. For the second dataset, the errors of the localised shapes along the sequences were again compared to the ground truth; however, the initial shape Z_{t-1} for each step was taken to be the reconstructed and localised shape at the previous step.

3 Results

Figure 5 shows the results of the catheter shape reconstructed and localised using the first data set with two catheter shapes at different bending shapes. The mean reconstruction and localisation errors of the catheter recovered from the optimal C-arm position were compared to the original C-arm view where the projection is taken. The results show an improvement in the catheter shape localisation with the optimal position. The errors reported for the C-arm position at 0° and 10° are the same since the original position was already optimal in that case and therefore the C-arm does not need to be rotated.

Reconstruction and localisation errors for the two sequences in the second dataset are shown in Table 1 for the left subclavian artery and aortic arch at both the original positions which were chosen to be 0° and 40° respectively and at the optimal C-arm positions estimated using the method. The large differences between the reconstruction and localisation errors for the optimal C-arm position and the fixed position prove that even with small but optimal rotation the catheter localisation can be achieved using a monoplane system. The results derived show that with this framework, the accuracy of 3D shape localisation is comparable to that of the conventional triangulation or 3D/2D registration based on biplane systems. However the method proposed is based on one single optimal view while biplane-based methods rely on stereo vision. The 3D recovery of the catheter shape using the proposed technique is shown in Figure 6.

4 Conclusions

A novel method for accurate 3D catheter shape reconstruction and localisation based on appearance priors and adaptive C-arm positioning has been proposed.

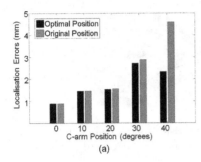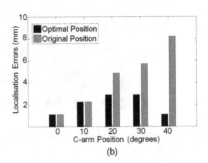

Fig. 5. The localisation errors of the two curved catheter shapes from the first data set. The results from the shape reconstruction and localisation at the optimal C-arm position are shown in black while those from original position are shown in grey.

Table 1. Reconstruction and localisation errors (in mm) for the left subclavian artery cannulation and the aortic arch pullback sequence

	Left Subclavian Artery					Aortic Arch			
Opt C-arm Position	1	2	3	4	5	1	2	3	4
2D Centreline Extraction (pixels)	0.81	0.89	0.89	0.69	0.52	0.66	0.69	0.68	0.73
3D Mean	0.53	2.40	1.45	1.17	2.69	1.52	2.78	4.14	5.98
3D StdDev	0.21	1.53	0.45	1.12	1.11	0.54	2.11	3.59	5.86
3D Tip	0.96	6.24	2.83	4.41	3.83	3.22	10.60	13.64	18.49
C-arm Position	0°	22°	10°	10°	10°	40°	40°	40°	0°
Fixed C-arm Position	1	2	3	4	5	1	2	3	4
2D Centreline Extraction (pixels)	0.81	1.10	0.86	0.95	1.00	0.66	0.69	0.68	0.78
3D Mean	0.53	2.95	3.66	8.79	7.71	1.52	2.78	4.14	7.30
3D StdDev	0.21	2.67	1.06	0.79	0.68	0.54	2.11	3.59	6.89
3D Tip	0.96	9.59	5.45	8.81	6.16	3.22	10.60	13.64	22.24
C-arm Position	0°	0°	0°	0°	0°	40°	40°	40°	40°

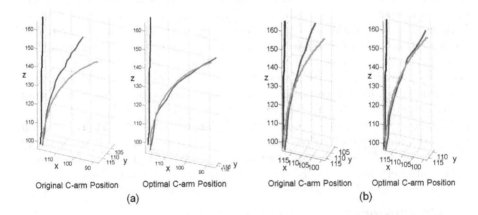

Fig. 6. Two catheter shapes (a) and (b) localised from the original C-arm position and from the optimal C-arm position. The initial 3D position of the catheter Z_{t-1} is shown in blue, the ground truth in green and the recovered 3D catheter shape Z_t in red.

It utilises fluoroscopic images alone to calculate the optimal C-arm rotation to best capture the 3D catheter shape. The results from detailed phantom experiments show the potential of the method for 3D catheter tracking and shape reconstruction. The advantage of the method is that it is designed for widely available monoplane C-arm systems and does not require additional hardware. This facilitates efficient navigation through complex anatomies, ensuring speed, safety and minimal disturbance to the operation workspace during endovascular intervention.

Acknowledgments. The authors wish to thank Dr. Celia Riga for her contribution to this research.

References

1. Antoniou, G.A., Riga, C.V., Mayer, E.K., et al.: Clinical applications of robotic technology in vascular and endovascular surgery. J. Vasc. Surg. 53(2), 493–499 (2011)
2. Hoffmann, M., Brost, A., Jakob, C., Bourier, F., Koch, M., Kurzidim, K., Hornegger, J., Strobel, N.: Semi-automatic catheter reconstruction from two views. In: Ayache, N., Delingette, H., Golland, P., Mori, K. (eds.) MICCAI 2012, Part II. LNCS, vol. 7511, pp. 584–591. Springer, Heidelberg (2012)
3. Brost, A., Liao, R., Hornegger, J., Strobel, N.: 3-D respiratory motion compensation during EP procedures by image-based 3-D lasso catheter model generation and tracking. In: Yang, G.-Z., Hawkes, D., Rueckert, D., Noble, A., Taylor, C. (eds.) MICCAI 2009, Part I. LNCS, vol. 5761, pp. 394–401. Springer, Heidelberg (2009)
4. Van Walsum, T., Baert, S.A., Niessen, W.J.: Guide wire reconstruction and visualization in 3DRA using monoplane fluoroscopic imaging. IEEE Trans. Med. Imaging 24(5), 612–623 (2005)
5. Brückner, M., Deinzer, F., Denzler, J.: Temporal estimation of the 3D guide-wire position using 2D X-ray images. In: Yang, G.-Z., Hawkes, D., Rueckert, D., Noble, A., Taylor, C. (eds.) MICCAI 2009, Part I. LNCS, vol. 5761, pp. 386–393. Springer, Heidelberg (2009)
6. Serradell, E., Romero, A., Leta, R., et al.: Simultaneous correspondence and non-rigid 3D reconstruction of the coronary tree from single X-ray images. In: ICCV, pp. 850–857 (2011)
7. Liao, R., Tan, Y., Sundar, H., Pfister, M., Kamen, A.: An efficient graph-based deformable 2D/3D registration algorithm with applications for abdominal aortic aneurysm interventions. In: Liao, H., Eddie Edwards, P.J., Pan, X., Fan, Y., Yang, G.-Z. (eds.) MIAR 2010. LNCS, vol. 6326, pp. 561–570. Springer, Heidelberg (2010)
8. Papalazarou, C., Rongen, P.M., et al.: 3D catheter reconstruction using non-rigid structure-from-motion and robotics modeling. In: SPIE Medical Imaging, pp. 831620–831620. International Society for Optics and Photonics (2012)
9. Viola, P., Jones, M.: Rapid object detection using a boosted cascade of simple features. In: CVPR, vol. 1, p. I–511 (2001)
10. Baert, S.A.M., Viergever, M.A., Niessen, W.J.: Guide-wire tracking during endovascular interventions. IEEE Trans. Med. Imaging 22(8), 965–972 (2003)
11. Palágyi, K., Kuba, A.: Directional 3D thinning using 8 subiterations. In: Bertrand, G., Couprie, M., Perroton, L. (eds.) DGCI 1999. LNCS, vol. 1568, pp. 325–336. Springer, Heidelberg (1999)

Uncertainty-Encoded Augmented Reality for Robot-Assisted Partial Nephrectomy: A Phantom Study

Alborz Amir-Khalili[1], Masoud S. Nosrati[2], Jean-Marc Peyrat[3],
Ghassan Hamarneh[2], and Rafeef Abugharbieh[1]

[1] University of British Columbia, Vancouver, Canada
[2] Simon Fraser University, Burnaby, Canada
[3] Qatar Robotic Surgery Centre, Qatar Science & Technology Park, Doha, Qatar

Abstract. In most robot-assisted surgical interventions, multimodal fusion of pre- and intra-operative data is highly valuable, affording the surgeon a more comprehensive understanding of the surgical scene observed through the stereo endoscopic camera. More specifically, in the case of partial nephrectomy, fusing pre-operative segmentations of kidney and tumor with the stereo endoscopic view can guide tumor localization and the identification of resection margins. However, the surgeons are often unable to reliably assess the levels of trust they can bestow on what is overlaid on the screen. In this paper, we present the proof-of-concept of an uncertainty-encoded augmented reality framework and novel visualizations of the uncertainties derived from the pre-operative CT segmentation onto the surgeon's stereo endoscopic view. To verify its clinical potential, the proposed method is applied to an *ex vivo* lamb kidney. The results are contrasted to different visualization solutions based on crisp segmentation demonstrating that our method provides valuable additional information that can help the surgeon during the resection planning.

1 Introduction

The emergence of robot-assisted interventions using medical robots (e.g. da Vinci Surgical System, Intuitive Surgical, Inc., Sunnyvale, CA, USA), has been shown to increase the accuracy and reduce the operative trauma associated with complex interventions. In partial nephrectomies, for instance, a crucial step is tumor identification during which the surgeon localizes the kidney tumor mass and identifies the resection margins. This step is important to properly plan and speed up the succeeding stage of tumor mass excision during which blood flow can only be safely obstructed for a limited time. More importantly, the accuracy of this step is necessary not only to preserve kidney function by sparing as much healthy tissue as possible, but also to avoid tumor recurrence by resecting all cancerous tissue.

The tumor identification step is usually performed with the help of multi-modal source of information at the surgeon's disposal: pre-operative scans (typically 3D CT and/or MR) and intra-operative data (2.5D stereo endoscopic data

C.A. Linte et al. (Eds.): MIAR/AE-CAI 2013, LNCS 8090, pp. 182–191, 2013.
© Springer-Verlag Berlin Heidelberg 2013

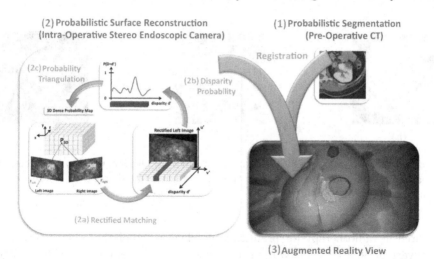

Fig. 1. Our uncertainty-encoded image-guidance framework consists of extracting 1) the probabilistic kidney/tumor boundaries from the CT volume prior to the operation and 2) the corresponding probabilistic surface information from the stereo endoscopic views intra-operatively using 2a) computational stereo matching techniques, 2b) converting matching weights into probability values, and 2c) triangulating the surface probabilities into the same domain as the CT. Finally, 3) we register the preoperative boundary uncertainties to the stereo endoscope using probabilistic surface reconstruction information and visualize the isoprobability contours onto the surgeon's console.

and, when available, laparoscopic 2D/3D ultrasound). Currently, these rich and complementary sources of information are just displayed on the surgeon's console in a tiled fashion (i.e. side-by-side) or even sometimes on a separate screen of a workstation nearby. These typical display setups require substantial additional effort from the surgeon to piece together a 3D mental map of the surgical scene that integrates all information together in order to localize the tumor and adjacent tissue. Hence, an augmented reality view, in which the endoscopic video stream is overlaid with highlighted kidney and tumor boundaries, can substantially reduce the effort required by the surgeon to achieve accurate and quick tumor excision.

To the best of our knowledge, all current methods rely on the visualization of a crisp segmentation only [1]. This renders the surgeon highly susceptible to the varying levels of confidence in what is overlaid on the screen. Segmentations are hardly ever 100% accurate for many possible reasons: graded decomposition [2], image acquisition artifacts, inter-expert segmentation variability, and fuzzy image segmentation [3,4]. These uncertainties can be important in subsequent analyses and decision-making [2,5].

In this paper, we propose to provide a visualization of uncertainties at the kidney and tumor boundaries as a visual cue to assist the surgeon in finding the optimal resection strategy. This is similar in concept to what is currently being

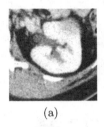
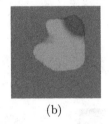
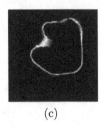

(a)   (b)   (c)

Fig. 2. Probabilistic pre-operative CT segmentation. (a) Original CT. (b) Membership probabilities of kidney (green), tumor (blue), and background (red). (c) Background boundary location probability (0 in black and 1 in white).

explored in radiotherapy for brain tumors when extrapolating glioma invasion with variable margins [6]. Our visual cues are derived from shape boundary uncertainties in the probabilistic segmentation of the pre-operative CT. This information is then registered to the endoscopic view as explained in Fig. 1. We apply our method to an *ex vivo* lamb kidney to create an uncertainty-encoded augmented reality view. We compare our results to standard guidance methods that use crisp segmentations and clearly demonstrate the benefits of our method and its utility for resection planning.

2   Methods

We first describe the probabilistic segmentation of the pre-operative CT that provides uncertainties about the boundary localization of kidney and tumor. Secondly, we perform a probabilistic 3D surface reconstruction from stereo endoscopy to which the probabilistic segmentation is directly registered.

2.1   Probabilistic Segmentation of Pre-operative CT Scans

The probabilistic segmentation of the pre-operative CT is based on the random walker segmentation algorithm [4,7] that generates membership probabilities of three manually seeded regions: background (BG: red), kidney (KD: green), and tumor (TM: blue) (Fig. 2b).

We denote the resulting multi-label probabilistic CT segmentation by:

$$P_{seg}^{CT} : \Omega \subset \mathbb{R}^3 \to \mathbf{p} \in \mathcal{S}^2 \ ,$$

where $\mathbf{p} = [p_{BG}, p_{KD}, p_{TM}]$ belongs to the simplex of order 2, and Ω is the spatial domain of the CT. From this multi-label probabilistic segmentation, we can extract the membership probability map of background P_{BG}^{CT}, kidney P_{KD}^{CT} and tumor P_{TM}^{CT} regions.

We also compute the likelihood $P_{surface}^{CT}$ of the *surface* union of kidney and tumor in the pre-operative CT (Fig. 2c) by combining the membership probabilities of being *inside* the kidney P_{KD}^{CT} and inside the tumor P_{TM}^{CT} as follows:

$$P_{surface}^{CT} = 1 - \frac{|(P_{KD}^{CT} + P_{TM}^{CT}) - 0.5|}{0.5} . \tag{1}$$

2.2   Probabilistic Stereo-Endoscopic Surface Reconstruction

We propose an extension of traditional computational stereo techniques of surface reconstruction from a single crisp surface [8] to a probabilistic representation of surfaces in 3-space.

Dense Matching of Left and Right Stereo Images. Using polar rectification [9] with the camera calibration parameters, the 2D dense matching of left and right stereo images is simplified to a 1D matching along parallel epipolar lines in the left and right rectified images. We use the normalized cross correlation (NCC) ratio on greyscale images as a matching similarity metric. This metric has the advantage of being less prone to changes in illumination. In contrast with current state-of-the-art methods, e.g. [10,11,12], instead of computing one set of robust and optimal matches, we retain *all* possible matches with their associated disparity (displacement $d \in \mathbb{Z}$ between matching points along the same horizontal line of the recitified images) and similarity measure ($c \in [-1, 1]$).

Construction of a 3D Probabilistic Voxel Map. In order to facilitate the pre-op to intra-op registration detailed in Section 2.3, we first create a 3D probabilistic voxel map in which each voxel stores the probability of being at the surface of the stereo endoscopic scene. To achieve this, we compute the disparity probability values by converting the NCC profile $\mathbf{c} = [c_1, c_2, \cdots, c_{N_d}]$ computed previously at every pixel $(u, v) \in \Omega_{2D} \subset \mathbb{R}^2$ in one of the rectified images for different disparities $d \in \mathcal{D} = \{d_1, d_2, \cdots, d_{N_d}\}$, where N_d is the total number of disparities. Basically, the NCC profiles are stacked into a 3D correlation map:

$$NCC_{3D}^{stereo} : (u, v, d_i) \in \Omega_{3D} \rightarrow c_i \in [-1, 1] \tag{2}$$

and converted into a 3D probabilititistic voxel map using the Gibbs measure as follows:

$$P_{3D}^{stereo}(u, v, d_i) = \frac{\exp\left(-\beta \left(\max_d \left(NCC_{3D}^{stereo}(u, v, d)\right) - NCC_{3D}^{stereo}(u, v, d_i)\right)\right)}{W(\beta)} , \tag{3}$$

where $W(\beta) = \sum_d \exp\left(-\beta \left(\max_d \left(NCC_{3D}^{stereo}(u, v, d)\right) - NCC_{3D}^{stereo}(u, v, d_i)\right)\right)$ is the partition function, and β is a free parameter.

Finally, the 3D position of each matched pair of points in the stereo views is triangulated with the camera projection matrices to transform P_{3D}^{stereo} into a probabilistic voxel map $P_{surface}^{stereo}$ in real world 3D space:

$$P_{surface}^{stereo} : (x, y, z) \in \Omega_{3D} \rightarrow [p, 1 - p] \in \mathcal{S}^1 , \tag{4}$$

where $p \in [0, 1]$ is the likelihood of a surface at voxel (x, y, z) in real world 3D space.

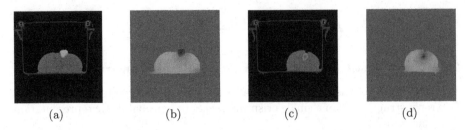

| (a) | (b) | (c) | (d) |

Fig. 3. Transverse slices of CT volume depicting our *ex vivo* lamb kidney phantom with (a) an exophytic and (c) an endophytic artificial tumor. (b) and (d) are probabilistic Random Walker segmentations of (a) and (c), respectively. Tumor labels are colored blue, kidney is colored green, and the background is red.

2.3 Registration of Stereo Camera and CT

We initialize the registration of the CT to the stereo camera in a semi-automatic manner using manually matched landmarks between the original CT, left and right camera views. In this first step, we use a similarity transformation to model the combination of (1) a rigid transformation to cope with different reference frames between stereo camera and CT acquisitions and (2) a global scaling to cope with ambiguities resulting from possible camera calibration errors. The resulting transformation is then refined with an automatic similarity registration of $P^{CT}_{surface}$ to $P^{stereo}_{surface}$ obtained respectively from (1) and (4). Finally, a non-linear registration step of these two volumes with a B-Spline transformation model is performed to cope with deformations occurring between the pre-operative CT acquisition and the surgical scene. We used `elastix` [13] with the sum of squared differences (SSD) similarity metric for the two last automatic registration steps.

3 Results

3.1 Materials

For validation purposes, we fabricated an *ex vivo* phantom using a lamb kidney and implanted artificial tumors inside it. Different materials (chewing gum and olive pit) were used to emulate low and high contrast kidney-tumor boundaries within the CT. The chewing gum was placed on the surface of the kidney to emulate a partially exophytic tumor/cyst (Fig. 3a) and the olive pit was planted deep inside the kidney (close to the renal pelvis) representing a completely endophytic tumor (Fig. 3c).

A 16 slice Siemens Somatom CT scanner was used to acquire a high resolution CT volume of the phantom. The resulting volume is composed of 130 (0.600 mm thick) transverse slices of 512×512 pixels (0.215 mm pixel spacing). Stereo endoscopy data was captured with a calibrated da Vinci S system at full HD 1080i resolution.

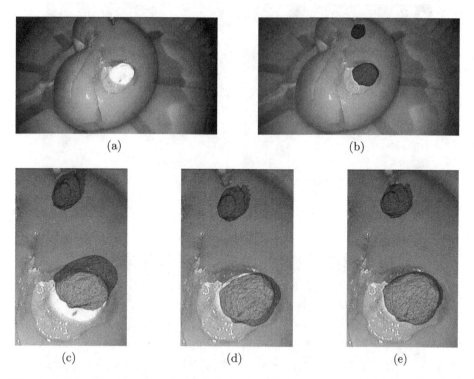

Fig. 4. Results of registration: (a) Original left stereo camera view, (b) final registered crisp mesh of the tumors (blue) projected on top of the image. Close-up views depicting intermediate results of the registration: (c) pose estimation, (d) automatic similarity transformation, and (e) non-rigid registration.

3.2 *Ex vivo* Lamb Kidney Study

The Random Walker segmentation algorithm was applied with manual seeding of each label in the CT volume. The probabilistic labeling corresponding to the two simulated tumors is illustrated in Fig. 3b and 3d. Note that the diffusion of uncertainties in the endophytic case is more visible compared to the exophytic tumor; this is a direct result of weaker contrast (CT intensity values: difference in pit/gum composition) at the kidney-tumor boundary. We were careful to keep the distances between the manually placed seeds and the visible boundaries constant to decrease the influence of seed placement on the resulting segmentations.

As illustrated in Fig. 4a, our phantom is quite smooth and lacks unique features on its surface. This results in a largely uncertain reconstruction from our stereo matching algorithm, which in turn causes the registration to be sensitive to the initial pose estimation. Successful registration was achieved after estimating the pose (Fig. 4c) using only four manually selected corresponding landmarks. The outcome of the registration was verified visually (Fig. 4) by projecting the kidney and tumor surfaces on both left and right endoscopy views. A small error

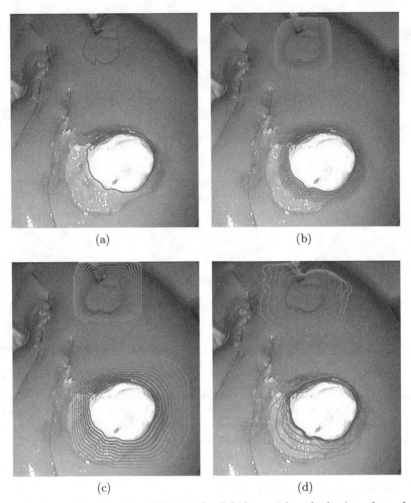

(a)   (b)

(c)   (d)

Fig. 5. Augmented reality view of *Ex vivo* lamb kidney with endophytic and exophytic artificial tumors showing different visualization scenarios: (a) crisp contour of projected mesh, (b) isotropic 2D diffusion of the crisp contour, (c) 2D projections of the crisp mesh dilated in 3D by 1 mm increments, (d) 2D projections of 3D isoprobabilities from 0.5 to 0.15. Contours range from the most probable boundary (red) to the most conservative boundary (green).

in alignment (< 1 mm) is observed in the resulting registration, this is due to the error in reconstruction which is attributed to lack of texture on the phantom.

In order to verify the usefulness of probabilistic boundary visualization, we present four visualization scenarios. In the **first case** (Fig. 4b), we generate a crisp mesh model of the tumor by thresholding the probabilistic segmented CT volume to extract the most probable kidney-tumor boundary. In our **second case**, we project the previously generated mesh onto a 2D plane (normal to the camera) and extract its contour (Fig. 5a). This particular approach does

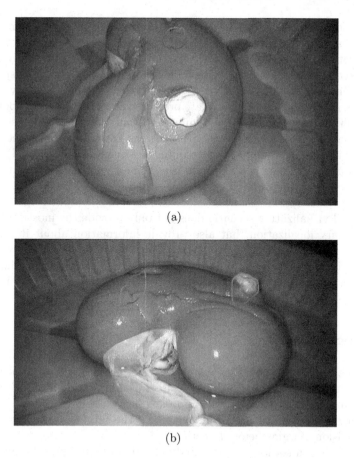

(a)

(b)

Fig. 6. (a) Top and (b) side views of *ex vivo* lamb kidney augmented with uncertainty-driven tumor boundary localization. Uncertainty is encoded into the tumor boundary ranging from certain (green) to uncertain (red).

not provide the surgeon with much additional information. Without any visible information (e.g. in the endophytic case) the surgeon's confidence regarding the visualized crisp boundary is, at best, changing isotropically away from the contour (as emulated in Fig. 5b). **Third case**, we isotropically dilate the 3D thresholded volume of the tumors by 1 mm increments and overlay the corresponding projected 2D contours (Fig. 5c). The resulting 2D contours dilate anisotropically as they are influenced by the orientation and shape of the tumor in 3-space. **Fourth case**, we propose thresholding the probabilistic volume at increasingly conservative confidence intervals instead of isotropic dilation to obtain isoprobability contours (Fig. 5d). In this case, we are essentially guiding the dilation of resection boundaries using the underlying uncertainty information extracted during the probabilistic segmentation of the CT. These results are consistent with our initial observation that the diffusion of uncertainties are greater in the endophytic case (pit/gum difference).

We presented the four cases to expert urology surgeons. The general consensus was that the information presented in the fourth case (Fig. 5d) is promising. A valid critique was made regarding the number of contours being overlayed on the endoscopy view: it obstructs the kidney more than the simple crisp solution (Fig. 5a). In order to address this problem, we present a complimentary visualization scenario in which uncertainties are projected onto a single crisp contour. We accomplish this by computing the minimum distance between the most probable contour and the most conservative one at every location of the most probable contour (distance from inner-most to outer-most contours in Fig. 5d). A lower distance implies a higher confidence in the boundary localization as it indicates a sharper edge in the probability map. We then transform these distances into a relative color map and use it to color-code the crisp contour (Fig. 6).

This final visualization scenario does not only provide the most probable tumor boundary localization, but also provide information about its local confidence. This visualization can guide the surgeon to quickly identify the best (most confident) place to start the resection. During the resection, the surgeon can always opt for the fourth case to see exactly how the uncertainty is diffused spatially.

4   Conclusion

We proposed a framework that enables extraction and registration of probabilistic data from two complimentary sources of information available in robot-assisted surgical interventions. Our approach provides the confidence in the resulting augmented information which can help the surgeon during the localization of excision margins before resection.

The novel visualization we presented is a proof of concept. The next step is to validate our experiments on clinical data and more realistic *ex vivo* phantoms with agar-based tumors of varying intensities, shapes and sizes [14]. We plan to conduct in-depth summative usability tests in addition to more formative usability tests to fully validate the integration of our uncertainty encoded visualization techniques into the clinical workflow. In the near future we aim to automate the initialization (pose estimation) steps and facilitate real-time operation of this framework. Although in this paper we presented uncertainty encoding from pre-operative CT, we will be taking advantage of other intra-operative sources of uncertainty to improve the confidence at the localized boundary while new data is acquired during the resection.

Acknowledgement. The authors would like to thank Dr. Abdulla Al Ansari and Dr. Osama Al-Alao for their expert opinion and assistance with the data acquisition. This publication was made possible by NPRP Grant from the Qatar National Research Fund (a member of the Qatar Foundation). The statements made herein are solely the responsibility of the authors.

References

1. Pratt, P., Mayer, E., Vale, J., Cohen, D., Edwards, E., Darzi, A., Yang, G.-Z.: An effective visualisation and registration system for image-guided robotic partial nephrectomy. Journal of Robotic Surgery, 1–9 (2012)
2. Udupa, J., Grevera, G.: Go digital, go fuzzy. Pattern Recognition Letters 23(6), 743–754 (2002)
3. Zhang, Y., Brady, M., Smith, S.: Segmentation of brain MR images through a hidden markov random field model and the expectation-maximization algorithm. IEEE Transactions on Medical Imaging 20(1), 45–57 (2001)
4. Grady, L.: Random walks for image segmentation. IEEE Transactions on Pattern Analysis and Machine Intelligence 28(11), 1768–1783 (2006)
5. Warfield, S., Zou, K., Wells, W.: Simultaneous truth and performance level estimation (STAPLE): An algorithm for the validation of image segmentation. IEEE Transactions on Medical Imaging 23(7), 903–921 (2004)
6. Konukoglu, E., Clatz, O., Bondiau, P., Delingette, H., Ayache, N.: Extrapolating glioma invasion margin in brain magnetic resonance images: suggesting new irradiation margins. Medical Image Analysis 14(2), 111–125 (2010)
7. Sinop, A.K., Grady, L.: A seeded image segmentation framework unifying graph cuts and random walker which yields a new algorithm. In: ICCV, pp. 1–8 (2007)
8. Hartley, R., Zisserman, A.: Multiple view geometry in computer vision, 2nd edn. Cambridge Univ. Press (2004)
9. Pollefeys, M., Koch, R., Van Gool, L.: A simple and efficient rectification method for general motion. In: ICCV, pp. 496–501 (1999)
10. Stoyanov, D., Scarzanella, M.V., Pratt, P., Yang, G.-Z.: Real-time stereo reconstruction in robotically assisted minimally invasive surgery. In: Jiang, T., Navab, N., Pluim, J.P.W., Viergever, M.A. (eds.) MICCAI 2010, Part I. LNCS, vol. 6361, pp. 275–282. Springer, Heidelberg (2010)
11. Bernhardt, S., Abi-Nahed, J., Abugharbieh, R.: Robust dense endoscopic stereo reconstruction for minimally invasive surgery. In: Menze, B.H., Langs, G., Lu, L., Montillo, A., Tu, Z., Criminisi, A. (eds.) MCV 2012. LNCS, vol. 7766, pp. 254–262. Springer, Heidelberg (2013)
12. Röhl, S., Bodenstedt, S., Suwelack, S., Kenngott, H., Müller-Stich, B., Dillmann, R., Speidel, S.: Real-time surface reconstruction from stereo endoscopic images for intraoperative registration. In: Proc. SPIE, vol. 7964, p. 796414 (2011)
13. Klein, S., Staring, M., Murphy, K., Viergever, M., Pluim, J.: Elastix: A toolbox for intensity based medical image registration. IEEE Transactions on Medical Imaging 29, 196–205 (2010)
14. Huber, J.S., Peng, Q., Moses, W.W.: Multi-modality phantom development. IEEE Transactions on Nuclear Science 56(5), 2722–2727 (2009)

Quantized Local Edge Distribution: A Descriptor for B-mode Ultrasound Images

Wing-Yin Chan, Yim-Pan Chui, and Pheng-Ann Heng

Department of Computer Science and Engineering
The Chinese University of Hong Kong
{wychan,ypchui,pheng}@cse.cuhk.edu.hk

Abstract. This paper presents an illumination invariant, histogram equalization invariant, rotation-robust and spatially stable texture descriptor for B-mode ultrasound images. We design a new edge-encoding descriptor that captures edge distributions of ultrasound textures. The distribution of edges categorized by their strength forms a signature of a specific textural pattern. Oriented edges are first quantized into different levels of salience according to local contrast and then aggregated to polar bins. A distance function that incorporates with our descriptor for effective texture comparison is introduced. The performance of the proposed descriptor is evaluated by various experiments.

Keywords: B-mode ultrasound image, image descriptor, edge statistic.

1 Introduction

B-mode ultrasound imaging is a widely available imaging modality. It is obtained by detecting the envelope of received back-echoes from a transducer. Ultrasound wave would attenuate in organs, be scattered by scatterers and be reflected upon acoustic boundaries. Scattered waves arrive at the transducer with random phase differences, superimpose together to produce stochastic patterns. Irregular tissue boundaries and tissue-dependent attenuation rates result in varying back-echo strengths and inconsistent illumination conditions.

An image descriptor represents the underlying features within a region of interest of an image. It is critical in many applications, including segmentation, classification, image retrieval, interest point detection, etc. The success of these applications relies on the coding and the extraction of image features. Feature coding and extraction in ultrasound images is particularly challenging due to the speckle rich property. A descriptor that captures textural patterns and be robust to imaging artifacts is always desirable.

In this work, we introduce a new type of edge encoding texture descriptor which is sufficiently distinctive to identify textural difference and robust to unavoidable artifacts inherited from the ultrasound imaging process. Our approach transforms an input patch into a set of (polar) orientated edge histograms. Oriented edges are quantized into salience levels according to local contrast. The encoded feature vector is invariant to illumination changes and histogram-based

C.A. Linte et al. (Eds.): MIAR/AE-CAI 2013, LNCS 8090, pp. 192–200, 2013.
© Springer-Verlag Berlin Heidelberg 2013

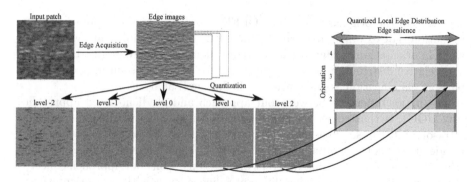

Fig. 1. Illustration of the QLED generation process. Edge images from multiple orientations are extracted from the input patch. Edges are quantized according to both local and global information. A collection of the distribution of edge salience from multiple orientations becomes a signature of the input patch.

operations, robust to rotation and spatially stable. We also provide a distance function which incorporates with our descriptor for effective texture comparison. We call our descriptor: Quantized Local Edge Distribution(QLED) descriptor.

2   Related Work

Recently, many approaches have been proposed to describe speckle patterns in ultrasound textures. These approaches mainly fall into two categories, distribution estimation [1,2,3] and edge encoding [4,5,6]. Distribution estimation approaches adopt various statistical models for the distribution of envelope intensity like Rayleigh distribution [1] or Nakagami distribution [2,3]. Distribution estimation approaches detect image local mean, variance or distribution parameters as feature descriptions and thus, are sensitive to histogram transformation or contrast enhancement. Edge encoding approaches focus on the occurrence of local edges or gradients and encode features in conjunction with positions, orientations and scales. Famous approaches include Local Binary Pattern(LBP) [7,5,6], Gray-Level Co-occurrence Matrix(GLCM) [8,4] and Histogram of Oriented Gradients(HOG) [9]. Distribution-based approaches sacrifice neighborhood information; edge encoding approaches do not capture high level information. There lacks a descriptor which considers both neighborhood relationships and high level information, and is robust to imaging artifacts.

3   Method

Figure 1 illustrates the work flow of generating a QLED descriptor. An ultrasound texture patch is decomposed into a set of edge images along different orientations. Edges along the same orientation are quantized into levels. The distribution of those quantized edges, having different salience levels, forms a signature of the original input. The QLED descriptor gives comprehensible information. For example, majority of the edges in orientation 1 are weak edges while in orientation 3, edges with different salience levels are evenly distributed. The relative distribution forms a feature vector which is useful in texture comparison, classification, segmentation or higher level analysis.

The major difference between our approach and gradient-based approaches (say HOG), is that edges are being processed instead of gradients. Note that ultrasound textures are basically interactions of point spread functions, the magnitude of gradients are often too small and unstable. Moreover, HOG gives a distribution of gradients among different orientations, while our approach concerns the distribution of edges among different salience levels within an orientation.

3.1   Edge Acquisition

We aim at identifying the textural pattern exhibits within a region of interest by capturing the distribution of oriented edges. The first stage is to record the relationships between neighboring pixels. Given an image patch I, $I(x, y)$ represents the pixel intensity located at (x, y). For any pixel, the intensity difference E between $I(x, y)$ and its' neighbor is defined as:

$$E_\alpha(x, y) = I(x + \delta cos(\alpha), y + \delta sin(\alpha)) - I(x, y) \tag{1}$$

where α is the concerned orientation at a small distance (δ). Edge properties are cyclic symmetric, therefore concerning the orientations between $0° - 180°$ is enough. This step eliminates histogram shifts as we only consider relative pixel intensities. The orientation resolution is controlled by the number of sampling orientation (P) that is $\alpha = (\alpha_1, \alpha_2, \ldots, \alpha_P)$. A patch is decomposed into P edge images, each contains edge information along a single orientation.

3.2   Edge Quantization

One characteristic appearance of ultrasound speckle patterns is the ripple-like texture. Microscopic view of these ripples is a collection of edges with various strengths. The distribution of them would be a powerful feature to discriminate speckle patterns. Previous researches [10,11] have demonstrated that thresholding on the histogram of edge magnitude is a practical metric of edge salience. Based on this idea, we quantize the strength of edges into salience levels according to the distribution of edge strength and local contrast. We set a constant quantization level λ to be the first κ percentile of the edge magnitude histogram plus a term related to the dynamic range of local intensity. We formulate the quantization as finding an intensity level of histogram threshold (λ) followed by quantizing the edges :

$$\arg\min_{\lambda \in [0-255]} \frac{\sum_{n=0}^{\lambda} H(n)}{\sum_{n=0}^{255} H(n)} - \kappa \tag{2}$$

$$S_\alpha = sign(E_\alpha) * \lfloor \frac{\|E_\alpha\|}{\lambda + t(I_{max} - I_{min})} \rfloor \qquad (3)$$

where $H(.)$ is the histogram of the magnitude of extracted edges, S_α is the quantized pattern containing the salience level of edges along orientation α and t is a parameter to control the impact from the dynamic range of the input patch. The parameter κ is set to the 30th percentile and t is set to 0.15.

3.3   Quantized Edge Binning

A quantized pattern shows the occurrence of interested edges represented by salience levels. The next step is to compute the distribution of these quantized edges for effective description. The frequency counts for each salience level are computed. To cope with indefinite input patch size, we normalize the frequency counts with the total number of pixels involved. Note that the computation of edges is not well defined in patch boundaries, those areas are trimmed and do not contribute. We define $C_\alpha(l)$ as the frequency counts for quantization level l at orientation α:

$$C_\alpha(l) = \frac{no.\ of\ pixels\ in\ S_\alpha = l}{total\ no.\ of\ pixels\ in\ patch} \qquad (4)$$

Finally, the QLED descriptor is generated by computing weighted components among orientation neighbors which are labeled with the same salience level. This can reduce aliasing effect due to discrete sampling in the first step. We accumulate Gaussian weighted distribution vectors in the polar direction.

$$Q_p(l) = \sum_{i=1}^{P} w_p(\alpha_i)C_{\alpha_i}(l)$$

$$w_p(\alpha_i) = \frac{1}{\sigma\sqrt{2\pi}} exp(-\frac{(\alpha_i - \alpha_p)^2}{2\sigma^2}) \qquad (5)$$

If rotational invariant is required, we may rotate the indices to a reference order. It is convenient to define the reference order according to the frequency counts of the non-salient entries ($l = 0$). The distribution vectors would be re-ordered such that the first vector would have the largest ratio of non-salient edges.

$$Q_{\hat{p}} = Q_{[(p+r)\ mod\ P]+1}$$

$$where\ Q_{\hat{p}=1}(0) \geq Q_{\hat{p}}(0),\ \forall p, \hat{p} \in \{1, 2, \ldots, P\} \qquad (6)$$

4   QLED Distance Measure

Image descriptors are usually high dimensional. A distance function is necessary for similarity measurement between descriptions. The QLED descriptor is of P-by-$(2L + 1)$ dimension, where L is the highest quantization level. Rather than computing an Euclidean distance between two high dimensional descriptors, we estimate the *difference in degree of disparity of edge salience*. The degree of disparity of edge salience is measured by high order moments of the QLED description. As we are not interested in the balance between the rising edges' salience and the falling edges' salience, but the disparity of the edges' salience, we take only the *even* moments. The distance between two QLED description is defined as

$$Distance(Q^1, Q^2) = \sum_n^P \sum_p \frac{1}{P} \cdot \sum_l^L \frac{|Q_p^1(l) - Q_p^2(l)| \cdot l^n}{L^n} \tag{7}$$

where $Q^1, Q^2 \in QLED$ and $n = 2, 4, 6...$ are the order of moments taken into consideration. Each term is normalized by a denominator, having the maximum possible difference in degree of disparity along an orientation among two descriptions. Taking such a normalization value would equalize the impact introduced by different order of moments, however this is not the only normalizing strategy. In practice, we consider up to the 6th moment.

5   Experiments

We conduct a series of experiments to demonstrate the feature extraction power of the QLED descriptor under various situations. Our experiments are designed to imitate real life applications. We compare our descriptor with two common and powerful texture descriptors, LBP and GLCM. In our implementation, the distance of two GLCM descriptions is computed as the Euclidean distance between two feature vectors formed by the {*Angular second moment, Contrast, Correlation*}, same as the definition in the original work [8]. LBP feature is obtained by finding neighbor relationship with parameters $P = 8, R = 1$. LBP labels are rotated to the minimum representation. LBP histograms are clamped to prevent domination. Distance of two LBP descriptions is computed by finding

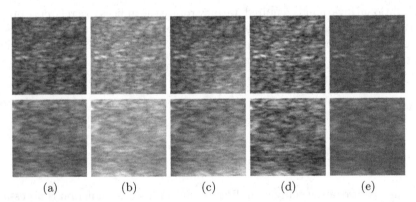

(a)   (b)   (c)   (d)   (e)

Fig. 2. Input patches. (Top row) Patch I, (Bottom row) Patch II. (a) Original, (b) Illuminated, (c) Locally illuminated, (d) Histogram stretched, (e) Histogram compressed.

Table 1. The measured distance between patches using QLED (lower is more similar)

I, σ^2	Dist.	I(a)	I(b)	I(c)	I(d)	I(e)	II(a)	II(b)	II(c)	II(d)	II(e)
0.34, 0.0076	I(a)	0.000	0.000	0.040	0.000	0.002	0.152	0.152	0.189	0.153	0.161
0.51, 0.0076	I(b)	-	0.000	0.040	0.000	0.002	0.152	0.152	0.189	0.153	0.161
0.41, 0.0132	I(c)	-	-	0.000	0.044	0.037	0.120	0.120	0.145	0.120	0.128
0.40, 0.0147	I(d)	-	-	-	0.000	0.023	0.153	0.153	0.189	0.154	0.162
0.32, 0.0022	I(e)	-	-	-	-	0.000	0.130	0.130	0.167	0.131	0.139
0.43, 0.0061	II(a)	-	-	-	-	-	0.000	0.000	0.037	0.000	0.009
0.63, 0.0061	II(b)	-	-	-	-	-	-	0.000	0.037	0.000	0.009
0.50, 0.0101	II(c)	-	-	-	-	-	-	-	0.000	0.036	0.035
0.40, 0.0155	II(d)	-	-	-	-	-	-	-	-	0.000	0.008
0.37, 0.0020	II(e)	-	-	-	-	-	-	-	-	-	0.000

Table 2. The measured distance using different descriptors (lower is more similar)

	Same Textural Pattern		Different Textural Pattern	
	I(a)-I(d)	II(a)-II(c)	I(a)-II(b)	I(d)-II(e)
GLCM (0-1)	0.118	0.141	0.105	0.241
$LBP_{8,1}$ (0-1)	0.000	0.006	0.003	0.003
QLED (0-1)	0.000	0.037	0.152	0.162

the inverse of the correlation between two histograms: $1 - corr(H^1_{LBP}, H^2_{LBP})$. The number of sampling orientation P of our QLED descriptor is set to 4. In this way, the angular sampling interval of QLED is equal to that of LBP, ensuring a fair comparison.

5.1 Illumination Variance

In this experiment, two patches are extracted from different tissues in a liver scan. We apply post-processing techniques, make variants of them, and compare their relative differences. Figure 2(a) (top and bottom) shows the two original patches followed by their variants. It is often the case that the region of interest occupies certain space in ultrasound scans. The illumination condition is unpredictable and the time gain compensation setting may not be evenly tuned. Therefore, a robust description of textural features is essential to dealing with uneven average intensities. As listed in Table 1, the distances between Patch I and its variants remain consistently low, while the distances between Patch I and variants of Patch II are consistently at a higher level. This demonstrates that the QLED descriptor together with the distance function can discriminate patches consistently under various conditions.

Table 2 shows a comparison between LBP, GLCM and QLED. Since GLCM does not focus on illumination invariant, the measured distances are not stable. One can not draw any reasonable conclusion to distinguish similar patterns from different patterns based on the measured distance given by GLCM. Both QLED and LBP show absolute resistant to histogram equalization (Case:I(a)-I(d)). In case of local illumination changes, the distance of similar patches (Case:II(a)-

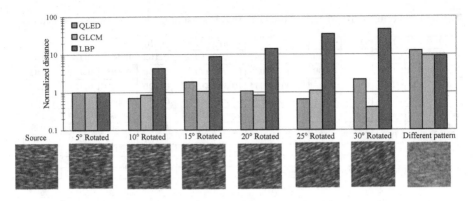

Fig. 3. An analysis of rotational robustness of descriptors. A 'source' patch is compared to its rotated counterparts. The rotation is ranged from 5° to 30°. A 'different pattern' is also compared as reference. The measured distances are normalized by the distance between the source and the 5° rotated patch.

II(c)) given by LBP is double to the distance between two different textural patterns. It happened that the illumination variation was so strong that some neighbor relationships had changed, the LBP label, as a consequence, changed. Successive values of LBP histogram do not bear any meaning and thus the change in measured distance is unpredictable. Compared to QLED, the distance changes slightly upon illumination variation, but is still much smaller than value between different textural patterns.

5.2   Rotational Variance

In clinical scans, textures vary upon scan directions. Here, we conduct another experiment to test for rotational variance. We artificially compound a set of ultrasound textural patches with gradual increase in rotation (5° − 30°) (Fig. 3 bottom). We compare the source patch with its rotated counterparts. GLCM is designed to be a strong rotation invariant descriptor. LBP is robust to rotation but not absolutely invariant in some data sets [7]. This test is challenging as the degree of textural rotation is smaller than the angular sampling intervals of all 3 types of descriptors involved.

We test the robustness of descriptors' resistant to rotation changes but, at the same time, remain sensitive to textural changes. We compute the distance between the source and other patches using 3 descriptors. The distances are normalized by the measured distance of the least rotated patch for easy comparison. Ideally, if a descriptor is robust to rotational changes, the normalized distance of all rotated patches to the source patches should be very similar. If the normalized distance increases upon texture rotation, its robustness is low. A plot of the measured distance between patches using 3 types of descriptors is shown in figure 3. (The actual measured distances for all the 3 descriptors are low.) Both QLED and GLCM show a distance close to 1 for the $10°, 15°, 20°, 25°, 30°$

rotated patches. The relatively larger distances (~10 times) between the source and the *different patten* patch also demonstrate that QLED and GLCM do not sacrifice textual sensitivity to obtain rotational invariance. For the LBP descriptor, the measured distance increases upon further rotation. Some of the measured distances are even higher than the distance to the *different patten* patch. One possible explanation is that the degree of rotation of those patches is less than the angular sampling interval such that the label rotation scheme of LBP fails to provide rotational invariance.

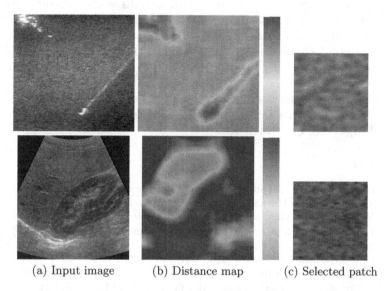

(a) Input image   (b) Distance map   (c) Selected patch

Fig. 4. An experiment on two clinical images. The patches in (c) (red squares in (a)) are compared with all pixels in the corresponding image. The textural distance is shown in the color-coded distance map in (b). Shades from green to red indicate increasing dissimilarity.

5.3   Experiment on B-mode Images

In the two previous experiments, we examine patches and their variants. Those situations are elementary compared to clinical images. In this experiment, we chose two complete B-mode images to demonstrate the capability of our descriptor(Fig. 4). The first one is a scan of jelly phantom with a biopsy needle inserted. On the upper left corner, there are air bubbles of previous insertion tracks, thus demonstrating a different texture. The second image is a scan of kidney scanned with a curved probe, stated in [12]. The images formed by curved probes are said to be *rotated* or *deformed* on the two sides, and are considered as very challenging for texture descriptors. Figure 4(b) shows the resultant distance maps. Similar textures are roughly indicated by the overlaid green color. Note that the distance maps are smooth and transitions can be found on boundaries rather than abrupt and unstable values. This property is potentially helpful to classification and segmentation problems.

6   Conclusion

In this work, we present a texture descriptor for B-mode ultrasound images and a corresponding distance function for texture comparison. We capture local edges and quantize them into different salience levels. The distribution of edge salience is shown to be a powerful feature to distinguish ultrasound textures. We also demonstrate simple applications of the QLED descriptor. Future works includes generalization of sampling resolution and quantization strategy. Application of QLED descriptor to more complicated classification and segmentation problems is favorable.

Acknowledgment. The work described in this paper was supported by a grant from the Research Grants Council of Hong Kong under General Research Fund scheme (Project No. CUHK412510).

References

1. Shankar, P.M.: A general statistical model for ultrasonic backscattering from tissues. IEEE Trans. on Ultrason., Ferroelect. and Freq. Control 47(3) (2000)
2. Bouhlel, N., Sevestre-Ghalila, S.: Nakagami markov random field as texture model for ultrasound rf envelope image. Computers in Biology and Medicine 39(6) (2009)
3. Wachinger, C., Klein, T., Navab, N.: Locally adaptive nakagami-based ultrasound similarity measures. Ultrasonics 52(4), 547–554 (2012)
4. Kim, N., Amin, V., Vilson, D., Rouse, G., Udpa, S.: Ultrasound image texture analysis for characterizing intramuscular fat content of live beef cattle. Ultrason. Imaging 20(3), 191–205 (1998)
5. Iakovidis, D.K., Keramidas, E.G., Maroulis, D.: Fuzzy local binary patterns for ultrasound texture characterization. In: Campilho, A., Kamel, M.S. (eds.) ICIAR 2008. LNCS, vol. 5112, pp. 750–759. Springer, Heidelberg (2008)
6. Liao, S., Law, W.K., Chung, C.S.: Dominant local binary patterns for texture classification. Trans. on Img. Proc. 18, 1107–1118 (2009)
7. Ojala, T., Pietikainen, M., Maenpaa, T.: Multiresolution gray-scale and rotation invariant texture classification with local binary patterns. IEEE Trans. on PAMI 24(7), 971–987 (2002)
8. Haralick, R.M., Dinstein, Shanmugam, K.: Textural features for image classification. IEEE Trans. on Systems, Man, and Cybernetics (3), 610–621 (1973)
9. Dalal, N., Triggs, B.: Histograms of oriented gradients for human detection. In: CVPR, pp. 886–893 (2005)
10. Rosin, P.L.: Edges: Saliency measures and automatic thresholding. In: Machine Vision and Application, pp. 139–159 (1997)
11. Qian, R., Huang, T.: A two-dimensional edge detection scheme for general visual processing. Pattern Recognition 1, 595–598 (1994)
12. Treece, G.M., Prager, R.W., Gee, A.H., Berman, L.: Fast surface and volume estimation from non-parallel cross-sections, for freehand three-dimensional ultrasound. Medical Image Analysis 3(2), 141–173 (1999)

Registration of Preoperative Liver Model for Laparoscopic Surgery from Intraoperative 3D Acquisition

Jordan Bano[1,2], Stéphane A. Nicolau[1], Alexandre Hostettler[1],
Christophe Doignon[2], Jacques Marescaux[1], and Luc Soler[1,3]

[1] IRCAD, Virtual-Surg, Strasbourg, France
[2] ICube (UMR 7357 CNRS), University of Strasbourg, France
[3] IHU, Institut Hospitalo-Universitaire, Strasbourg, France
jordan.bano@gmail.com

Abstract. Augmented reality improves the information display during intervention by superimposing hidden structures like vessels. This support is particularly appreciated in laparoscopy where operative conditions are difficult. Generally, the displayed model comes from a preoperative image which does not undergo the deformations due to pneumoperitoneum. We propose to register a preoperative liver model on intraoperative data obtained from a rotational C-arm 3D acquisition. Firstly, we gather the two models in the same coordinate frame according to anatomical structures. Secondly, preoperative model shape is deformed with respect to the intraoperative data using a biomechanical model. We evaluate our method on two in vivo datasets and obtain an average error of 4 mm for the whole liver surface and 10 mm for the vessel position estimation.

Keywords: registration, liver, laparoscopy, intraoperative, augmented reality.

1 Introduction

Laparoscopic surgery is a well-know technique that can replace open surgery to improve patient healthcare. However, this kind of surgery is difficult to achieve due to the loss of 3D depth and tactile perceptions during intervention. Augmented reality has been proposed to display structures like liver vessels or tumours that are usually hidden on the video [8,9,13]. This information is usually coming from an image acquired before the intervention and thus without pneumoperitoneum. This gas injection, that creates a working space for surgeons, highly modifies viscera shape and particularly the liver which undergoes deformations over several centimeters [5] and are extremely difficult to simulate [6,7] (cf. Fig. 1). Therefore, it is mandatory to update the preoperative model shape for augmented reality based guidance applications. Obviously, this update can be done only if intraoperative information of the critical structures is available.

C.A. Linte et al. (Eds.): MIAR/AE-CAI 2013, LNCS 8090, pp. 201–210, 2013.
© Springer-Verlag Berlin Heidelberg 2013

Practically, such information can be provided by organ surface acquisition (using an optical technique) or by intraoperative 3D acquisition (using a rotational C-arm like Zeego SIEMENS). Although rotational C-arms are currently not routinely integrated in surgical rooms, such a set-up begins to be more and more available in hospitals [11,12,14].

In this paper, we propose an approach to update the shape of a preoperative model of the liver using information extracted from an intraoperative 3D volume acquired with a rotational C-arm. To our knowledge, it is the first time that a non-rigid registration of a preoperative 3D model on an intraoperative data acquired after pneumoperitoneum has been evaluated in vivo, in the context of laparoscopic surgery.

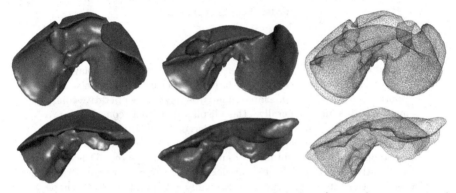

Fig. 1. One can see the porcine liver surface mesh before (resp. after pneumoperitoneum) in the left column (resp. middle column). The two meshes in wireframe (on the right) outline the important deformations that porcine liver undergoes due to pneumoperitoneum: the anterior part shifts down and the left lobe moves toward the left in the abdominal cavity.

Related Work. Vagvolgyi et al. [1] proposed to register a preoperative model of the kidney on an intraoperative surface reconstruction computed from a stereo endoscope. Firstly, a rigid alignment is performed using interactively selected landmarks, refined by an ICP registration. Secondly, a deformation is applied so that the preoperative model fits the reconstructed surface using a mass spring model. The same kind of method is applied for open surgery application, based on a two-step registration (rigid and non-rigid) using surface information from an optical system [3,10,2]. Despite realistic results, no quantitative evaluation was provided on their patient data.

In our context, all these methods cannot provide a good global accuracy. Indeed, the liver undergoes important motion and compression in the anteroposterior direction, but, even if we know the position of the anterior intraoperative part of the liver, the posterior part position remains unknown. One can clearly see in Fig. 1 that an alignment of anterior faces of preoperative and intraoperative liver cannot guarantee a proper registration of the posterior liver part, mainly because of the compression, which makes anterior and posterior parts closer. Without introperative information of the posterior part, it seems extremely difficult to foresee the liver shape.

Based on this information, we propose a three-step registration method to update the liver preoperative shape from a quick analysis of an intraoperative 3D acquisition. We highlight that our method does not rely on the intraoperative image quality, which is usually poor due to low dose parameters and inserted instruments or trocars, and quite common with rotational C-arm. Moreover, the acquired volume must not necessarily contain the whole liver but a reasonable part of its anterior surface, the spine and the portal vein entry for the initial alignment step of our method.

Firstly, we describe our three-step registration and the data that we have to extract from intraoperative images (cf. Sec. 2). Secondly, we will present the evaluation of our method on two porcine data sets showing that such an approach can provide an updated 3D model with an accuracy within 3 mm for liver surface and 10 mm for vessels (cf. Sec. 3).

2   Method

Our registration is composed of three intraoperative steps. Firstly, a global rigid registration is proposed to align the posterior part of the liver shape of both models in the same space using spine and portal vein entry positions. Then, we compute a matching between the two anterior surfaces using an interactive tool based on geodesic distance analysis. Finally, this matching is used to update the preoperative model shape from a biomechanical simulation engine.

2.1   Pre-processing of Data Input

The liver and critical structures (vessels and tumours) are segmented on the preoperative acquisition by experts using semi-automatic tools and corresponding surface meshes are computed (M_P being the preoperative liver model in this paper). A volume mesh Vm_P is also computed for the liver with the CGAL library (http://www.cgal.org), which is required for the biomechanical deformation step.

We assume that the liver posterior part does not undergo deformations due to pneumoperitoneum (cf. Fig. 2). This assumption seems quite reasonable since analysis of two pairs of 3D acquisitions of pigs (before and after pneumoperitoneum) shows that shape deformation in this part is small. Indeed, ICP rigid registration of the posterior part leads to surface registration errors of 1 mm on average. The spine undergoes a little deformation during gas injection and can thus be used as a landmark to estimate the liver posterior part position. Segmentation of the spine is done automatically with a threshold of the intraoperative medical image and by keeping the largest connected component. However, the liver can slide a little along the spine (cranio-caudal direction) although it is attached to vena cava and aorta. Relying on spine registration only is thus not sufficient and a further translation is necessary. We decided to use the main portal vein bifurcation, visible in both preoperative and intraoperative images to compute this translation.

For the non-rigid registration step, the anterior surface of the liver in the intraoperative image M_I is necessary and segmented (cf. Fig. 3): firstly, we threshold the air (around -1000 HU) and we compute the two main connected components which are the air around the patient and the air in the abdominal cavity. Then, we keep the part of tissue (between 100 HU and 210 HU) which is connected to the air in the abdominal cavity only. The other viscera such as stomach and bowels are also extracted with this method. Thus, a manual step is required to delineate the liver area only on the surface model. The mesh curvature close to liver boundaries, allows an easy visual identification (and could be automatized in the future).

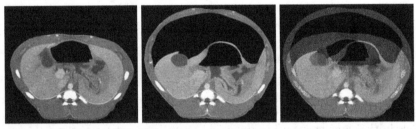

Fig. 2. One can see that the posterior part of the liver is not much deformed after pneumoperitoneum. On the left: the image before pneumoperitoneum, on the right: the image after pneumoperitoneum. The left image was rigidly registered according to the spine position and the portal vein entry point. On both images, we highlight in yellow the liver posterior part. One can see on the right image that the liver shape remains almost identical after pneumoperitoneum.

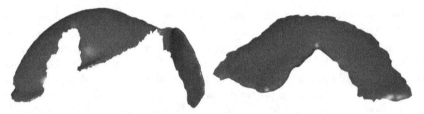

Fig. 3. On both figures, one can see the anterior part of the liver after pneumoperitoneum extracted with our method.

2.2   Rigid Registration Using Anatomical Landmarks

In this step, we rigidly register the preoperative and the intraoperative model using the spine position and the portal vein entry point. A first ICP rigid registration is performed between both meshes of the spine. The translation of this rigid registration is then refined using a manual identification of the portal vein entry point in both 3D images, easily identified despite the low quality of the C-arm acquisition (cf. Fig. 4).

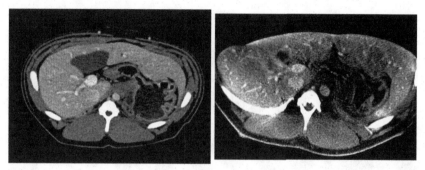

Fig. 4. One can see the preoperative CT (on the left) and the C-arm 3D acquisition (on the right). The bifurcation of the portal vein we use to refine the translation is highlighted with a red cross.

2.3 Vertex Matching between M_P and M_I

In the previous step, the preoperative model M_P was rigidly registered on M_I so that when superimposed, their posterior part is on top of each other. The next step is the computation of the vertex matching between anterior parts of M_P and M_I. This matching step is performed using geodesic distances on meshes between vertices and relevant anatomical landmarks.

These landmarks are manually identified and matched on both meshes. We call a geodesic distance map GDM_L the set of geodesic distances between each mesh vertex and a landmark L. The geodesic distance is the length of the shortest path along the mesh between two vertices and is computed with the *geodesic* library (http://code.google.com/p/geodesic/). We assume that the geodesic distance of a vertex V_P to a landmark on M_P is approximately the same as the distance between the corresponding vertex V_I and the matched landmark on M_I (cf. Fig. 5). Practically, three GDM associated to three landmarks are sufficient to compute all vertex matches.

For each vertex V_I, we compute its anatomical corresponding V_C on M_P which minimizes the following criteria:

$$V_C = \underset{V_k \in M_P}{\arg\min} \sum_{L_I^j, L_P^j \in LandmarkSet} ||(GDM_{L_I^j}(V_I) - GDM_{L_P^j}(V_k))|| \bullet \delta,$$

$$\text{where } \delta \text{ is a normalized weight: } \delta = \frac{[GDM_{L_I^j}(V_I)]^{-1}}{\sum_{i \in [0;NbLandmark]}[GDM_{L_I^i}(V_P)]^{-1}} \quad (1)$$

(which increases when V_I is close to the landmark L_I^j)

2.4 Biomechanical Deformation

The resulting matches provide a displacement field of the liver anterior surface. A biomechanical model is then used to interpolate this field on the liver inner

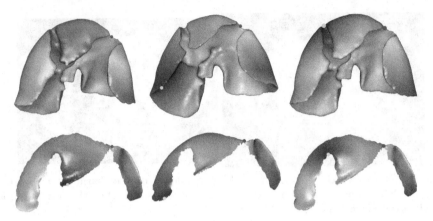

Fig. 5. One can see the preoperative liver mesh M_P (top row) and the liver anterior part after pneumoperitoneum M_I (bottom row) obtained from the method in Sec. 2.1. Colours on each mesh illustrate the geodesic distance of each vertex to a landmark (the yellow point). Blue vertices are close to the landmark and red ones are far. One can see that anatomically matched vertices have approximately the same colour (the red point is an example).

part. The volume mesh of the preoperative mesh is associated with a finite element model for soft tissue deformation. M_P and this volume mesh are mapped together: each vertex of M_P is associated with a tetrahedron of Vm_P. Thus, if a displacement is applied on a vertex of M_P, a corresponding displacement is propagated to the associated tetrahedron of Vm_P using the transpose of the Jacobian of the mapping. In a same way, the vessel mesh is mapped with Vm_P: when Vm_P is deformed, the vessels are also deformed. We assume that the liver posterior part is not deformed during pneumoperitoneum, thus, the posterior vertices of M_P are fixed (cf. Fig. 6). The deformation of M_P is finally performed by adding springs between the matched points with a stiffness selected empirically so that M_P overlaps M_I (cf. Fig. 6).

The biomechanical parameters used for the finite element model are Young's modulus and Poisson ratio. These parameters represent the elasticity and compressibility properties of the liver. We choose realistic values found in literature for Young's modulus (15 kPa found in [4]). The Poisson ratio is equal to 0.35 to allow slight volume compression or dilation. Indeed, it happens that the volume of the liver slightly changes during pneumoperitoneum.

3   Evaluations on Porcine Data

Our evaluation is performed on data from two pigs: a pair of 3D volume data sets has been acquired with contrast agent before and after pneumoperitoneum for both pigs. For the first pair, the pig stayed on the same CT table, so that the rigid registration based on spine was not necessary (only translation had to be estimated). For the second pair, the pig was moved from a CT to a Zeego

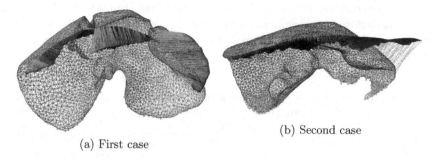

(a) First case   (b) Second case

Fig. 6. One can see the two meshes before our biomechanical deformation using SOFA for the two cases. The source mesh is in red and each of its vertices is pulled to match with its matching vertex on the target blue mesh using springs (in green). The fixed points in the posterior part are in pink.

C-arm: preoperative data has been acquired with CT and intraoperatively after pneumoperitoneum on Zeego.

The evaluation requires a ground truth: segmentation of the liver (M_F) and its vessels on the intraoperative acquisition is performed for both cases. We evaluate the registration accuracy of our method on the liver surface and the simulated vessel positions: we compare our registration results with the segmentation of the intraoperative acquisition. The biomechanical simulation is performed using the FEM from the SOFA engine (http://www.sofa-framework.org/).

We highlight that the ground truth liver segmentation was done fully manually on Zeego image due to the acquisition quality: image intensity values in the liver are extremely inhomogeneous due to artefacts.

On average, our method requires about 5 minutes, including all the interactive steps: intraoperative segmentation (1 min), rigid registration (1 min), vertex matching (2 min) and biomechanical deformation (1 min). This duration is a reasonable delay for the surgeon, although it should be reduced to 1 min to be totally accepted in the clinical workflow.

3.1   Evaluation of the Mesh Surface Position

We compare our computed surface mesh M_R with the full intraoperative mesh M_F. We provide a colour scheme for M_R which illustrates the distance between it and M_F. This colour scheme is done by computing the distance between each triangle T_R of M_R and the mesh M_F (i.e. the length of the orthogonal projection of the gravity center G of T_R on the closest triangle of M_F). The contribution of each triangle is weighted according to its area size.

We obtain a mean error within 4 mm for the whole liver in both cases. As a reference we compute the distance between the two input meshes just after the rigid registration and the mean error is 6 mm (for more details cf. Tab.1 and Fig. 7). We also compute the distance before rigid registration for the first case, as the images were acquired within a short delay in the same CT-scan.

The main errors are in the cranial part of the liver. Indeed, the diaphragm is also deformed during pneumoperitoneum which causes deformation of several millimeters, which are difficult to predict since they cannot be easily segmented in the intraoperative images.

Table 1. The distance between each triangle of M_R and the ground truth segmentation is computed and sorted in four groups. Each group contains a quartile of the triangle total number weighted by its area size. The distance is between M_R and M_F: before registration (1), after rigid registration (2) and after non-rigid registration (3).

Colour range	First case (mm)			Second case (mm)	
	(1)	(2)	(3)	(2)	(3)
Blue to Turquoise	0 - 3.4	0 - 1.4	0 - 1.0	0 - 2.9	0 - 1.2
Turquoise to Green	3.4 - 6.2	1.4 - 3.4	1.0 - 2.5	2.9 - 6.3	1.2 - 3.2
Green to Yellow	6.2 - 10.9	3.4 - 8.7	2.5 - 4.2	6.3 - 11.3	3.2 - 6.3
Yellow to Red	10.9 - 54.9	8.7 - 47.1	4.2 - 12.4	11.3 42.2	6.3 - 40.8
Mean ($\pm$ Std.Dev.)	6.0 ($\pm$ 7.2)	4.9 ($\pm$ 6.8)	2.3 ($\pm$ 2.4)	6.3 ($\pm$ 7.0)	3.6 ($\pm$ 4.6)

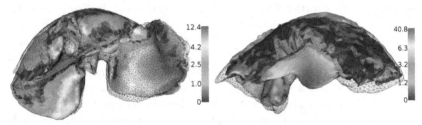

Fig. 7. One can see the results of our method on the liver surface of the examples illustrated in Fig. 1 with the ground truth in black wireframe. Both meshes are coloured according to Tab.1: the left one with the third column and the right one with the fifth column. For the second case on the right, one can see that the results are not very good on the middle part of the liver. In fact, during pneumoperitoneum, the middle liver lobe went to the right under the right lobe. This phenomenon also explains the average surface error of 3.6 mm . Our registration does not manage this kind of displacement for the moment.

3.2   Evaluation of the Vessel System

The evaluation of the vessel registration accuracy is performed on both cases (cf. Fig. 8). We compute the Euclidean distance between some vein bifurcations which have been manually selected. We obtain for the first case (resp. the second case), an average error of 17.5 mm $\pm$ 9.0 mm and maximum value 37.4 mm (resp. 14.8 mm $\pm$ 10.7 mm and maximum value 38.2 mm) without our registration and 10.3 mm $\pm$ 2.7 mm and maximum value 15.8 mm (resp. 10.8 mm $\pm$ 8.3 mm and maximum value 28.9 mm) after the non-rigid registration (cf. Fig. 8).

We have observed that the improvement of the non-rigid registration is less important for the second data set due to the lobe sliding phenomenon. Indeed, the non-rigid registration properly compensates for the lobe motion only if lobe surface is identified and matched on both preoperative and intraoperative images. On the second data set, since one lobe moved and is hidden below another one, we could not perform a proper surface matching. If we ignore this lobe in the error computation (the first error on the right histogram on Fig. 7), the average error decreases to 9 mm ± 2.5 mm. We believe that results should be better on human data since human liver is not composed of independent lobes and has less elastic properties.

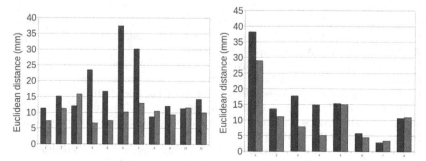

Fig. 8. One can see the Euclidean distance between vessel bifurcations after rigid registration (in blue) and after non-rigid registration (in orange). Each column represents the error of one bifurcation.

4 Conclusion

In this paper, we propose to update a preoperative shape model using intraoperative data from a 3D C-arm acquisition. Firstly, we have shown that a registration based on an anterior surface information only is insufficient to provide good accuracy. To overcome this issue, we have proposed to register the posterior part with the reasonable assumption that it remains rigid. The anterior part deformation is performed with a non-rigid registration corresponding to the anatomical area in the intraoperative image. Results show the feasibility of our approach. We are aware that our method requires manual steps (portal vein entry identification and landmark matching), but it seems reasonable for our clinicians. In fact, the main concern of surgeons is the registration error. Our method still has to be improved since surgeons consider that an acceptable guidance accuracy for deep structures is about 5 mm (for instance to show preoperative resection planning). In case we manage to obtain better intraoperative image quality, our work could be a very good initialization for intensity-based registration which may decrease the registration error of our method. We are currently working with radiologists on acquisition device parameters to improve the image quality.

Finally, we believe that our method can also be used with 3D reconstruction based on the endoscopic video. Indeed, the anterior surface we have segmented for our method is approximately what we can expect from a Structure-from-Motion method. If the endoscope is tracked using an optical tracking system as in [11], the table can be used as a reference to initialize the rigid registration up to a translation (along the table plane), that could be determined by a quick localization of the portal vein from the endoscopic view. This approach will also be tested in the future and integrated in an augmented reality software to visually assess the registration accuracy of our system.

Acknowlodgement. We are gareteful to IHU-Strasbourg for providing the Zeego acquisitions on pigs.

References

1. Vagvolgyi, B., et al.: Video to ct registration for image overlay on solid organs. In: Proc. Augmented Reality in Medical Imaging and Augmented Reality in Computer-Aided Surgery (AMIARCS), pp. 78–86 (2008)
2. Rucker, D.C., et al.: Nonrigid liver registration for image-guided surgery using partial surface data: A novel iterative approach. In: SPIE Medical Imaging, p. 86710B. International Society for Optics and Photonics (2013)
3. Cash, D.M., et al.: Compensating for intraoperative soft-tissue deformations using incomplete surface data and finite elements. IEEE Transactions on Medical Imaging 24(11), 1479–1491 (2005)
4. Samur, E., et al.: A robotic indenter for minimally invasive characterization of soft tissues. International Congress Series, vol. 1281, pp. 713–718 (2005)
5. Sanchez-Margallo, F.M., et al.: Anatomical changes due to pneumoperitoneum analyzed by mri: an experimental study in pigs. Surg. Radiol. Anat. 33(5), 389–396 (2011)
6. Bano, J., et al.: Simulation of pneumoperitoneum for laparoscopic surgery planning. In: Ayache, N., Delingette, H., Golland, P., Mori, K. (eds.) MICCAI 2012, Part I. LNCS, vol. 7510, pp. 91–98. Springer, Heidelberg (2012)
7. Bano, J., Hostettler, A., Nicolau, S.A., Doignon, C., Wu, H.S., Huang, M.H., Soler, L., Marescaux, J.: Simulation of the abdominal wall and its arteries after pneumoperitoneum for guidance of port positioning in laparoscopic surgery. In: Bebis, G., et al. (eds.) ISVC 2012, Part I. LNCS, vol. 7431, pp. 1–11. Springer, Heidelberg (2012)
8. Marescaux, J., et al.: Augmented-reality–assisted laparoscopic adrenalectomy. JAMA: The Journal of the American Medical Association 292(18), 2214 (2004)
9. Masamune, K., Sato, I., Liao, H., Dohi, T.: Non-metal slice image overlay display system used inside the open type MRI. In: Dohi, T., Sakuma, I., Liao, H. (eds.) MIAR 2008. LNCS, vol. 5128, pp. 385–392. Springer, Heidelberg (2008)
10. Clements, L.G., et al.: Organ surface deformation measurement and analysis in open hepatic surgery: method and preliminary results from 12 clinical cases. IEEE Transactions on Biomedical Engineering 58(8), 2280–2289 (2011)
11. Feuerstein, M., et al.: Intraoperative laparoscope augmentation for port placement and resection planning in minimally invasive liver resection. IEEE Transactions on Medical Imaging 27(3), 355–369 (2008)
12. Shekhar, R., et al.: Live augmented reality: A new visualization method for laparoscopic surgery using continuous volumetric computed tomography. Surgical Endoscopy, 1–10 (2010)
13. Nicolau, S.A., et al.: Augmented reality in laparoscopic surgical oncology. Surgical Oncology 20(3), 189–201 (2011)
14. Nozaki, T., et al.: Laparoscopic radical nephrectomy under near real-time three-dimensional surgical navigation with c-arm cone beam computed tomography. Surgical Innovation 19(3), 263–267 (2012)

Volume Visualization for Neurovascular Augmented Reality Surgery

Marta Kersten-Oertel, Simon Drouin, Sean J.S. Chen, and D. Louis Collins

McConnell Brain Imaging Center, MNI, McGill University, Montreal, Canada

Abstract. In neurovascular image-guided surgery, surgeons use pre-operative vascular data sets (from angiography) to guide them. They map information from angiography images onto the patient on the operating room table to localize important vessels. This spatial mapping is complex, time consuming and prone to error. We've developed an augmented reality (AR) system to visualize the pre-operative vascular data within the context of a microscope/camera image. Such an AR visualization enhances the surgeon's field of view with data that is not otherwise readily available (e.g., anatomical data beyond the visible surface or data about the flow of blood through the vessels), and it aids the surgeon to better understand the topology and locations of vessels that lie below the visible surface of the cortex. In this paper, we explore a number of different volume rendering methods for AR visualization of vessel topology and blood flow.

1 Introduction

Mixed reality visualizations have become a focus of research in the medical domain for surgical training, planning, diagnosis and guidance. The purpose of such visualizations is to improve the understanding of complex multimodal data within the context of the patient in the operating room (OR). In image-guided surgery (IGS) augmented reality (AR) visualization is achieved by introducing pre-operative virtual models of patient data onto the patient or into live images of the surgical field of view. To date, the most frequently used analyzed data representations of patient anatomy are simple surface or wireframe renderings of the data [7]. This, despite faster processors and graphics cards that allow for real-time rendering rates of volume rendered virtual data onto real world images. One advantage of using volume rendering for virtual data is that a larger number of visualization methods may be studied by appropriately tuning transfer functions. This in turn may allow for better depth and spatial perception, and more visually pleasing results.

In this work, we present a volumetric visualization method for augmented reality in neurovascular surgery. Understanding intra-operative vascular scenes is difficult for numerous reasons. In vascular neurosurgery, surgeons use an operating microscope that enables a magnified, more precise and clear view of the local region of interest. The microscope, however, provides no information as to the vessel anatomy below the surface. The burden is with the surgeon to best map

C.A. Linte et al. (Eds.): MIAR/AE-CAI 2013, LNCS 8090, pp. 211–220, 2013.

the rudimentary images on the navigation system to the patient lying on the table. This task is made more difficult due to the frequent repositioning of the surgical microscope during surgery and the lack of visible external anatomical landmarks because of the sterile draping of the patient. By registering the live microscope image (or a camera image) in the OR with pre-operative plans, models and data sets the surgeon can get a better understanding of the layout of the vessels beyond those seen only at the surface. In Fig. 1 on the left, we show IBIS (the Intra-operative Brain Imaging System navigation system) [4] with the current type of navigation view (the three cross planes of the pre-operative dataset plus the microscope image) used for neurosurgery at the Montreal Neurological Institute (Canada), on the right, we show the AR view which would replace the microscope image.

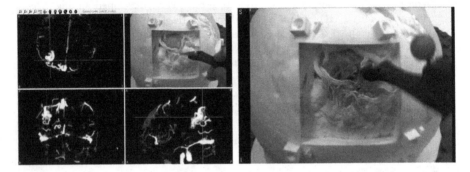

Fig. 1. *Left*: The navigation view used for neurosurgery at our institute, three cross planes of the segmented vessels from the pre-operative CTA dataset (coronal, sagital and axial) plus the microscope image). *Right*: We replace the microscope image with the AR view to aid understanding of the layout of the vessels beyond those seen on the cortical surface.

Cerebral vascular scene understanding is complex for several reasons. Two of these are: (1) difficulties in spatial and depth understanding of the vascular data due to the fact that many vessels overlap at many different depths and the large number of furcations and (2) difficulties in intra-operatively distinguishing between arteries and veins in vascular abnormalities (where both look red under the microscope). In this paper we address both of these issues by introducing different volume rendering techniques. *Scene de-cluttering*, which allows relevant information in terms of topologically close vessels to the neurovascular anomaly, is used for enhanced spatial understanding. The perceptive cue of aerial perspective (implemented as fog) is used to enhance relative depth perception of the vessels. *Colour-coding* of vessels based on flow information is used to differentiate between arteries and veins. Furthermore, to combine the vascular volumes with live images from the microscope and to ensure that the virtual objects are perceived as being within the patient rather than floating in front of the patient we use edges extracted from the microscope image as a depth cue. AR visualizations, which provide better spatial and depth understanding, as well as information as to blood flow within vessels, may reduce the amount of time required to locate specific vessels of interest, and may help to reduce the amount of resected tissue during surgery.

2   Background and Related Work

Arteriovenous malformations (AVMs) are abnormal collections of blood vessels. The central part of the AVM, or the nidus, is made up of abnormal vessels that are hybrids of true arteries and veins. AVMs are fed by one or more arteries (feeders), and are drained by one or more draining veins (drainers). These feeding and draining vessels often have weakened walls and therefore may leak or rupture. Neurosurgery for AVMs involves identifying the margins of the malformation and tying off or clipping the feeder vessels, obliterating the draining veins and removing or obliterating the nidus. A detailed understanding of the arterial inflow from feeders and venous drainage from drainers is therefore important for clinical evaluation and management of AVMs.

The use of techniques which aid the characterization of the pattern and distribution of feeders and drainers by quantification of the relative blood flow is necessary as it is not always trivial to identify whether a vessel is a feeding artery or an arterialized vein. By visualizing information from blood flow analysis in the vessels we can aid surgeons to intra-operatively distinguish between feeders and drainers. With the use of AR, we believe, we can aid surgeons by reducing the time to localize and identify important vessels during surgery by showing the vessels which are not visible when looking at the cortex through the surgical microscope and by colour coding vessels to help in differentiation.

A number of mixed reality systems have been developed for neurosurgery. Examples include: Edwards et al.'s [5] microscope-assisted guided interventions (MAGI) system, a stereoscopic microscope for neurosurgery and otolaryngology; Glossop et al.'s [6] projector based system for craniotomies; and Paul et al.'s [14] system that allows for both AR and AV visualization for neuronavigation. For more information about mixed reality surgical systems the reader is referred to the review by Kersten et al. [7].

To date few systems have used volumetric representations of virtual objects in mixed reality. In Kersten et al.'s review of the state of art in mixed reality IGS only about 1% of reviewed papers used volume rendering [7]. Systems that have used volumetric data rather than surface or wireframe representations include those developed by Bichlmeier et al.[2], Volonté et al. [19], Mischkowski et al. [12], Konishi et al. [10], Scheuering et al. [16], Suzuki et al. [17], Wieczorek et al. [18] and Yamaguchi et al. [20]. In our system we use volume rendered pre-operative angiography data as our virtual object because volume rendering allows for direct manipulation of visualization parameters. Furthermore, particular volume visualization methods which use perceptual cues have been shown to provide a good depth understanding of cerebral vasculature, in particular when compared to stereoscopic visualization [9].

3   Volume Rendering in Neurovascular AR

We developed a test development environment where we use a 3D printed nylon head phantom, in lieu of a patient, to study different AR visualization methods. Details about the system, including calibration and registration information, as well as the development of the phantom used for visualization studies can be found in Drouin *et al.* [4]. In this section, the system is described using the checklist for mixed reality system descriptions based on the DVV taxonomy [8].

3.1   Data

The visualized imaging data used in our system is comprised of CT or MR angiography and/or 3D X-ray angiography, depending on the data that is available for each patient. The 3D volumetric data is acquired pre-operatively and is volume rendered as a virtual object that is registered to live patient images of the cerebral cortex in the OR. In the following example we use: a combination arterial and venous-phase CT-DSA acquired using a Toshiba Aquilion ONE (Toshiba Medical Systems) with an isotropic 0.5mm resolution and two 3D X-ray angiography with selective vessel contrast injection acquired using the GE Advantx LC LP+ Biplane Angiographic System (GE Healthcare) with an isotropic 0.4mm resolution. In terms of prior-knowledge data, a 3D surface representation of a pointer may be rendered on the screen when used. We currently do not visualize any patient specific scores or derived data.

3.2   Visualization Processing

In order to extract the vessels from the angiography data, region growing with a pre-defined threshold was used. The segmented vascular data set was then volume rendered using a number of different visualization methods, mainly: vascular scene de-cluttering, feeder/drainer colour coding based on blood flow, and fog rendering for enhanced depth perception.

Combining Virtual Objects with the Camera Image. The goal of AR is to fuse a camera image that provides contextual information about the location of the surgical target with the pre-operative scans that provide precise information about the configuration of the surgical target. To this effect, our approach has been to modulate the opacity of the camera image to show more of the volume rendering in the region of the surgical target and more of the camera image elsewhere. Simply fading out transparency from the area around the surgical target presents a problem: the volume rendered image appears to be above the surface of the patient. Salient features, such as edges, extracted from the camera image have been used to provide better spatial and depth understanding in AR visualizations (e.g. Avery *et al.* [1] and Lerotic *et al.* [11]). In our work, we use the cue of occlusion: in the area around the surgical target where the camera image is made transparent to show the virtual object below the surface, we keep only the edges extracted from the camera image. To find those edges we use a Sobel operator which computes an approximation of the gradient of the image intensity function. The Sobel operator was implemented as a shader in OpenGL. Each pixel's rgb and alpha components are computed as follows:

$$(RGB\ component)\ I_{disp_i}.rgb = I_{cam_i}.rgb \qquad (1)$$

$$(Alpha\ component)\ I_{disp_i}.a = (1.0 - f) + (f * ||\overrightarrow{G_i}||) \qquad (2)$$

where I_{disp_i} is pixel i of the displayed image, I_{cam_i} is pixel i of the raw camera image, $\overrightarrow{G_i} = (G_{x_i}, G_{y_i})$ is computed with the standard 3x3 sobel kernel

$$G_x = \begin{bmatrix} 1 & 0 & -1 \\ 2 & 0 & -2 \\ 1 & 0 & -1 \end{bmatrix} * I_{cam_i}, G_y = \begin{bmatrix} 1 & 2 & 1 \\ 0 & 0 & 0 \\ -1 & -2 & -1 \end{bmatrix} * I_{cam_i} \qquad (3)$$

and factor f is used to fade out transparency starting from radius r_1 to radius r_2 around point $\overrightarrow{C}$ which is a projection of the surgical target in image space

$$f = \begin{cases} d < r_1 & 0.0 \\ r_1 < d < r_2 & \exp{-\frac{\left(\frac{d-r_1}{r_2-r_1}\right)^2}{.25}} \\ d > r_2 & 1.0 \end{cases} \qquad (4)$$

where $d = ||\overrightarrow{P} - \overrightarrow{C}||$, $\overrightarrow{P}$ is the image space coordinate of the pixel considered. Once I_{disp} is computed, it is combined with the volumetric data using OpenGL's alpha blending. Figure 2 illustrates the different steps involved in the computation of the final AR view.

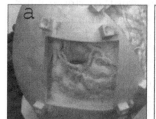 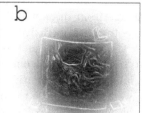 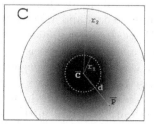

Fig. 2. (a) The original image. (b) The computed alpha channel ($I_{disp_i}.a$). (c) Representation of the variables involved in the computation of the alpha channel.

De-cluttering. Vascular data is complex in terms of the number of vessels that overlap in depth and the many furcations of the vessels. Visualization of vessels, therefore, may involve de-cluttering (selectively removing details) of vessels, to show the most relevant vessels at a given point in surgery. We can determine and visualize topologically close vessels to an AVM by using a level-set front propagation method which is seeded at the AVM nidus [3]. A transfer function is then used to fade out vessels so that further vessels from the nidus become more and more transparent. In Fig. 3 (a) we show the pre-operative dataset. In (b) the vascular volume is rendered as a virtual object with the real camera image. The large amount of vessels makes it difficult to understand the spatial layout of the vessels, furthermore, not all vessels are relevant to the surgery. We therefore allow selective viewing of vasculature close to the AVM nidus, making distant vessels transparent (Fig. 3 (c)).

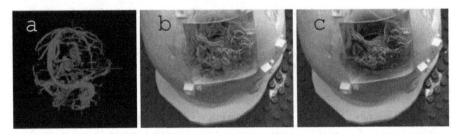

Fig. 3. (a) The pre-operative vascular data (combination of MRA, CT DSA and X-ray angiography. (b) Combined virtual vascular volume with real camera image. (c) Combined virtual vascular volume using de-cluttering based on distance from AVM.

Colour-Coding Flow. Neurosurgery for AVMs involves identifying the margins of the malformation and tying off or clipping the feeder vessels, obliterating the draining veins and removing or obliterating the nidus. The task of differentiating between veins and arteries is difficult and can be complicated by the fact that the paths of vessels leading into the nidus are tortuous and may not conform to the standard topology or known anatomical locations. Clipping the wrong vessels may cause the AVM to rupture or cut-off blood flow to other regions of the brain. Therefore, a detailed understanding of the arterial inflow from feeders and venous drainage from drainers is crucial for management of AVMs. In order to aid surgeons to intra-operatively differentiate between feeding and draining vessels we use Chen et al.'s[3] method for vessel labelling based on level-set front propagation. In this method a curve of the level set is evolved based on the intensities in an image. By propagating the level-set front through the vessels in the raw images, we are able to use the algorithm to determine the path of blood flow in the vessels. Vessels are colour coded based on the labels, as arteries (coloured red), veins (coloured blue), or as being within the nidus (coloured purple) as in Fig. 4.

Fog. Depth perception and spatial understanding of angiography data is complex due to the fact that many vessels overlap at different depths and there is a lack of perceptual cues available for scene understanding. Kersten *et al.* [8] found that aerial perspective (implented as fog) was one of the best cues for relative depth perception of vascular volumes for both novices and surgeons. Here, we examine the use of fog in the context of an AR visualization (Fig. 5).

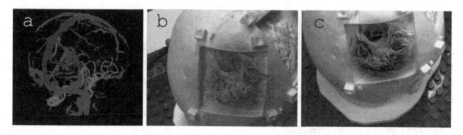

Fig. 4. (a) A colour labelled flow map with feeders (red), drainers (blue) vessels, and nidus (purple). (b) Coloured labelled vessels as virtual object combined with the camera image. (c) AR scene with colour labelled and de-cluttered vascular volume.

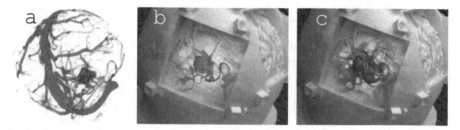

Fig. 5. (a) Volume rendering with fog used as a cue for distance; further vessels exhibit less contrast than those closer to the viewer. (b) Volume rendered vessel AR scene with fog. (c) Volume rendered AR scene with vessels rendered based on flow (red for feeding vessels, blue for draining vessel, and purple for nidus).

3.3   View

The *perception location* of our system is a monitor. As *display*, we use a flat screen digital monitor, allowing for greater control of what type of data is displayed and what processing can be done on both the virtual objects and on the live camera image. Furthermore, by using the display of the navigation system as the perception location we can provide the surgeon not only with information as to what is below the surface but with the context of the information, i.e. how the entire vascular volume relates to the anatomy in the area of resection.

In terms of *interactions*, the user can control the radius of the transparent circle which shows the vessels beyond the visible surface of the cortex. Users can control the location of the center of the circle. Furthermore, the user may interact with the augmented reality visualization by turning on and off the camera image, rotating the scene, and tuning the transfer function of the volume.

4   Results

We presented our system to a number of neurosurgeons and the neuronavigation team at the Montreal Neurological Institute (Canada). The neuronavigation team develop plans and visualizations for image-guided surgery. As well as giving demos of the system to two neurosurgeons specializing in neurovascular surgery, we asked a number of neurosurgeons to fill out an online questionnaire on the perceived usefulness of the different visualization methods in the context of image-guided neurosurgery. They rated the techniques on a Likert scale from 1 to 5 (where 5 was that the method would be very useful and 3 they were unsure of the method's usefulness). We also asked for comments on the different visualization techniques. The questionnaire can be seen online at: http://tinyurl.com/pjmhdq6.

The neuronavigation team evaluated all of the visualizations as beneficial to navigation in comparison to the currently used navigation system (Table 1).

Table 1. Results of the online questionnaire. Experts rated the different visualization techniques on a Likert scale from 1 to 5 (5 very useful, 3 unsure). Coding: DR=Decluttered Red, CR=Cluttered red; DC-C=Decluttered Colour-coded; C-CC=Cluttered Colour-coded; FR=Fog Red; FC-C=Fog Colour-coded; Fav R=Favourite of red images; Fav C-C=Favourite of Colour-coded images.

Occupation	DR	CR	DC-C	C-CC	FR	FC-C	Fav R	Fav C-C
Neuronavigation	3	4	4	4	3	3	DR	CC-C
Neuronavigation	5	5	5	5	5	5	DR	DC-C
Neurosurgeon	2	3	4	4	3	3	FR	C-C
Neurosurgeon	4	2	2	3	3	3	DR	DC-C
Neurosurgeon	4	1	3	3	4	4	DR	DC-C
Neurosurgeon	4	1	4	3	2	3	DR	C-C
Neurosurgeon	4	2	3	4	4	3	DR	DC-C
Average for neurosurgeons	4.2	2	3.6	4	3.6	3.6		

On average, the neurosurgeons found that decluttered red vessels (4.2) and visualizing flow to and from the nidus (4) were most helpful and would be most useful intra-operatively. The colour coding was found useful whether the scene was cluttered or de-cluttered suggesting that for better organized visualizations (i.e. colour coding), more information could be viewed and deciphered by the viewer. Fog (both red and colour coded) and decluttered colour-coding was on average found to be somewhat useful (3.6). In general the ratings varied greatly across the neurosurgeons.

One of the neurosurgeons specializing in neurovascular surgery commented that in the OR surgeons move the surgical microscope around in order to benefit from the motion parallax cue. Therefore, they could imagine moving the camera from our system around to help them visualize the nidus and its relationship with all the vessels. Specifially, the surgeon stated that: "watching the relative movement of the deeper vessels to those located more superficially" would allow them "to best position [themselves] over the surgical corridor leading most directly to the vessel(s) of interest."

5 Conclusions and Future Work

We have presented an AR reality neuronavigation system and explored different volume rendering visualization techniques for vessel identification and localization as well as spatial understanding of vasculature. We found that the results varied greatly between neurosurgeons. This suggests that performance tests on tasks may be better suited and more conclusive for visualization evaluations. Surgeon's individual preferences for different types of visualzations may not correspond to what makes them more efficient or aids them in surgical tasks.

At the same time we received very positive feedback from both neurosurgeons and the neuronavigation team and will be bringing our AR system into the OR in the coming weeks. In particular, we will need to study how the visualization methods work with real images of the cortex.

The next step of this work will involve experiments in the lab and studies in the OR which look at if and when AR visualization is useful for neurovascular surgery. Furthermore, we will also examine the posibility of injecting information from our visualization into the microscope to limit surgical workflow disruptions.

Acknowledgements. The authors would like to thank all of the participants in our study. We would also like to thank Dr. David Sinclair and Kelvin Mok for the vascular data sets, for initial discussions about this work and for providing valuable insights into neurovascular visualization problems.

References

1. Avery, B., Sandor, C., Thomas, B.: Improving Spatial Perception for Augmented Reality X-Ray Vision. In: IEEE Virtual Reality Conference (VR 2009), pp. 79–82 (March 2009)
2. Bichlmeier, C., Ockert, B., Heining, S.M., Ahmadi, A., Navab, N.: Stepping into the operating theater: ARAV – augmented reality aided vertebroplasty. In: ISMAR, pp. 165–166 (2008)
3. Chen, S.J.S., Kersten-Oertel, M., Drouin, S., Collins, D.L.: Visualizing the path of blood flow in static vessel images for image guided surgery of cerebral arteriovenous malformations. In: Proc. of SPIE Medical Imaging: Image-Guided Procedures, Robotic Interventions, and Modeling, 8316308316 (February 2012)
4. Drouin, S., Kersten-Oertel, M., Chen, S.J.-S., Collins, D.L.: A Realistic Test and Development Environment for Mixed Reality in Neurosurgery. In: Linte, C.A., Moore, J.T., Chen, E.C.S., Holmes III, D.R. (eds.) AE-CAI 2011. LNCS, vol. 7264, pp. 13–23. Springer, Heidelberg (2012)
5. Edwards, P., Hawkes, D., Hill, D., Jewell, D., Spink, R., Strong, A., Gleeson, M.: Augmentation of reality using an operating microscope for otolaryngology and neurosurgical guidance. J. Image Guid. Surg. 1, 172–178 (1995)
6. Glossop, N., Wang, Z.: Projection augmented reality system for computer-assisted surgery. In: CARS, vol. 1256, pp. 65–71 (2003)
7. Kersten-Oertel, M., Jannin, P., Collins, D.L.: The state of the art of visualization in mixed reality image guided surgery. Computerized Medical Imaging and Graphics 37(2), 98–112 (2013)

8. Kersten-Oertel, M., Jannin, P., Collins, D.L.: DVV: A Taxonomy for Mixed Reality Visualization in Image Guided Surgery. IEEE Transactions on Visualization and Computer Graphics 18(2), 332–352 (2012)
9. Kersten-Oertel, M., Chen, S.J.S., Collins, D.L.: A Comparison of Depth Enhancing Perceptual Cues for Vessel Visualization in Neurosurgery. CARS 7(1), 166–167 (2012)
10. Konishi, K., Hashizume, M., Nakamoto, M., Kakeji, Y., Yoshino, I., Taketomi, A., Sato, Y., Tamura, S., Maehara, Y.: Augmented reality navigation system for endoscopic surgery based on three-dimensional ultrasound and computed tomography: Application to 20 clinical cases. In: CARS, vol. 1281, pp. 537–542 (2005)
11. Lerotic, M., Chung, A.J., Mylonas, G.P., Yang, G.Z.: pq-space Based Non-Photorealistic Rendering for Augmented Reality. In: Ayache, N., Ourselin, S., Maeder, A. (eds.) MICCAI 2007, Part II. LNCS, vol. 4792, pp. 102–109. Springer, Heidelberg (2007)
12. Mischkowski, R.A., Zinser, M.J., Kübler, A.C., Seifert, U., Zöller, J.: Clinical and experimental evaluation of an augmented reality system in craniomaxillofacial surgery. In: CARS, vol. 1281, pp. 565–570 (2005)
13. Osborn, A.: Diagnostic Cerebral Angiography, 2nd edn. Lippincott Williams & Wilkins (1999)
14. Paul, P., Fleig, O., Jannin, P.: Augmented virtuality based on stereoscopic reconstruction in multimodal image-guided neurosurgery: methods and performance evaluation. IEEE T. Med. Imaging 24(11) (2005)
15. Ropinski, T., Steinicke, F., Hinrichs, K.: Visually supporting depth perception in angiography imaging. In: Butz, A., Fisher, B., Krüger, A., Olivier, P. (eds.) SG 2006. LNCS, vol. 4073, pp. 93–104. Springer, Heidelberg (2006)
16. Scheuering, M., Schenk, A., Schneider, A., Preim, B., Greiner, G.: Intraoperative augmented reality for minimally invasive liver interventions. In: SPIE Med. Imag., vol. 5029, pp. 407–417 (2003)
17. Suzuki, N., Hattori, A., Tanoue, K., Ieiri, S., Konishi, K., Tomikawa, M., Kenmotsu, H., Hashizume, M.: Scorpion shaped endoscopic surgical robot for NOTES and SPS with augmented reality functions. In: Liao, H., Eddie Edwards, P.J., Pan, X., Fan, Y., Yang, G.-Z. (eds.) MIAR 2010. LNCS, vol. 6326, pp. 541–550. Springer, Heidelberg (2010)
18. Wieczorek, M., Aichert, A., Kutter, O., Bichlmeier, C., Heining, R., Euler, E., Navab, N.: GPU-accelerated rendering for medical augmented reality in minimally-invasive procedures. In: BVM (2010)
19. Volonté, F., Pugin, F., Bucher, P., Sugimoto, M., Ratib, O., Morel, P.: Augmented reality and image overlay navigation with osirix in laparoscopic and robotic surgery: not only a matter of fashion. J. Hepatobiliary Pancreat. Sci. 18, 506–509 (2011)
20. Yamaguchi, S., Ohtani, T., Yatani, H., Sohmura, T.: Augmented reality system for dental implant surgery. In: Shumaker, R. (ed.) VMR 2009. LNCS, vol. 5622, pp. 633–638. Springer, Heidelberg (2009)

Reinforcement Learning Based Model Selection and Parameter Estimation for Pharmacokinetic Analysis in Drug Selection

Fei Gao[1], Jingjia Xu[1], Huafeng Liu[2,1], and Pengcheng Shi[1]

[1] Golisano College of Computing and Information Sciences,
Rochester Institute of Technology, Rochester, NY, 14623, USA
[2] State Key Laboratory of Modern Optical Instrumentation, Zhejiang University,
Hangzhou, 310027, China

Abstract. Selecting effective drug candidate is a crucial procedure in drug discovery and development. Dynamic Positron Emission Tomography (dPET) is an ideal imaging tool for pharmacokinetic analysis in drug selection, because it offers possibilities to tract the whole procedure of drug delivery and metabolism when the drug is radio-labeled properly. However, various challenges remain: 1) the kinetic models for drugs are generally very complicated and selecting a proper model is very difficult, 2) solving the kinetic models often needs special mathematical considerations, 3) dPET imaging suffers from poor spatial and temporal resolutions, 4) blood sampling is required in pharmacokinetic analysis, but it is very hard to generate an accurate one. In this paper, we propose a reinforcement learning based model selection and parameter estimation method for pharmacokinetic analysis in drug selection. We first utilize several physical constraints to select the best possible model from a bank of models, and then estimate the kinetic parameters based on the selected model. The method highly improves the accuracy in model selection and can estimate corresponding kinetic parameters even with an inaccurate blood sampling. The quantitative accuracy of our method is tested by experiments using digital phantom and Monte Carlo simulations. Furthermore, 3 cases of patient studies on model selection and parameter estimation are also provided to show the potentials to reduce drug development cycle and save money for the pharmaceutical industry.

1   Introduction

In drug discovery and development, the procedure of drug selection is full of challenging issues. Kelloff et al. show that more than 90% of all new oncology drugs fail in the late stages of development because of inadequate activity and difficulties in determining their efficacy [1]. Quantitative pharmacokinetic analysis with dynamic Position Emission Tomography (dPET) imaging now plays a promising role as determinants of in vivo drug action to help select drug candidate. Fast and accurate pharmacokinetic analysis with rapid information feedback in the

C.A. Linte et al. (Eds.): MIAR/AE-CAI 2013, LNCS 8090, pp. 221–230, 2013.
© Springer-Verlag Berlin Heidelberg 2013

early stage of drug discovery and development is critical to obtain the in vitro and in vivo drug properties[2][3].

dPET is an imaging method to monitor the spatiotemporal distribution of an injected radiotracer and reflect its cellular level changes. This feature makes dPET an excellent tool to facilitate pharmacokinetic analysis by tracking the whole procedure of drug delivery and metabolism[4]. With the dPET acquisition data, compartmental analysis forms the basis for tracer kinetic modeling[5]. A typical procedure of pharmacokinetic analysis by dPET imaging include, firstly, setting up a working hypothesis of the target enzyme or receptor for a particular disease, secondly, establishing suitable models (or surrogate markers) to test biological activities, and at last, screening the new drug molecules for biological activities. In this procedure, model selection by dPET has seldom been studied because of various scientific challenges, for example, 1) the kinetic models for drugs are generally very complicated, when facing a new biomarker (new drug), it is hard to determine which model will work best, 2) accurately solving these complicated models always needs special mathematical considerations, 3) although we can always use more complicated models to represent certain biological activity, the computational cost increase significantly due to the complex of the model, which cause a burden for the early drug discovery. 4) measurement data from dPET suffers from poor spatial and temporal resolutions, especially the first several time frames, 5) blood sampling is required in pharmacokinetic analysis but it is very hard to generate an accurate one[6].

In this paper, we propose a reinforcement learning based method which combines model selection and parameter estimation for pharmacokinetic analysis by dPET. Machine learning in image processing and analysis is growing rapidly[7]. Of various machine learning methods, reinforcement learning is meant to be a general approach to learn from interactions[8]. It is a control method which presents a robust mechanism for goal directed decision making. Unlike supervised learning methods, no examples of desired behavior are provided during training, instead, behavior is guided through positive or negative reinforcements[9]. Therefore, this method do not require a large training dataset, and is especially suitable for preclinical drug selection and pharmacokinetic analysis with only limited data sets[10]. Additionally, as a control mechanism, the method can solve the complicated kinetic models with noisy dPET acquisition data. Furthermore, the method can inherently deal with disturbances during blood sampling.

Most models can be decomposed into a set of compartments, so we first define a model bank which consists of basic compartment models. Then we design the method to be able to first choose the most suitable model from the model bank for the measurement data, and then estimate the kinetic parameters based on the selected models. Since in clinical routines, an accurate blood sampling is very difficult to get, we also test our method with both an accurate input function and an inaccurate one. Quantitative analysis is conducted using digital phantom and Monte Carlo simulations. Furthermore, 3 cases of patient studies are also provided to show the potentials to reduce drug development cycle and save money for the pharmaceutical industry.

2   Method

2.1   Drug Kinetic Models

Drug kinetic models include simple drug transport model, which generally contains equal or less than three compartments and can be solve directly, and complicated biological models, which can contain up to twenty compartments and generally requires prior knowledge to solve[5]. Most complicated models with many compartments can usually be decomposed into a combination of simple models with less than four compartments. In our study, we build a model bank which consist of 6 basic models with less than four compartments. The model bank shown in Fig.1 includes two compartment blood flow model (Model 1), standard two tissue three compartment Phelps 4K model with reversible target tissue (Model 2) and Sokoloff 3K model with irreversible target tissue (Model 3), three tissue five parameter bertoldo model (Model 4), standard three tissue four compartment model (Model 5 and Model 6). More complicated models with more compartments and parallel models with multiple injections can be extended from aforementioned standard models [11][12].

All six models can be represented by a set of differential equations with corresponding kinetic parameters $K = \{k_1, k_2 \cdots k_n\}$, where n is the number of kinetic parameters. Here we utilize Model 2 as an example to demonstrate our method. Model 2 can be represented by first-order differential equations

$$\frac{dC_F(t)}{dt} = k_1(t)C_P(t) + k_4(t)C_B(t) - (k_2(t) + k_3(t))C_F(t) \tag{1}$$

$$\frac{dC_B(t)}{dt} = k_3(t)C_F(t) - k_4(t)C_B(t) \tag{2}$$

The measurement of dPET is the combination of radiotracer in plasma C_P, non-specific binded radiotracer C_F and specific binded radiotracer C_B through

$$C_{PET} = (1 - V_b) \cdot (C_F + C_B) + V_b \cdot C_P \tag{3}$$

$$Y = DC_{PET} + e \tag{4}$$

where V_b is the blood volume fraction, Y is measured projection data , D is the system probability matrix, and e is the noises during acquisition. Eqn.(4) can be represented by a more general time-dependent form for all models as

$$Y(t) = DX(K, t) + e(t) \tag{5}$$

2.2   Temporal-Difference Reinforcement Learning

Temporal Difference reinforcement learning (TD Learning) is a combination of Monte Carlo ideas and dynamic programing[8][9]. Therefore, like Monte Carlo methods, TD Learning can learn from raw experiences without pre-defined models, and like dynamic programing, TD learning can update its estimations based

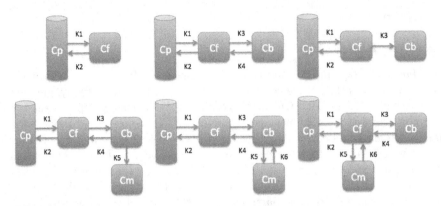

Fig. 1. Compartment models. Model 1-6, from left to right, from top to bottom.

on a part of learning outcomes rather than the final outcome. These features are especially suitable for model selection and noisy dPET data. Regardless of model, when we have an initial K, we define an action set a, which contains $2n$ components, $\{a_1^+, a_1^-, a_2^+, a_2^-, \cdots a_n^+, a_n^-, \}$, the subscript corresponds to the kinetic parameter, the superscript represents increasing (+) or decreasing (-) that kinetic parameter by certain amount during estimation. We derive the TD Learning algorithm for model selection and parameter estimation from the classic one as shown in $Algorithm 1$. Details will be shown in next subsection.

2.3   Model Selection and Parameter Estimation Process

Model Selection. As shown in the algorithm, reinforcement learning acts according to the rewards, we define three rewards based on physical constraints for model selection. The combination of three rewards is able to exclude non-matching models fast, which can improve the computational efficiency, and reduce the disturbances from the noises in low count dPET data. By denoting K' as the estimated kinetic parameters after selecting an action from a,

1. *Reward 1*: We compare the measured total counts in each time frame of measurement data Y and estimated total counts with K'.

$$MSE(TotalCounts(Y(t)), TotalCounts(DX(K',t))) < Threshold1 \quad (6)$$

2. Reward 2: We compare the first order difference of Time Activity Curve (TAC) from measurement data Y and TAC curve estimated with K'.

$$MSE(Difference(TAC(Y)), Difference(TAC(DX(K',t)))) < Threshold2 \quad (7)$$

3. Reward 3: This is an optional reward, if there is priori knowledge from clinical data available, they are learned together through a 2-hidden layer neural network (NN), and then used as a reference for estimated K'.

$$MSE(NN(Y), K') < Threshold3 \quad (8)$$

where MSE is the operation to calculate the mean squared error. When each reward criterion is met, we have a reward $(rew = +1)$, otherwise, $(rew = -1)$. Then we accumulate all rewards by eligible trace Q-Learning [8] as shown in the *Algorithm*1

$$Q(K, a) \leftarrow Q(K, a) + \alpha[rew_{m+1} + \gamma Q(K_{m+1}, a_{m+1}) - Q(K, a)] \qquad (9)$$

where α, γ are learning parameters, which control the width and depth of learning. Proofs in [8] show that α and γ mostly affect the convergence speed, and have only limited effect on learning accuracy after convergency. By setting proper learning parameters, all the states will be traversed through all actions in Monte Carlo/TD learning, the possible solutions are reflected by positive accumulated rewards. After iterations, the action with biggest positive rewards will be the final result. Here we choose both α and γ to be 0.1 as suggested in the book[8]. Q is the value function in the Q-Learning, which stores all the rewards, and m represents iteration steps.

Then the algorithm is applied to every model in the model bank, with each estimated K' from the maximum in Q, we calculate the *Bias* between estimated TAC (TAC_e) and true TAC (TAC_m) from measurement data for each model by $Bias = \frac{1}{T} \sum \frac{\|TAC_m - TAC_e\|}{TAC_m}$, where T is number of time frames. The model with the lowest *Bias* in the model bank will be the selected model by our method.

Parameter Estimation. When using **Algorithm 1** to choose model, simultaneously calculated K' will be the initial parameter for that model. Furthermore, the kinetic parameter can also be calculated with a refined action set a_{ref} containing smaller increasing or decreasing amount using *Algorithm*1.

Algorithm 1. Model Selection and Parameter Estimation by TD Learning

Initialize Q(K,a) arbitrarily
Initialize K
Repeat until convergency
    Randomly choose one action from a
    Repeat for all steps
        Take action a, generate K', observe reward *rew* using defined criteria
        Choose a' from K' derived from Q
        Accumulate all rewards using Eqn. 9
        K ← K'
    End
End
Select the maximum in Q, corresponding K is the estimated K

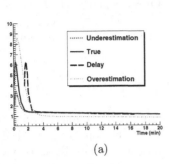
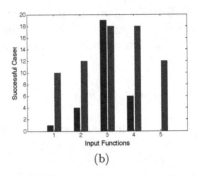

(a)   (b)

Fig. 2. (a) Input functions (b) Success rate of model selection by Fitting method(left & blue) and our method(right & red). Input function 1-5: highly underestimation, disturbed underestimation, perfect input function, disturbed overestimation, highly overestimation.

3   Experiments and Results

3.1   Experiment Settings

In order to evaluate the quantitative accuracy of the proposed method, our first experiment starts with Zubal phantom and Monte Carlo simulations. One slice of the phantom is shown in Fig. 3 (a). The input function used here is Feng input, $C_P^{FDG}(t) = (A_1t - A_2 - A_3)e^{-\lambda_1 t} + A_2e^{-\lambda_2 t} + A_3e^{-\lambda_3 t}$. The base values of the parameters λ_i and A_i selected here are $A_1 = 28\mu Ci/mL/min$, $A_2 = 0.75\mu Ci/mL$, $A_3 = 0.70\mu Ci/mL$, $\lambda_1 = 4.1339min^{-1}$, $\lambda_2 = 0.01043min^{-1}$ and $\lambda_3 = 0.1191min^{-1}$. In our experiments, we test 5 cases of input function, perfect input function, disturbed input function with 20% error (both overestimation and underestimation), and highly overestimated and underestimated input function with 50% error. A demonstration of overestimation, underestimation and delayed injection is shown in Fig. 2 (a). For each input function test, we simulate 4 cases with each model, so there are totally 120 cases for 6 models.

The TAC are calculated based on the dynamic acquisition procedure that consists of 29 frames: 6×5sec, 2×15sec, 6×0.5min, 3×2min, 2×5min and 10×10min. The acquisition data is treated by random correction, normalization, scatter correction, attenuation sequentially. The results are estimated by both weighted Levenberg-Marquardt fitting method and our method for comparison.

3.2   Experiment Results

Currently, there are still no well-accepted methods to perform model selection, researchers either predefine several models and then compare their statistical results from several studies, or generate the model from a large set of clinical experimental studies. All these efforts need relatively a longer study cycle and more funds. The method we are proposing is a feasibility study for fast identifying the models. The accuracy of our method is validated by predefined ground

Table 1. Model selection results. NA is "Not Applicable" (i.e. The model is early excluded by our combined reward defined in Sec 2.3).

	Model1	Model2	Model3	Model4	Model5	Model6
DataSet 1	0.0962	NA	NA	NA	NA	NA
DataSet 2	0.8116	0.1695	NA	0.2721	NA	NA
DataSet 3	0.9250	NA	0.6175	0.7801	0.6828	NA
DataSet 4	0.5177	NA	0.5394	0.1426	NA	NA
DataSet 5	NA	NA	0.6316	0.2546	0.1483	NA
DataSet 6	0.8608	0.4677	NA	0.3530	NA	0.2752

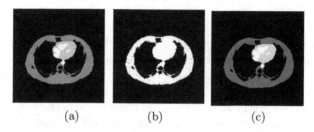

(a)   (b)   (c)

Fig. 3. Parametric image by (a) Ground Truth (b) Fitting (c) Our method

truths from Monte Carlo studies and clinical common understandings. The results are also compared with commonly used model fitting methods in Monte Carlo studies.

Table.1 shows the model selection results of 6 selected cases. Dataset 1-6 are the simulation results based on Model 1-6. Dataset 1-3 are estimated with overestimated input function, while Dataset 4-6 are estimated with underestimated input function. The results show the model selection calculation by our methods. The lowest biases clearly show the selected models in each case. And Fitting method fails in nearly all highly overestimated or underestimated cases. For the total 120 cases, we summarize the model selection results and show them in Fig.2 (b), the results are classified by input function types. The statistical results further shows fitting method will only work when the input function can be well estimated, while our method can still maintain a good selection results with even highly over- or under-estimated input function. That is important since the overestimations and underestimations in input functions are very normal in clinical practices.

As we mentioned in the method section, besides model selection, our method can also estimate the kinetic parameters. Fig.3 shows one example of estimated parametric images, which is based on DataSet 2 in Table.1. 3 Region of Interests (ROIs) are first selected in heart, muscle and body surface, and then the kinetic parameters are estimated by both Fitting method and our reinforcement learning method. The Fitting method reflects the overestimation in the image while

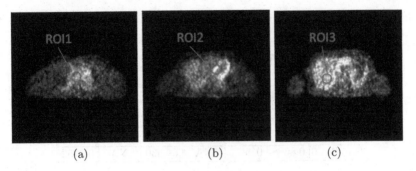

Fig. 4. (a) Case 1 (b) Case 2 (c) Case 3

our method can still reconstruct the correct kinetic parameters. Because of the limitation of pages, we could not cover all the aspects of comparison, however, the results listed above proved the ability of our method to correctly select the model and estimate the kinetic parameters.

Currently, there are still no well-accepted methods to perform model selection, researchers either predefine several models and then compare their statistical results from several studies, or generate the model from a large set of clinical experimental studies. All these efforts need relatively a longer study cycle and more funds. What we are proposing is a feasibility study for fast identifying the models. The accuracy of our method is validated by predefined ground truths from Monte Carlo studies and clinical common understandings.

3.3 Real Patient Experiments

We study three cases of real patient dPET scans. Fig. 4 shows the 3 cases, the first case is the scan of patient thorax, a ROI is defined in the normal muscle region, the second case studies a ROI in the heart region, and the third case is with a ROI in the liver. The dPET scans are performed on our PET scanner, the dynamic data set consists of 40 time frames: 20×0.5min, 15×1min and 5×2min. The input function is estimated by fitting the reconstructed dynamic images. This input function is equal to a disturbed one affected by noises in reconstructed images. The model selection results are shown in Table.2. The results of model selections are consistent with suggestions from clinical studies. ROI 1 is normal tissue and Model 3 is mostly used. ROI 2 is near the left ventricular and highly affected by the blood flow, so the blood flow model (Model 1) is most suitable. For ROI 3, clinical results had shown the necessity and importance of estimation of K4 in liver cancer, and our method correctly choose the right Model 2 (Phelps 4K model). In all 3 studies, the non-applicable models are excluded successfully. The estimated kinetic parameters are shown in Table.3.

Table 2. Model selection results. NA is "Not Applicable".

	Model1	Model2	Model3	Model4	Model5	Model6
Case 1	1.5901	1.4248	1.1735	1.6549	1.5558	NA
Case 2	0.7963	NA	NA	0.9482	NA	NA
Case 3	1.3809	1.0721	1.6025	1.2169	NA	NA

Table 3. Estimated kinetic parameters for 3 cases. NA is "Not Applicable".

	K1	K2	K3	K4	K5	K6
Case 1	0.0960	0.1540	0.0375	NA	NA	NA
Case 2	0.1080	0.0838	NA	NA	NA	NA
Case 3	0.0400	0.0620	0.0145	0.0015	NA	NA

4   Conclusion

We present a reinforcement learning based model selection and parameter estimation method for pharmacokinetic analysis. The method can choose the most suitable model from the model bank for the measurement data, and then estimate the kinetic parameters based on the selected models. Both Monte Carlo simulation and real patient studies show the ability of our method to accurately select the proper model from the model bank and then estimate the kinetic parameters under noisy low-count dPET acquisition data and inaccurate input function.

References

1. Kelloff, G.J., Sigman, C.C.: Cancer Biomarkers: Selecting the Right Drug for the Right Patient. Nature Reviews Drug Discovery 11(3), 201–214 (2012)
2. Willmann, J.K., Van Bruggen, N., Dinkelborg, L.M., Gambhir, S.S.: Molecular Imaging in Drug Development. Nature Reviews Drug Discovery 7(7), 591–607 (2008)
3. Catafau, M., Bullich, S.: Molecular Imaging PET and SPECT Approaches for Improving Productivity of Antipsychotic Drug Discovery and Development. Current Medicinal Chemistry 20(3), 378–388 (2013)
4. Bhattacharyya, S.: Application of Positron Emission Tomography in Drug Development. Biochem. Pharmacol. 1, e128 (2012)
5. Gunn, R.N., Gunn, S.R., Cunningham, V.J.: Positron Emission Tomography Compartmental Models. Journal of Cerebral Blood Flow & Metabolism 21(6), 635–652 (2001)
6. Gunn, R.N., Gunn, S.R., Turkheimer, F.E., Aston, J.A., Cunningham, V.J.: Positron Emission Tomography Compartmental Models: A Basis Pursuit Strategy for Kinetic Modeling. Journal of Cerebral Blood Flow & Metabolism 22(12), 1425–1439 (2002)
7. Wang, S., Summers, R.: Machine Learning and Radiology. Medical Image Analysis 16, 933–951 (2012)

8. Sutton, R.S., Barto, A.G.: Reinforcement Learning: An Introduction, vol. 1. Cambridge Univ. Press (1998)
9. Wiering, M., van Otterlo, M.: Reinforcement Learning: State-of-the-Art, vol. 12. Springer (2012)
10. Strauss, L.G., Pan, L., Cheng, C., Haberkorn, U., Dimitrakopoulou-Strauss, A.: Shortened Acquisition Protocols for the Quantitative Assessment of the 2-Tissue-Compartment Model Using Dynamic PET/CT 18F-FDG Studies. Journal of Nuclear Medicine 52(3), 379–385 (2011)
11. Kelly, C.J., Brady, M.: A Model to Simulate Tumour Oxygenation and Dynamic [18F]-Fmiso PET Data. Physics in Medicine and Biology 51(22), 5859 (2006)
12. Gao, F., Liu, H., Jian, Y., Shi, P.: Dynamic Dual-Tracer PET Reconstruction. In: Prince, J.L., Pham, D.L., Myers, K.J. (eds.) IPMI 2009. LNCS, vol. 5636, pp. 38–49. Springer, Heidelberg (2009)

Delineating 3D Angiogenic Sprouting in OCT Images via Multiple Active Contours

Ting Xu[1], Fengqiang Li[2], Duc-Huy T. Nguyen[3], Christopher S. Chen[3,4], Chao Zhou[2], and Xiaolei Huang[1]

[1] Department of Computer Science and Engineering, Lehigh University, Bethlehem, PA 18015, USA
[2] Department of Electrical and Computer Engineering, Lehigh University, Bethlehem, PA 18015, USA
[3] Department of Chemical and Biomolecular Engineering, University of Pennsylvania, Philadelphia PA 19104, USA
[4] Department of Bioengineering, University of Pennsylvania, Philadelphia PA 19014, USA

Abstract. Recent advances in Optical Coherence Tomography (OCT) has enabled high resolution imaging of three dimensional artificial vascular networks in vitro. Image segmentation can help quantify the morphological and topological properties of these curvilinear networks to facilitate quantitative study of the angiogenic process. Here we present a novel method to delineate the 3D artificial vascular networks imaged by spectral-domain OCT. Our method employs multiple Stretching Open Active Contours (SOACs) that evolve synergistically to retrieve both the morphology and topology of the underlying vascular networks. Quantification of the network properties can then be conducted based on the segmentation result. We demonstrate the potential of the proposed method by segmenting 3D artificial vasculature in simulated and real OCT images. We provide junction locations and vessel lengths as examples for quantifying angiogenic sprouting of 3D artificial vasculature from OCT images.

Keywords: Angiogenesis, Curvilinear Network, Active Contours, Optical Coherence Tomography.

1 Introduction

Angiogenesis, a process where new vessels form from existing vasculature, relies on a series of highly coordinated events. During angiogenic sprouting, some of the most fundamental questions in vascular biology concern how endothelial cells coordinate to build branching tubular networks, which appear to be morphologically different in a tissue-specific manner. The molecular mechanisms to pattern tissue-specific vascular networks remain largely unknown.

Previously, the angiogenic process has been observed, manipulated and studied using confocal microscopy [1]. In this paper, we present an alternative approach in which the 3D angiogenic process is monitored using OCT images.

C.A. Linte et al. (Eds.): MIAR/AE-CAI 2013, LNCS 8090, pp. 231–240, 2013.
© Springer-Verlag Berlin Heidelberg 2013

Optical Coherence Tomography (OCT) is a non-invasive 3D optical imaging modality which provides 3D reconstructional images of biological tissues with micro-scale image resolution [2]. OCT can be used to monitor the angiogenic sprouting morphogenesis with millimeter penetration depth, which is better than that of confocal microscopy. We also show that image analysis of OCT image data can provide quantitative information about the angiogenic system, thus gives insights into how the system works.

Delineating blood vessels is the first step toward quantitative study of the angiogenic process. Quantification of angiogenic vasculature by segmentation methods has been reported using binarization [3] and skeletonization [4] or using explicit models such as generalized cylinder [5] or super-Gaussian functions [6]. Compared to our proposed method, [5] does not provide topological information such as junction locations of the vasculature network. There is a large literature for 3D vessel segmentation in imaging modalities such as MRA or CTA [7]. [8] extracted centerlines of arteries in CTA/MRA by a minimal path method, where user inputs of starting and ending points for the path is required. In contrast, our method can extract the centerlines without the need of manual initialization. We found there has been no work on the segmentation and quantification of 3D angiogenesis from OCT images, which suffer from heavy speckle noise, non-uniform intensities and gaps in the vessels. These present a more challenging case in which some traditional methods like skeletonization followed by binarization do not work well.

In this work we use open parametric active contours or "Snakes" [9], which can explicitly take into account the linear nature of the vessels. As a variant of the original "Snakes", Stretching Open Active Contours (SOACs) [10] are open curves that adapt under the influence of image forces as well as stretching forces exerted at both tips. SOACs have been successfully applied to the segmentation of microtubules [11], tracking of actin filaments [12], and tracing axons [13].

Multiple active contours that elongate and merge with one another have been used to segment networks of actin filaments in 2D TIRFM images [14]. The approach is good for images with high noise. Here we present an extension and significant modification of the multiple SOACs method to address the more challenging issues that arise in 3D OCT and demonstrate its potential by results on both simulated and real OCT images.

2   Methods

Stretching Open Active Contours with an adaptive stretching force (Sect. 2.1) are first initialized automatically by identifying intensity ridge points in 3D (Sect. 2.2). Initial SOACs then evolve sequentially according to a specific set of rules to handle overlap (Sect. 2.3). The result is a network of SOACs. Finally, we locate vessel junctions and extract the optimal vessel network topology by applying smoothness constraints on SOAC segments across junctions (Sect. 2.4).

2.1 SOAC with Adaptive Stretching Force

A SOAC, $r(s), s \in [0, L]$, where s is the arc length parameter and L is its length, is an open-ended parametric active contour with stretching force applied at its two tips (Fig. 1). The image force applied on the curve makes it conform to desired image features when the model elongates. The stretching force is defined as [14]:

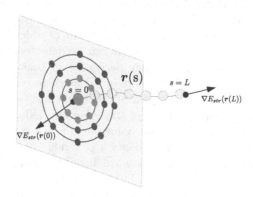

Fig. 1. Illustration of a Stretching Open Active Contour (SOAC) with adaptive stretching forces applied at its two tips. Local foreground and background intensities are estimated by the evenly distributed green and red samples, respectively, on the perpendicular plane of the end tangential.

$$\nabla E_{str}(r(s)) = \begin{cases} -\dfrac{r'(s)}{|r'(s)|} \cdot F(s), & \text{if } s = 0, \\ \dfrac{r'(s)}{|r'(s)|} \cdot F(s), & \text{if } s = L, \\ 0, & \text{if } 0 < s < L \end{cases} \qquad (1)$$

where E_{str} is the stretching energy and $F(s)$ is the magnitude of stretching force determining the elongation of a SOAC.

Unlike previous methods where $F(s)$ are determined globally [10,12,14], we define it here to be proportional to the image contrast local to the SOAC tips:

$$F(s) = \frac{I_f(r(s)) - I_b(r(s))}{I_f(r(s))} = 1 - \frac{I_b(r(s))}{I_f(r(s))}, \qquad s = 0, L \qquad (2)$$

where $I_f(r(s)|_{s=0,L})$ and $I_b(r(s)|_{s=0,L})$ are the local foreground and background intensity at tips, respectively. This definition can avoid under-segmentation of dim vessels and over-segmentation of bright ones in the presence of foreground and background intensity variations.

We found that an effective way to estimate $I_f(r(s)|_{s=0,L})$ and $I_b(r(s)|_{s=0,L})$ is to sample local intensities around the tips and then compute the average of the intensity samples. Specifically, samples are drawn uniformly on concentric circles from the plane $r'(s) \cdot (x - r(s))|_{s=0,L} = 0$, where x is the spatial variable in the image coordinates. The tip itself and those samples that lie on circles of radii less than R_{near} are for local foreground intensity estimation, while samples that lie on circles of radii between R_{near} and R_{far} are for local background intensity estimation (Fig. 1).

2.2   Automatic Initialization of Multiple SOACs

Here we extend the automatic initialization in [14] to 3D. We can initialize SOACs on the centerlines of vessels by locating 3D intensity ridge points. We define a ridge point in axis k to be the image location of which intensity is locally maximum along axis $k, k = 0, 1, 2$. Thus it can be detected by looking for the plus-to-minus sign change in the image derivative in that axis direction [15]. Then we identify candidate SOAC points in 3D as ridge points in at least two axis directions. Specifically, we define a SOAC candidate point *along* x axis as a point that is a ridge point *in* both of the other two axis directions, namely, y and z. Similarly, a SOAC candidate point *along* y is a ridge point in both x and z, and a SOAC candidate point *along* z is a ridge point in both x and y directions. Next, candidate SOAC points are linked to form initial SOACs.

In order to avoid ambiguities when linking SOAC candidate points, we initialize SOACs separately along each axis direction. That is, locally connected candidate points along x are linked to form an initial SOAC along x, and the process is repeated to form SOACs along y and z. The constructed initial SOACs are redundant but they will become a concise representation of the vascular network after their sequential evolution.

2.3   Sequential Evolution of Multiple SOACs

Initialized SOACs will evolve until convergence, one after another, in a sequential manner. We introduce schemes to keep the converged network of SOACs free of overlap.

Detecting general overlap for the current evolving SOAC involves calculating the Euclidean distance from each point of the SOAC to each points of all converged SOACs, and overlaps are all sets of consecutive points of which the distance is less than a threshold d_e. Detecting general overlap after each iteration is too expensive which would dramatically slow down the sequential evolution. If, otherwise, this is done after all the SOACs have converged, then the more redundant initial SOACs are, the more computation have been wasted when SOACs extend onto foregrounds that have already been extracted, leading to many duplicate segmentation.

Here we adopt a balanced strategy. We divide overlaps into *end overlap* and *non-end overlap*. The former, usually caused by SOAC elongation, is the overlap that starts from the end points of the evolving SOAC. Eliminating *end overlap* timely can prevent aforementioned duplicate segmentation. Detecting *end overlap* can be done efficiently because we essentially check from two tips only, and stop at the first non-overlap point. We check this type of overlap after each iteration so that it is nearly a $O(1)$ operation[1]. The latter, *non-end overlap*, is more general than *end overlap* thus more expensive to detect, and is done once after convergence. *Non-end overlap* is usually caused by SOAC body drifting in the presence of weak edges.

2.4 Correcting the Topology of SOAC Network

The network of converged SOACs may not be topologically correct because SOACs evolve one after another, those SOACs that start early have a better chance to extend along multiple branches. When they elongate across intersections of branches, artificial corner may occur.

To retrieve a topologically correct network, we use the fact that the artificial vascular network typically involves straight vessels crossing one another or side branches forming off straight vessels. Using the recorded connectivity information, we first cut the SOACs at each junction into "SOAC segments" so that no SOACs extend across any junctions. Short SOAC segments are discarded. Next we construct an undirected graph $G = (V, E)$, where V is the set of vertices which are end points of SOAC segments. For any two vertices, u, v, we have an edge $(u, v) \in E$ if $\|u - v\|_2 < d_g$, d_g is a distance threshold. Once we have the graph G, we apply connected components analysis in G to detect clusters of vertices, where each cluster represents a junction. More specifically, let one connected component be denoted by C, and $|C|$ be the number of vertices in C, then C is a junction if $|C| > 1$, with $|C|$ being the degree of the junction; otherwise it corresponds to a dangling vessel end.

We define the smoothness between a pair of end points as the angle between the tangential vectors of SOAC segments at the two end points. For each detected junction, we recursively link up the smoothest pair of end points across it, until all pairs are linked or the angle between current smoothest pair does not satisfy a threshold θ. All the SOAC segments that are linked up become part of one longer SOAC.

3 Experimental Results

We validate the proposed method quantitatively using simulated vessel images with ground truth. For real OCT images, we evaluate our results qualitatively because of lack of ground truth. Moreover, the junctions and vessel lengths are presented as examples of quantification based on the segmentation results.

3.1 Validation on Simulated Vascular Images

The goal of testing on simulated 3D vascular network is to quantify the accuracy and robustness of our method. We use one of our segmentation result (a SOAC network) for an OCT image to generate the simulated images. The set of known SOACs serve as the ground truth for validation.

---

[1] The only exception is when the evolving SOAC is totally redundant so the entire sequence of points are checked.

Generation of Simulated Images. We generated simulated images using a real OCT image segmentation result, which serves as the skeleton of the simulated vessels. A clean simulated image was generated by diffusing these skeletons with a Gaussian kernel of $\sigma = 3$ voxels in each direction. Let the real OCT image be $I_{oct}(\boldsymbol{x})$ and its corresponding segmentation result (i.e. the ground truth) be $\boldsymbol{r}_{gt}(s)$. The clean image $I_{clean}(\boldsymbol{x})$ is computed as

$$I_{clean}(\boldsymbol{x}) = [a \cdot (W(\boldsymbol{x}) \cdot I_{oct}(\boldsymbol{x})) + b] * G_{\sigma_f}(\boldsymbol{x}) \tag{3}$$

where $W(\boldsymbol{x})$ is a window function,

$$W(\boldsymbol{x}) = \begin{cases} 1, & \text{if } \boldsymbol{x} \in \boldsymbol{r}_{gt}(s) \\ 0, & \text{otherwise} \end{cases} \tag{4}$$

The scale and shift factor a and b is used for scaling up the intensity and generating a constant background, respectively. The clean image is then corrupted by a multiplicative speckle noise thus the noisy image $I_{noise}(\boldsymbol{x})$ [16]:

$$I_{noise}(\boldsymbol{x}) = I_{clean}(\boldsymbol{x}) \cdot Y \tag{5}$$

where $Y \sim \Gamma(\frac{1}{\sigma_\Gamma^2}, \sigma_\Gamma^2)$ is a random variable of Gamma distribution. Both noisy and clean images are 8-bit. We vary b from 0 to 9 and set $\sigma_\Gamma = 0.5, 1$. This combination gives 20 simulated images of different degradation quantified by the Peak Signal-to-Noise Ratio (PSNR) between I_{noisy} and I_{clean}.

Results and Evaluation. We measure *vertex error* and *Hausdorff distance* between resultant SOACs $\{\boldsymbol{r}_c(s)\}$ and the ground truth $\{\boldsymbol{r}_{gt}(s)\}$. Here we treat all computed SOAC points as one set R_c and all ground truth points as another set R_{gt}. The vertex error is defined similar to "error per face" in [17],

$$d_V(R_c, R_{gt}) = \frac{1}{2|R_c|} \sum_{\boldsymbol{x}_c \in R_c} \min_{\boldsymbol{x}_{gt} \in R_{gt}} \|\boldsymbol{x}_c - \boldsymbol{x}_{gt}\| + \frac{1}{2|R_{gt}|} \sum_{\boldsymbol{x}_{gt} \in R_{gt}} \min_{\boldsymbol{x}_c \in R_c} \|\boldsymbol{x}_{gt} - \boldsymbol{x}_c\| \tag{6}$$

and the Hausdorff distance between R_c and R_{gt} is

$$d_H(R_c, R_{gt}) = \max\{ \max_{\boldsymbol{x}_c \in R_c} \min_{\boldsymbol{x}_{gt} \in R_{gt}} \|\boldsymbol{x}_c - \boldsymbol{x}_{gt}\|, \max_{\boldsymbol{x}_{gt} \in R_{gt}} \min_{\boldsymbol{x}_c \in R_c} \|\boldsymbol{x}_{gt} - \boldsymbol{x}_c\|\} \tag{7}$$

An example segmentation result for one of the simulated images is shown in Fig. 2. The d_V-PSNR and d_H-PSNR curves for these 20 simulated images are plotted in Fig. 3, which shows the segmentation error (in terms of vertex error and Hausdorff distances) is very low on simulated images with PSNR greater than 25dB. Comparing the three results in Fig. 4 shows that the number of false positives drastically decreases as PSNR increases. Common SOAC parameters [14] used for both simulated and experimental images are set as follows: viscosity coefficient $\gamma = 2$ for controlling the step size for SOAC evolution; first order continuity weight $\alpha = 0.01$ for controlling SOAC's tension; second order continuity weight $\beta = 0.01$ for controlling SOAC's rigidity; image force weight $k_{img} = 1$; stretching force weight $k_{str} = 0.01$. The junction smoothness threshold $\theta = 2\pi/3$.

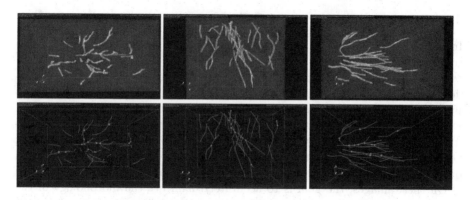

Fig. 2. Three orthogonal views of a simulated image (upper row) and its segmentation result shown in same view (lower row). Note SOACs (Magenta) are shown with the detected junction points (Green).

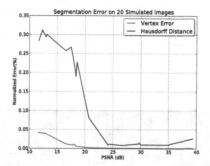

Fig. 3. d_V-PSNR and d_H-PSNR curve. The error is in fraction of the length of the diagonal of the image volume.

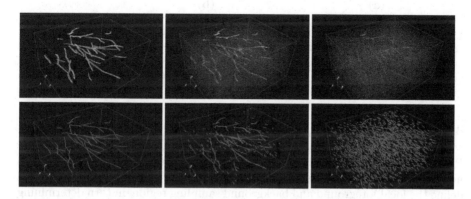

Fig. 4. Comparison of results on images with different PSNR values. First column: PSNR = 26.6dB (image same as in Fig. 2). Second column: PSNR = 16.5dB. Third column: PSNR = 12.3dB. Note the different number of false positives introduced.

3.2 Results on Experimental OCT Images

In our experiment, we tested our algorithm on images acquired using a custom spectral-domain OCT system. The system was developed using a supercontinuum light source, which enabled $1.5\mu m$ axial resolution in tissue. A 175-degree conical lens [18,19] was used in combination with a 10× objective to provide an extended depth-of-field of $200\mu m$ and a traverse resolution of $2.3\mu m$. Data acquisition was performed at 20,000 A-scans/s with over 100 dB sensitivity. 3D OCM images were acquired on the artificial blood vessel device [1] with voxel size $1.0 \times 1.0 \times 1.0\mu m$. Because we do not have ground truth, we perform qualitative evaluation for results on experimental images.

On these images, the goal is to accurately delineate the morphology of the vascular network and identify vessel junction points. Figure 5 shows one result of applying our method. The output includes multiple SOACs, each representing an individual vessel in the vascular network. The length of each SOAC is used to estimate the length of the vessel. For each SOAC, we have densely sampled points on the curve as well as image intensity along the curve. From these we can compute distributions of orientation, curvature, and intensity along the vessels. Besides the geometry and intensity information, we also have the junction locations identified (green spheres) and the connectivity information among vessels.

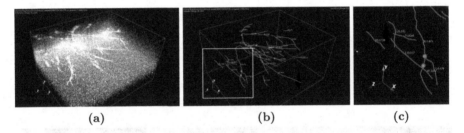

(a)   (b)   (c)

Fig. 5. Example segmentation results on an experimental OCT image. Image size is $480 \times 300 \times 600$. (a) an OCT image of artificial vascular network; (b) Resultant SOACs and junction points (green spheres); (c) a zoomed-in view of a portion of the extracted network (the area enclosed by the white square in (b)). Estimated vessel lengths (Unit: μm) are displayed as text labels.

4 Discussion and Conclusion

Parameter tuning is often needed when different kinds of experimental images need to be analyzed. One useful parameter is the pair of R_{near} and R_{far}, which define the local foreground and background sampling region, in turn determining how much a SOAC is stretched. R_{near} and R_{far} needs to be set according to the vessel scale.

In summary, we proposed a novel method for analyzing OCT images of the angiogenic process. The method is based on a network of SOACs, where we introduce new initialization method in 3D, regularization for sequential evolution, and topology correction for the converged SOAC network. With the ability to obtain morphological and topological quantification of in vitro vessels, this algorithm together with molecular perturbations will provide insights into the molecular mechanisms that regulate vascular patterning both in developmental and pathological vasculature. In our future work we will include optimization of parameters and estimation of vessel radius in the framework.

Acknowledgments. This work is supported by NIH grant R01GM098430 and R00-EB010071 and Lehigh Start-Up Fund.

References

1. Nguyen, D.H.T., Stapleton, S.C., Yang, M.T., Cha, S.S., Choi, C.K., Galie, P.A., Chen, C.S.: Biomimetic model to reconstitute angiogenic sprouting morphogenesis in vitro. Proceedings of the National Academy of Sciences 110(17), 6712–6717 (2013)
2. Huang, D., Swanson, E., Lin, C., Schuman, J., Stinson, W., Chang, W., Hee, M., Flotte, T., Gregory, K., Puliafito, C., et al.: Optical coherence tomography. Science 254(5035), 1178–1181 (1991)
3. Blacher, S., Devy, L., Burbridge, M., Roland, G., Tucker, G., Noël, A., Foidart, J.M.: Improved quantification of angiogenesis in the rat aortic ring assay. Angiogenesis 4(2), 133–142 (2001)
4. Niemisto, A., Dunmire, V., Yli-Harja, O., Zhang, W., Shmulevich, I.: Robust quantification of in vitro angiogenesis through image analysis. IEEE Transactions on Medical Imaging 24(4), 549–553 (2005)
5. Abdul-Karim, M.A., Al-Kofahi, K., Brown, E.B., Jain, R.K., Roysam, B.: Automated tracing and change analysis of angiogenic vasculature from in vivo multiphoton confocal image time series. Microvascular Research 66(2), 113–125 (2003)
6. Tyrrell, J.A., Mahadevan, V., Tong, R.T., Brown, E.B., Jain, R.K., Roysam, B.: A 2-d/3-d model-based method to quantify the complexity of microvasculature imaged by in vivo multiphoton microscopy. Microvascular Research 70(3), 165–178 (2005)
7. Lesage, D., Angelini, E.D., Bloch, I., Funka-Lea, G.: A review of 3d vessel lumen segmentation techniques: Models, features and extraction schemes. Medical Image Analysis 13(6), 819–845 (2009)
8. Çetingül, H.E., Gülsün, M.A., Tek, H.: A unified minimal path tracking and topology characterization approach for vascular analysis. In: Liao, H., Eddie Edwards, P.J., Pan, X., Fan, Y., Yang, G.-Z. (eds.) MIAR 2010. LNCS, vol. 6326, pp. 11–20. Springer, Heidelberg (2010)
9. Kass, M., Witkin, A., Terzopoulos, D.: Snakes: Active contour models. International Journal of Computer Vision 1, 321–331 (1988)
10. Li, H., Shen, T., Smith, M., Fujiwara, I., Vavylonis, D., Huang, X.: Automated actin filament segmentation, tracking and tip elongation measurements based on open active contour models. In: IEEE International Symposium on Biomedical Imaging: From Nano to Macro, ISBI 2009, June 28-July 1 2009, pp. 1302–1305 (2009)

11. Nurgaliev, D., Gatanov, T., Needleman, D.J.: Chapter 25 - automated identification of microtubules in cellular electron tomography. In: Cassimeris, L., Tran, P. (eds.) Microtubules: in Vivo. Methods in Cell Biology, vol. 97, pp. 475–495. Academic Press (2010)

12. Smith, M.B., Li, H., Shen, T., Huang, X., Yusuf, E., Vavylonis, D.: Segmentation and tracking of cytoskeletal filaments using open active contours. Cytoskeleton 67(11), 693–705 (2010)

13. Wang, Y., Narayanaswamy, A., Tsai, C.L., Roysam, B.: A broadly applicable 3-D neuron tracing method based on open-curve snake. Neuroinformatics 9, 193–217 (2011)

14. Xu, T., Li, H., Shen, T., Ojkic, N., Vavylonis, D., Huang, X.: Extraction and analysis of actin networks based on open active contour models. In: 2011 IEEE International Symposium on Biomedical Imaging: From Nano to Macro, March 30-April 2, pp. 1334–1340 (2011)

15. Chang, S., Kulikowski, C., Dunn, S., Levy, S.: Biomedical image skeletonization: A novel method applied to fibrin network structures. Studies in Health technology and Informatics 84(2), 901–905 (2001)

16. Lehmann, G.: Noise simulation. The Insight Journal (July 2010)

17. Narayanaswamy, A., Dwarakapuram, S., Bjornsson, C., Cutler, B., Shain, W., Roysam, B.: Robust adaptive 3-D segmentation of vessel laminae from fluorescence confocal microscope images and parallel GPU implementation. IEEE Transactions on Medical Imaging 29(3), 583–597 (2010)

18. Leitgeb, R.A., Villiger, M., Bachmann, A.H., Steinmann, L., Lasser, T.: Extended focus depth for fourier domain optical coherence microscopy. Optics Letters 31(16), 2450–2452 (2006)

19. Bolmont, T., Bouwens, A., Pache, C., Dimitrov, M., Berclaz, C., Villiger, M., Wegenast-Braun, B.M., Lasser, T., Fraering, P.C.: Label-free imaging of cerebral-amyloidosis with extended-focus optical coherence microscopy. The Journal of Neuroscience 32(42), 14548–14556 (2012)

The Role of Augmented Reality in Training the Planning of Brain Tumor Resection

Kamyar Abhari, John S.H. Baxter, Elvis S. Chen, Ali R. Khan, Chris Wedlake, Terry Peters, Roy Eagleson, and Sandrine de Ribaupierre

Robarts Research Institute
Western University, London, ON, Canada

Abstract. The environment in which a surgeons is trained profoundly effects their preferred method for visualizing patient images. While classical 2D viewing might be preferred by some older experts, the new generation of residents and novices has been raised navigating in 3D through video games, and are accustomed to seeing 3D reconstructions of the human anatomy. In this study, we evaluate the performance of different groups of users in 4 different visualization modalities (2D planes, orthogonal planes, 3D reconstruction and augmented reality). We hypothesize that this system will facilitate the spatio-visual abilities of individuals in terms of assessing patient-specific data, an essential requirement of many neurosurgical applications such as tumour resection. We also hypothesize that the difference between AR and the other modalities will be greater in the novice group. Our preliminary results indicate that AR is better or as good as other modalities in terms of performance.

Keywords: Augmented Reality, Neurosurgical Training, Tumour Resection, Surgical planning.

1 Introduction and Clinical Motivation

Brain cancer is among the least survivable types of cancers with a five-year relative survival rate of 35% [1]. It is estimated that 2,800 Canadians and 23,000 Americans were diagnosed with primary brain tumours in 2012, resulting in 1,800 and 13,700 deaths respectively [2][1]. Compared to alternative courses of treatments, surgical resection of a tumour is the most recommended option [3]. Pre-operative planning of tumour resection interventions involves identifying optimal surgical pathways and specifying surgical entry points based on a number of criteria, geared towards minimizing post-surgery complications. Surgeons often make use of multiple views of the brain to plan brain tumour resection. Older surgeons are often trained with axial planes only (CT-scan and later MRI), whereas the younger generation of experts are trained with tri-planar views of axial, sagittal, and coronal images sampled from 3D MRI datasets. However, with advancements in technology, medical students and residents are now accustomed to 3D reconstructed structures. Furthermore, they are able to interact with these 3D neuroanatomical structures in a Virtual Reality (VR) environment using the

C.A. Linte et al. (Eds.): MIAR/AE-CAI 2013, LNCS 8090, pp. 241–248, 2013.
© Springer-Verlag Berlin Heidelberg 2013

same skills employed when playing 3D video games. For a surgeon to be able to determine a desirable surgical approach for a procedure, visualizing the location of the lesion is essential. Classically, they form a mental image of the lesion within the skull from the 2D MRI images using their anatomical knowledge and spatial reasoning abilities. There are a number of factors to take into account in determining an optimal path for the brain tumour resection, one being the distance between the entry point on the skull and the tumour. Minimizing this distance would minimize the surgical path and as a result, the amount of tissue cut during the procedure. Another consideration, however, is to estimate the longest axis of the tumor - since if the tumour is retracted along this axis, there will be minimal disruption to tissues adjacent to the tool. Another consideration which is often the most important is the location of major pathways and eloquent areas that control functions such as speech, motion, vision, etc. Disruption to these areas during surgery can lead to postoperative deficits in the patient. Most surgical institutions in developed countries possess neuronavigational systems, which enables surgeons to load the images, reconstruct them in 3D, choose their trajectory, and confirm that their approach does not interact with major vessels, eloquent areas or take an unfeasibly deep path. Unfortunately, many developing countries do not have access to this expensive technology. In addition, this system does not account for brain shift, and is prone to technical and user errors. It is therefore essential for a trainee to be able to identify the ideal surgical approach for a tumor using anatomical landmarks. Augmented Reality (AR) enables the overlay of virtual information onto an image of the patient's body in the OR. This can help with surgical planning, and can also serve as a training tool. In our case, we have developed a system to assist junior trainees to identify the locations of eloquent areas, white matter tracts, and the tumour in the brain. AR thereby provides intuitive visualization of the brain and facilitates trainee interaction with the different structures. Although, many AR systems have been developed for neurosurgical applications [4]-[9], only few studies have been conducted to evaluate the usability and efficacy of such systems compared to other modalities. In this paper, we evaluate an AR-based surgical training platform to determine how a user performs as the function of visualization mode. Our main hypothesis is that the benefit of AR would improve the performance of all users during the task of determining the optimal surgical approach.

2   Materials and Methods

2.1   Material

A previously developed surgical training AR system was extended for the purpose of these experiments. Our AR system was based on off-the-shelf AR eyewear (Vuzix 920AR) with twin displays/cameras, as well as a head phantom and a stylus. The Vuzix eyewear as well as the head phantom and the stylus were tracked with an optical tracking system (Polaris, NDI, Canada). To control the experimental variables such as the location and orientation of the longest axis of the tumor, and its proximity to eloquent areas, 28 segmented tumor samples

(DTI challenge workshop, MICCAI, 2010-11) were placed in different regions of the brain by an expert to create realistic and clinically relevant scenarios. In addition to the tumors, we also incorporated functional areas (extracted from functional MRI datasets) of the motor cortex representing the peripheral limbs, as well as the visual cortex, the language areas, and the hippocampus (short term memory). Tractography of major fasciculi (white matter tracts of neurons in the brain, connecting two functional areas) were also incorporated within the volume: uncinate fasciculus (connecting the orbitofrontal cortex to the temporal lobe and limbic system - associated with emotion regulation, cognition, declarative memory and face recognition/memory and its lesion associated with different psychiatric disorders), Meyer's loop (prolongation of the optic tracts essential for vision), arcuate fasciculus (connecting the Wernicke and Broca language areas) as well as the corticospinal tracts (descending fibers from the motor areas to the spinal cord enabling movements in the face, trunk and limbs). A total of 112 different scenarios were created and displayed randomly to the subjects. In order to operationalize a comparison between different visualization modes, images containing the MRI of the brain (anatomical T1 image), segmented tumour, eloquent areas, and white matter tract were displayed in 2D (axial, coronal and sagittal planes - Fig. 1-a), orthogonal planes (XP - Fig. 1-b), 3D (Fig. 1-c) and AR (Fig. 1-d).

2.2   Participants

3 expert neurosurgeons with >5 years of practice, 4 intermediate (residents and fellow) with >2 years of training and 4 novices (graduate students) with no neurosurgical experience participated in this study.

2.3   Methodology

Participants were asked to identify the longest axis of the tumour as well as the shortest path from the surface of the cortex to the tumour. For the longest axis task (LA), subjects were asked to align the stylus with the longest axis of the tumour. For the shortest distance task (SD), they were asked to place the tip of the stylus on the appropriate location on the head phantom. Each experiment involved 64 trials [1] (32 trials per task) in which the patient MR volume randomly selected from the database and displayed in the 4 different modalities described earlier. The display of these modalities - as well as the task performed- was counterbalanced between and within subjects to correct for the effect of training and fatigue (e.g. Fig. 2). The response time (RT), the location of the stylus (in SD), and orientation (in LA) were recorded for every trial. The RT was the time elapsed between the time at which subjects start scrolling through the images and the time at which subject indicated their desired point/angle.

---

[1] 48 trials for one of our experts.

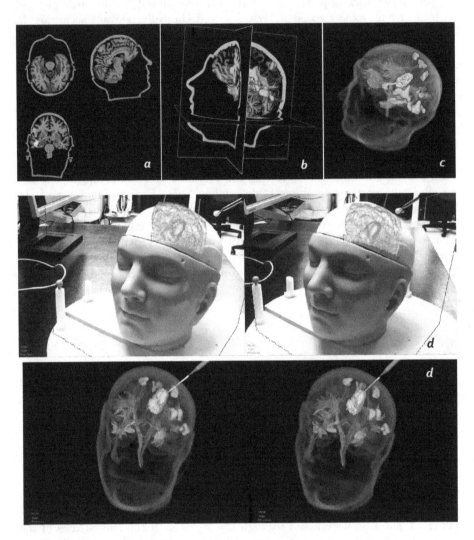

Fig. 1. Different Visualization Modalities: a) 2D, b) XP, c) 3D, and d) AR

3D → XP → AR → 2D → 2D → AR → XP → 3D

Fig. 2. An example illustrating the order of modalities visualization

2.4   Analysis

The recorded location/orientation of the stylus was compared to the longest axis of the segmented tumour determined using geometrical Principal Components Analysis (i.e. the primary eigenvector). For the shortest distance, the gold standard was computed by finding the shortest possible distance from the surface of the tumour to the surface of the cortex (Inaccessible points of entry such as face, ears, and neck were excluded in this process) The index of performance was calculated in accordance with Fitts' methodology, respecting the tradeoff between speed and accuracy [10]. The index of performance is the product of their speed (the reciprocal of time, i.e. $\frac{1}{RT}$) multiplied by the Index of Difficulty of the task (i.e. the logarithm of the probability that they could perform the task by luck). In other words, the Index of Performance (Ip) can be determined using the following formulas:

$$I_p|LA = \frac{1}{RT} \log_2 \frac{\mu_R}{R_{error}}, R_{error} = \text{Rotational Error}$$

$$I_p|SD = \frac{1}{RT} \log_2 \frac{\mu_T}{T_{error}}, T_{error} = \text{Translational Error}$$

Note that in above formula μ_R is the mean error angle if chosen randomly and is equal to 57° (1 radian). On the other hand, μ_T is computed for each individual case using a Monto-Carlo simulation. This is done by distributing random points on the surface of the skull and finding the mean shortest distance to the tumour.

3   Results and Discussion

3.1   Longest Axis

The I_p for the LA task is depicted in Fig. 3. By looking at the I_p, it becomes apparent that in all modalities but AR, experts outperform both trainees and novices, particularly in 2D. In case of AR, however, novices performed as accurate as experts but with higher variation. A multivariate ANOVA test indicated that only the mode of visualization was significant ($p=0.02$ <0.05) but not the expertise. No significant interaction effect between visualization method and expertise was observed. Post-hoc analysis using the Tukey test revealed that subjects' level of performance (i.e. I_p) was significantly higher in AR compared to 2D and XP ($\mu_{AR}=.093$, $\mu_{3D}=.066$, $\mu_{2D}=.045$, $\mu_{XP}=.035$).

3.2   Shortest Distance

The I_p for the SD task is illustrated in Fig. 4. Similar to LA, the index of performance for experts was higher than both intermediate residents and novices (in case of 2D, intermediate performed equally well but significantly better than novices). A multivariate ANOVA test indicated that both the mode of visualization and expertise were significant (Mode: $p=0.001$ <0.05, Expertise: $p=0.005$

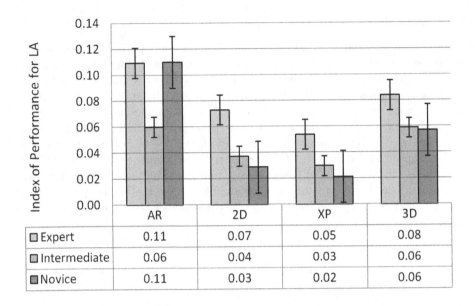

Fig. 3. Index of Performance for the task of longest axis

<0.05). No significant interaction effect between visualization method and expertise was observed. Post-hoc analysis using Tukey test showed that a) experts were significantly better than novices, and b) subjects' level of performance (i.e. Ip) was significantly higher in AR and 3D compared to XP ($\mu_{AR}=.085$, $\mu_{3D}=.073$, $\mu_{2D}=.055$, $\mu_{XP}=.040$).

4   Conclusion

Perceiving the spatial relationships between relevant structures such as tumours and eloquent areas is necessary for successful neurosurgical pre-operative planning. The usability of such percepts is heavily influenced by the mode of visualization and interaction within the neurosurgical planning environment. Most experts (>5 years of experience) were trained at a time when 3D reconstructions of brain images were scarce and therefore accustomed to interpreting 2D images. CT imaging was classically presented as axial slices, while MRI images as orthogonal slices (axial, coronal, and sagittal canonical views). Experts are able to interpret 3D structures, identify anatomical landmarks in order to plan for the approach, and measure those landmarks on the skin before starting surgery after viewing only 2D images. The new generation of trainees, however, who started their residency training in neurosurgery over the past 6 years, has been trained using 3D models of the brain. They also have been trained to use neuronavigation systems for most neurosurgical procedures. Therefore, while they are still used to looking at 2D images to prepare their approaches, they tend to

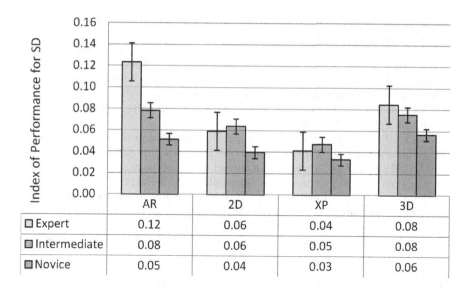

	AR	2D	XP	3D
□ Expert	0.12	0.06	0.04	0.08
▨ Intermediate	0.08	0.06	0.05	0.08
▨ Novice	0.05	0.04	0.03	0.06

Fig. 4. of Performance for the task of shortest distance

rely more on new technology to help them in their planning. In any case, our preliminary results show that all subjects with a neurosurgery background performed better than novices in all visualization modalities to identify the shortest distance and longest axis [2]. Nevertheless, AR was shown to be superior to other modalities (or equally good) in terms of performance. XP, on the other hand, was significantly slower for everyone, and most subjects reported anecdotally that they did not feel comfortable working in that modality. In addition, experts were impressed by the functionality of the AR. Future studies need to include more expert neurosurgeons and intermediate subjects. In addition, our novices comprised of graduate students who have participated in our previous studies and are used to working with MRI images. Thus, a new group of novices will be recruited to act as nave subjects.

Acknowledgments.

References

1. American Cancer Society: Cancer Facts and Figures. American Cancer Society, Atlanta (2012) (available online. last accessed December 12, 2012)
2. Canadian Cancer Statistics, produced by Canadian Cancer Society, Statistics Canada, Provincial/Territorial Cancer Registries, Public Health Agency of Canada (2012) (available online. last accessed December 12, 2012)

---

[2] with the exception of AR for identifying the longest axis where novices performed better than intermediate subjects.

3. National Cancer Institute (NCI) booklet (NIH Publication No. 09-1558) (available online. posted April 29, 2009)
4. Azimi, E., Doswell, J., Kazanzides, P.: Augmented reality goggles with an integrated tracking system for navigation in neurosurgery (2012)
5. Drouin, S., Kersten-Oertel, M., Chen, S.J.-S., Collins, D.L.: A realistic test and development environment for mixed reality in neurosurgery. In: Linte, C.A., Moore, J.T., Chen, E.C.S., Holmes III, D.R. (eds.) AE-CAI 2011. LNCS, vol. 7264, pp. 13–23. Springer, Heidelberg (2012)
6. Mahvash, M., Besharati Tabrizi, L.: A novel augmented reality system of image projection for image-guided neurosurgery. Acta Neurochirurgica, 1–5 (2013)
7. Mitha, A.P., et al.: Simulation and augmented reality in endovascular neurosurgery: Lessons from aviation. Neurosurgery 72(suppl. 1), A107–A114 (2013)
8. Yudkowsky, R., et al.: Practice on an augmented reality/haptic simulator and library of virtual brains improves residents' ability to perform a ventriculostomy. Simulation in Healthcare 8(1), 25–31 (2013)
9. Shamir, R.R., et al.: Trajectory planning with Augmented Reality for improved risk assessment in image-guided keyhole neurosurgery (2011)
10. Fitts, P.M.: The information capacity of the human motor system in controlling the amplitude of movement. J. Exp. Psychol. 47(6), 381–391 (1954)

Matching Functional Connectivity Patterns for Spatial Correspondence Detection in fMRI Registration

Zhenyu Tang[1,2], Di Jiang[1,2,3], Hongming Li[1,2], and Yong Fan[1,2,*]

[1] Brainnetome Center, Institute of Automation, Chinese Academy of Sciences,
Beijing 100190, China
[2] National Laboratory of Pattern Recognition, Institute of Automation,
Chinese Academy of Sciences, Beijing 100190, China
[3] Department of Mathematics, Zhejiang University, Hangzhou 310027, China
yfan@nlpr.ia.ac.cn, yong.fan@ieee.org

Abstract. A novel method is proposed to match functional connectivity patterns represented by graphs for spatial registration of fMRI data. Different from existing functional connectivity pattern based registration methods that detect corresponding functional units across different subjects by minimizing their difference in functional connectivity strength, our method adopts a graph representation to characterize functional connectivity information among all voxels in fMRI data of each subject, then detects spatial correspondence between subjects using graph matching. To integrate information of both functional connectivity strength and spatial relations, the graph representation of functional connectivity information of fMRI data models each voxel as one graph node and connects each pair of graph nodes with an edge weighted by their functional connectivity strength measure, estimated as correlation coefficient between their functional signals. To make the graph matching computationally feasible, an iterative matching strategy with stochastic resampling is proposed to match graphs of spatially distributed local functional connectivity patterns and subsequently to drive the image registration iteratively. The proposed method has been validated by registering resting state fMRI data of 20 healthy subjects. The validation experiment results have demonstrated that our method can achieve improved inter-subject functional consistency. A comparison experiment result has further indicated that the proposed method can achieve better performance than existing methods.

Keywords: fMRI registration, graph matching, functional connectivity pattern.

1 Introduction

Functional Magnetic Resonance Imaging (fMRI) has been widely utilized in studies of neuroscience and neuropsychiatric disorders for investigating the brain's function

---

* Corresponding author.

C.A. Linte et al. (Eds.): MIAR/AE-CAI 2013, LNCS 8090, pp. 249–257, 2013.
© Springer-Verlag Berlin Heidelberg 2013

architecture and function alternations due to diseases in vivo. To facilitate voxel-wise statistical analysis of fMRI data from multiple subjects, spatial alignment of fMRI data from different subjects is required as a preprocessing step. The spatial alignment of fMRI data is typically achieved by registering their corresponding Structural MRI (sMRI) data and using resulting mapping fields to align the fMRI data. However, brain functional units are not necessarily aligned with the brain anatomical structure consistently across different subjects due to inter-subject functional variability [1].

Recently, several methods have been proposed for fMRI data registration based on the fMRI data themselves [2-4]. A method proposed in [2] directly used the functional signal at each voxel as features to detect corresponding functional units by maximizing correlation coefficient of inter-subject functional signals in fMRI data for achieving inter-subject cortical surface registration. However, such a method can only be used for task-oriented fMRI data, not suitable for registering resting-state fMRI data due to that resting state functional signals across different subjects are not always synchronic. Several studies have proposed to detect corresponding functional units across different subjects by maximizing similarity of functional connectivity patterns for spatial alignment of fMRI data. In [3], the spatial alignment of inter-subject cortical surfaces was achieved by maximizing similarity of correlation matrices of functional signals of the whole cortical surfaces, each encoding one subject's whole brain functional connectivity pattern. A spectral embedding method was used in [4] to extract features from the whole brain correlation matrix of functional signals and the extracted features of different subjects were matched using a point set registration algorithm to compute mapping field. However, the features of different subjects extracted using the spectral embedding are not directly comparable, and ad hoc techniques had to be adopted to make the features invariant to rotation, order and sign of individual coordinate axes [4]. In [5, 6] local functional connectivity pattern was defined for each voxel and estimated as a probability distribution of correlation coefficients between functional signals of voxels within a local region of the voxel considered. All the available functional connectivity pattern based registration methods do not explicitly take into consideration the spatial relationship of functional connectivity information among different functional units.

To integrate information of both functional connectivity strength and spatial relations, we propose to detect corresponding functional units by matching graph based functional connectivity patterns for fMRI data registration. In particular, each fMRI data is presented by a graph that encodes the whole brain functional connectivity information, containing both connectivity strength and spatial relationship in the fMRI data. In such a graph, voxels are regarded as graph nodes that are connected with edges weighted by functional connectivity measures between the connected graph nodes. The spatial correspondence detection between the two fMRI data of different subjects is then solved by graph matching [7, 8]. Both synthetic fMRI data and resting-state fMRI data of 20 subjects were used to evaluate our method and evaluation results demonstrated that our method can improve the inter-subject functional consistency.

2   Methods

2.1   Graph Representation of Functional Connectivity Pattern

Given a subject's fMRI data, its whole brain functional connectivity information is characterized by a graph $G = (V, E)$, where V is a set of graph nodes modeling all gray matter voxels $(v_1, ..., v_n)$, and $E = \{e_{x,y} | x, y = (1, ..., n)\}$ is a set of graph edges that connect all possible pairs of nodes. Each graph edge $e_{x,y}$ is weighted by functional connectivity strength, estimated as the Pearson Correlation Coefficient (PCC) between functional signals at two nodes connected by the edge. Since the symmetric property of the PCC, the graph is undirected.

2.2   Correspondence Detection by Graph Matching with Topological Constraint

Given two graphs $G_1(V_1, E_1)$ with m nodes and $G_2(V_2, E_2)$ with n nodes, the objective of graph matching is to determine correspondence of nodes as well as edges of the two graphs, i.e., finding an assignment matrix $\boldsymbol{S} \in \{0,1\}^{m \times n}$, in which $\boldsymbol{S}_{i,j} = 1$ if node v_i in G_1 corresponds to node v_j in G_2, under the one-to-one constraint: $\sum_{j=1}^{n} \boldsymbol{S}_{i,j} \leq 1$ $(i = 1, ..., m)$ and $\sum_{i=1}^{m} \boldsymbol{S}_{i,j} \leq 1$ $(j = 1, ..., n)$. The graph matching problem can be formulated as

$$s = \arg\max(s^T \boldsymbol{W} s),$$
$$s.t. \ s \in \{0,1\}^{mn}, \ \sum_{j=1}^{n} S_{(i-1) \times n + j} \leq 1, (i = 1, ..., m) \quad , \quad \sum_{i=1}^{m} S_{(i-1) \times n + j} \leq 1, (j = \quad (1)$$
$$1, \quad n)$$

where s is a column vector obtained by concatenating each row of $\boldsymbol{S}$, and $\boldsymbol{W}$ is an $mn \times mn$ affinity matrix. In particular, diagonal and non-diagonal elements of $\boldsymbol{W}$ describe node-to-node correspondence and edge-to-edge correspondence between two graphs, respectively. Since the functional signals in resting state fMRI data of different subjects are typically not synchronous, especially for resting state fMRI data, the graph matching of functional connectivity patterns can only rely on the edge-to-edge correspondence. Therefore $\boldsymbol{W}_{i,i} = 0, i = 1, ..., mn$ and the edge-to-edge affinity is computed as

$$\boldsymbol{W}_{i,j} = exp\left(-\left(\alpha|e_{a,b}^1 - e_{c,d}^2| + \beta\frac{|\|\vec{ab}\| - \|\vec{cd}\||}{\|\vec{ab}\| + \|\vec{cd}\|}\right)\right), \quad (2)$$
$$a = \lfloor i/n \rfloor, b = \lfloor j/n \rfloor, c = i \bmod n, d = j \bmod n,$$

where $e_{a,b}^1$ and $e_{c,d}^2$ are edge weights calculated by the Pearson Correlation Coefficient (PCC) between functional signals at two nodes connected by the edge in G_1 (nodes v_a and v_b, $a, b = 1, ..., m, a \neq b$) and G_2 (nodes v_c and v_d, c, $d = 1, ..., n, c \neq d$) respectively. $\|\vec{ab}\|$ and $\|\vec{cd}\|$ are lengths (in pixel) of the edges from node v_a to v_b and from v_c to v_d respectively. The operator $\lfloor x \rfloor$ rounds x to its nearest integer towards minus infinity. The optimization problem shown in Eqn. (1) is an Integer Quadratic Program (IQP). Since IQP is NP-hard, s is usually relaxed to have continuous values, i.e., $s \in [0,1]^{mn}$ so that approximate solutions can be obtained [7, 8]. In this study, we adopt the random walk based graph matching me-thod proposed in [7] for its accuracy and computational efficiency.

To achieve reliable matching, a topological constraint based on Jacobian deter-minant of the mapping vectors is applied as a hard constraint in the graph matching. In particular, once a solution of the graph matching is available, spatial mapping is determined for each voxel x, and Jacobian determinant $J(x)$ of the deformation field at voxel x can be calculated. If $J(x) < 0$ then the matched node is discarded. As illustrated in Fig. 1, there are two cases of matched nodes. Fig. 1 left shows the map-ping vectors with $J(.) > 0$ while Fig. 1 right gives an example where $J(.) < 0$. The mapping vectors are obtained from nodes falling in a region centered at the red point and their matched nodes in the other graph. Matched nodes are marked in the same color.

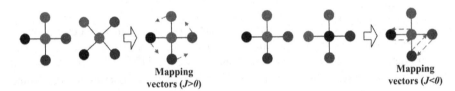

Fig. 1. Two cases of matched nodes and their corresponding mapping vectors (matched nodes in two graphs are in the same color). One mapping's Jacobian determinant is greater than zero (left), and the other is less than zero (right).

2.3   Dense Mapping Field Computation Using Iterative Graph Matching

Since the computational cost is high to matching the whole brain graphs of functional connectivity patterns, we solve the graph matching problem using a stochastic resam-ple strategy. In particular, graphs of functional connectivity patterns are built at even-ly distributed spatial locations in the brain to capture local functional connectivity patterns, and then graphs of local functional connectivity patterns are matched to es-tablish correspondence between subjects and drive the image registration iteratively.

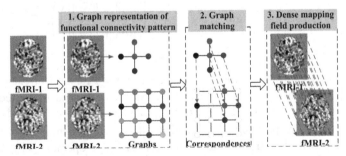

Fig. 2. Illustration of matching graph based connectivity pattern to achieve fMRI registration

Fig. 2 illustrates the whole process of our method for registering fMRI-1 (moving data) to fMRI-2 (fixed data). For the fMRI-1, a graph is constructed to capture a given voxel's local connectivity patterns within its neighborhood. The graph is constructed within a Region of Interest (ROI, marked as a red rectangle) centered at this voxel. The voxel and its neighboring voxels in the ROI are nodes of the graph and each edge is weighted by the Pearson Correlation Coefficient (PCC) of functional signals between its connected nodes. In the same way, graphs of local functional connectivity patterns can be constructed for each voxel in fMRI-2. Then the correspondence between voxels of the two fMRI data are established by matching corresponding graphs using graph matching algorithms [7, 8]. It is worth noting that for each graph in the moving data, the matched graph is searched in a graph at the same voxel position but with a larger ROI in the fixed data. Based on all matched graphs, a dense mapping field for registering the moving data to the fixed one can be produced. The graphs illustrated in Fig. 2 are based on 2D fMRI data examples and 4-connectivity for simplicity. In our method, all graphs are built on 3D fMRI data and fully connected.

To achieve robust and efficient fMRI data registration, we adopt an iterative graph matching strategy to perform the image registration iteratively. In particular, at each iteration step, a pre-defined number of voxels are randomly sampled in the Gray Matter (GM) of the moving fMRI data because meaningful functional signals are located in the GM. To achieve sub-voxel regional accuracy, the fixed fMRI data is up-sampled. For each pair of graphs at the same location in the moving and fixed fMRI data, the random walk based graph matching [7] with the topological constraint is used to establish spatial correspondence between their graph nodes. Such a procedure has been proved to be efficient and robust in non-rigid image registration [9]. Based on the corresponding voxels established by graphs, a dense mapping field can be obtained by composing updating mapping field derived from the matched graphs after each iteration step formulated as

$$d_{update}^r(x,y,z) = \sum_{i=1}^{n_c} d_i^r g_\sigma(p_i^r, x, y, z), x = 1, ..., w, y = 1, ..., h \; z = 1, ..., l,$$
$$d^r(x,y,z) = d^{r-1}\left(d_{update}^r(x,y,z)\right), \tag{3}$$

where d_{update}^r is the updating mapping field after the rth iteration, w, h and l are width, height and length of the fMRI data, d_i^r is the mapping vector obtained from matched graphs at the ith selected voxel located at position p_i^r, n_c is the pre-defined number of the selected voxels in each iteration, $g_\sigma(.)$ is the Gaussian kernel defining weight for d_i^r at the position (x,y,z), and d^r is the currently obtained dense mapping field that is applied to the moving image for achieving a better spatial initialization for the next iteration. The iterative process gradually improves the spatial alignment of corresponding functional units of the moving and fixed fMRI data. The iteration stops when converges, i.e., no significant change occurs in the resulting mapping field or the iteration excesses a pre-defined number.

3   Results

Our proposed method was tested using synthetic fMRI images and resting-state fMRI data of 20 subjects. We also compared our method with an fMRI registration method that characterizes local functional connectivity pattern for each voxel using a probability distribution of correlations between functional signals of the voxel and its neighboring voxels within a local region [5,6].

The synthetic fMRI data were used to intuitively demonstrate the capability of finding corresponding position between two images by matching graphs of functional connectivity patterns. Each synthetic fMRI image contains two different regions (a rectangle and a circle), pixels in the same region are assigned with the same fMRI signal extracted from a real fMRI data, as shown in Fig. 3 left. Fig. 3 right shows corresponding pixels in both images and their spatial relations detected by the proposed method.

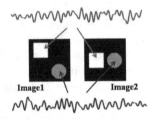 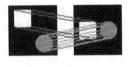

Fig. 3. Left: two synthetic fMRI images, each image contains two regions (a rectangle and a circle) and pixels in the same region are assigned with the same fMRI signal extracted from a real fMRI data. Right: corresponding pixels in both images and their spatial relations detected by the proposed method.

Our method was also validated based on a resting state fMRI dataset with 20 healthy subjects, obtained from http://fcon_1000.projects.nitrc.org (New York_b). All the image data were preprocessed by slice timing, head movement correction, band-pass filtering, and regressing out signals of white matter and cerebrospinal fluid. No spatial smoothing was applied to the images. In addition, to reduce huge computational workload and to accelerate the convergence speed, fMRI data of all subjects were initialized by corresponding mapping fields obtained by registering their corresponding sMRI data to the MNI152 space with a spatial resolution of 3×3×3 mm^3 using ANTS (http://www.picsl.upenn.edu/ANTS/) with a nonlinear registration model, namely SyN [10]. A mask image of the brain gray matter was generated to constrain the randomly selected voxels only in the gray matter area.

In our experiment, one fMRI data was randomly chosen as the fixed fMRI data (template) and the rest 19 fMRI data were registered to the template image. The fixed fMRI data was up-sampled by 2 folders to achieve sub-voxel registration accuracy. At each iteration step, 120 voxels were randomly selected and evenly distributed in the GM in the moving fMRI data. Since fMRI data have been initially registered by structural image registration in the preprocessing stage, for each selected voxel, a 3×3×3 voxels ROI centered at the voxel was used to construct a graph representing the functional connectivity pattern, while the graph for the voxel at the same position in the fixed fMRI data was constructed in an 11×11×11 voxels ROI.

To evaluate the inter-subject functional consistency of the resting state fMRI data before (initialized with mapping fields from sMRI registration) and after using our method, we performed an Independent Component Analysis (ICA) based analysis. Since the Default Mode Network (DMN) can be reliably detected in resting state fMRI data [11], we focused on the inter-subject consistency of DMNs of the 20 fMRI datasets. Particularly, the ICA was performed using GIFT for these 20 subjects before and after using our method, respectively [12]. The number of Independent Components (ICs) was set to 20 following GIFT's default settings. The DMN component was automatically identified by means of template matching. The subject specific DMNs were transferred to Z-score maps. Then t-tests across the subjects were performed based on the subject-specific Z-score maps for each of the two groups of functional images (before and after using our method). As shown in Fig. 4 left, the t values increased after the image data were registered using our method, indicating the improved inter-subject functional consistency. The differences between numbers of voxels larger than specific t value thresholds after and before using our method ($n_{after} - n_{before}$) further indicates that the proposed method improved inter-subject functional consistency as all the differences were positive (Fig. 4 right).

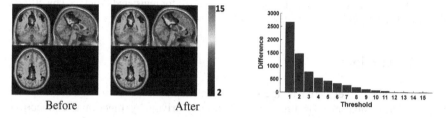

Fig. 4. Left: t-map of DMN before and after using our method. Right: The number of voxels with the difference ($n_{after} - n_{before}$) larger than each specific t value threshold.

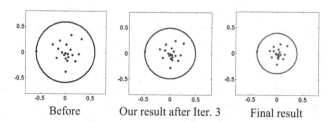

Fig. 5. Distribution of 20 DMNs obtained from data before using our method (left), our method after 3 iterations (middle) and final result (right). The DMNs are shown as 2D dots.

The inter-subject functional consistency of the 20 subjects before and after using our method was further assessed by pair-wise similarities of their DMNs. Specifically the distance between two subjects' DMN components is measured by their functional distance: 1.0 − Pearson Correlation Coefficient (PCC) between their DMNs. Then, the DMN components are projected onto the 2D space using Multi-Dimensional Scaling (MDS) according to their functional distances (Fig. 5). As shown in Fig. 5, the inter-subject functional distances across different subjects gradually decrease with the progression of our method.

We also obtained registration results for the same fMRI dataset using the method proposed in [5, 6], referred to as PDF-based registration method. We performed the same DMN based evaluation for the registered fMRI data. Fig. 6 shows the number of voxels larger than each specific t value threshold using the method (noted as PDF-based method) and our method, indicating our method can get better registration performance.

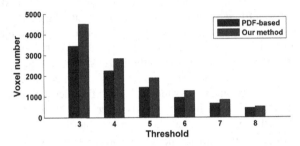

Fig. 6. Number of voxels in the DMN exceeding each specific t value threshold, determined by ICA on registered fMRI data. Then t value for each voxel was calculated by one sample t-tests across subjects based on the subject-specific Z-score maps for registered fMRI data by different methods, including PDF-based method and our method.

4   Discussions

We presented a novel fMRI image registration method that is directly based on the functional information. The image registration is driven by functional connectivity patterns that can overcome the problem of asynchrony of functional signals across different subjects. Different from the existing functional connectivity pattern based registration methods [3-6], we proposed a graph based representation to encode both the functional connectivity measures and their spatial information, which facilitates robust inter-subject spatial correspondence detection of the same functional units with spatial coherence. Such a representation of functional connectivity patterns is also generally applicable to both task-oriented and resting state fMRI data. The inter-subject spatial correspondence detection between different subjects can then be converted to the graph matching problem. Furthermore, to make the graph matching more robust and reliable, a topological constraint defined by the Jacobian determinant is added. To achieve an efficient image registration, an iterative graph matching strategy with stochastic resampling is introduced to perform the image registration that has been proved to be efficient and robust for non-rigid image registration [9]. The implementation of our method can be further improved by 1) adopting an adaptive size of ROI to construct graphs of localized functional connectivity patterns, and 2) considering the statistical significance of functional connectivity measures of functional signals in graph based representation of functional connectivity patterns.

The ongoing study is focusing on evaluating the proposed method by splitting the fMRI data into training and testing data along the time-dimension for cross-validation, and applying the method to datasets including both healthy subjects and patients. Furthermore, we will optimize the algorithm to accelerate the computation with the help of parallel computation.

Acknowledgement. This study was partially supported by the National Basic Research Program of China (973 Program) 2011CB707801, the National High Technology Research and Development Program of China (863 Program) 2012AA011603, the National Science Foundation of China (Grant Nos. 30970770, 91132707, 81271514, and 81261120419), and the Hundred Talents Program of the Chinese Academy of Sciences.

References

1. Ye, D.H., Hamm, J., Kwon, D., Davatzikos, C., Pohl, K.M.: Regional Manifold Learning for Deformable Registration of Brain MR Images. In: Ayache, N., Delingette, H., Golland, P., Mori, K. (eds.) MICCAI 2012, Part III. LNCS, vol. 7512, pp. 131–138. Springer, Heidelberg (2012)
2. Sabuncu, M.R., Singer, B.D., Conroy, B., Bryan, R.E., Ramadge, P.J., Haxby, J.V.: Function-based intersubject alignment of human cortical anatomy. Cerebral Cortex 20, 130–140 (2010)
3. Conroy, B., Singer, B., Haxby, J., Ramadge, P.: fMRI-Based Inter-Subject Cortical Alignment Using Functional Connectivity. Advances in Neural Information Processing Systems 22, 378–386 (2009)
4. Langs, G., Tie, Y., Rigolo, L., Golby, A., Golland, P.: Functional Geometry Alignment and Localization of Brain Areas. Advances in Neural Information Processing Systems 23, 1225–1233 (2010)
5. Jiang, D., Du, Y., Cheng, H., Jiang, T., Fan, Y.: fMRI Alignment Based on Local Functional Connectivity Patterns. In: SPIE Medical Imaging, San Diego, United States, vol. 831415 (2012), doi:10.1117/1112.911077
6. Jiang, D., Jiang, T.Z., Fan, Y.: Groupwise Fmri Registration Using Multi-Range Functional Connectivity Patterns. In: 2012 9th IEEEInternational Symposium on Biomedical Imaging (ISBI), pp. 1763–1766 (2012)
7. Cho, M., Lee, J., Lee, K.M.: Reweighted Random Walks for Graph Matching. In: Daniilidis, K., Maragos, P., Paragios, N. (eds.) ECCV 2010, Part V. LNCS, vol. 6315, pp. 492–505. Springer, Heidelberg (2010)
8. Leordeanu, M., Hebert, M.: A spectral technique for correspondence problems using pairwise constraints. In: ICCV (2005)
9. Klein, S., Staring, M., Pluim, J.P.W.: A Comparison of Acceleration Techniques for Nonrigid Medical Image Registration. In: Pluim, J.P.W., Likar, B., Gerritsen, F.A. (eds.) WBIR 2006. LNCS, vol. 4057, pp. 151–159. Springer, Heidelberg (2006)
10. Avants, B.B., Epstein, C.L., Grossman, M., Gee, J.C.: Symmetric diffeomorphic image registration with cross-correlation: evaluating automated labeling of elderly and neurodegenerative brain. Med. Image Anal. 12, 26–41 (2008)
11. Laird, A.R., Eickhoff, S.B., Li, K., Robin, D.A., Glahn, D.C., Fox, P.T.: Investigating the Functional Heterogeneity of the Default Mode Network Using Coordinate-Based Meta-Analytic Modeling. J. Neurosci. 29, 14496–14505 (2009)
12. Calhoun, V.D., Adali, T., Pearlson, G.D., Pekar, J.J.: A method for making group inferences from functional MRI data using independent component analysis. Hum. Brain Mapp. 14, 140–151 (2001)

Calibration and Stereo Tracking
of a Laparoscopic Ultrasound Transducer
for Augmented Reality in Surgery

Philip Edgcumbe[1], Christopher Nguan[3], and Robert Rohling[1,2]

[1] Department of Electrical and Computer Engineering,
University of British Columbia, Vancouver, BC, Canada
{edgcumbe,rohling}@ece.ubc.ca
[2] Department of Mechanical Engineering,
University of British Columbia, Vancouver, BC, Canada
[3] Department of Urologic Sciences,
University of British Columbia, Vancouver, BC, Canada
chris.nguan@urology.com

Abstract. Laparoscopic ultrasound is a useful adjunct for guidance in minimally invasive surgery. Tracking the location of the ultrasound transducer relative to the laparoscope would enable an augmented reality overlay of subsurface anatomical features on the surgeon's field of view. The accuracy of tracking is a critical aspect for such augmented reality guidance. We propose stereo tracking of visible markers on a new "pickup" laparoscopic ultrasound transducer and a direct transformation of the ultrasound image into the coordinates of a stereo laparoscope. We also suggest that ultrasound calibration be performed using a separate stereo camera system with a wide baseline. Such calibration is shown to improve point reconstruction accuracy from 3.1 mm to 1.3 mm.

Keywords: Ultrasound, Augmented Reality, Robotic Surgery.

1 Introduction

Minimally invasive surgery (MIS) offers significant advantages compared to open surgery. For example, incisions are smaller, there is less post-operative pain, and a shorter post-operative recovery. However, MIS procedures have disadvantages including: limited view of the surgical field, and reduction of surgical dexterity. Two technologies hold promise to help overcome these disadvantages. These are stereo laparoscopes which improve a surgeon's depth perception and laparoscopic ultrasound (LUS) which improve visualization of subsurface anatomical features. Industry has recognized the demand for stereo laparoscopes as represented firstly, by the inclusion of a stereo laparoscope with the da Vinci Surgical System (Intuitive Surgical, Sunnyvale, CA, UBC), [7] and secondly, by the development of stereo laparoscopes for non-robotic MIS such as the Viking 3DHD Vision System (Viking Systems, Westborough, MA, USA) and the Endoeye Flex 3D (Olympus, Shinjuku, Tokyo, Japan). There is growing interest in the use of

C.A. Linte et al. (Eds.): MIAR/AE-CAI 2013, LNCS 8090, pp. 258–267, 2013.
© Springer-Verlag Berlin Heidelberg 2013

stereo laparoscopy for standard laparoscopy and for tracking tools and instruments as part of an augmented reality system [8].

LUS improves surgical safety by allowing surgeons to visualize important anatomy beneath the organ surface. 82% of surgeons practicing endoscopy expect an increase in the use of LUS in the next 5-years [17]. To improve the accessibility and ease of interpretation of LUS, several research groups have developed augmented reality LUS systems by tracking the position of a LUS transducer. Offline ultrasound calibration must be performed to determine the transformation from the ultrasound image coordinate system to the LUS transducer marker coordinate system. During ultrasound calibration and during surgery, the accuracy of the tracking of the LUS transducer determines the overall accuracy of the augmented reality LUS system. Tracking of the LUS transducer has been achieved by robotic kinematics [13], optical tracking [9,12], electromagnetic tracking [3], and a combination of optical tracking and electromagnetic tracking [4]. An external base coordinate system, which must be used for tracking with robot kinematics, electromagnetic tracking and external optical tracking, makes tracking susceptible to error amplification due to the lever-arm effect. Maximizing the calibration accuracy is critical to these augmented reality systems.

One of our previous contributions to the field of robotic LUS was the development of a small "pick-up" LUS transducer that can be picked-up by the da Vinci robot and controlled by the surgeon at the da Vinci console [15]. BK Medical (Herlev, Denmark) sells a similar product called the ProART. In this paper we propose an augmented reality LUS system using the new pick-up LUS transducer [15] and stereo laparoscopy. Pratt et al. developed a similar augmented reality LUS system for mono laparoscopy and a pick-up LUS transducer [12]. They used the laparoscope to track the LUS transducer and eliminated the need for an external base coordinate system. This visual tracking of the LUS transducer offers the potential of higher accuracy due to a reduced lever-arm effect and a direct transformation from the ultrasound image to the camera via visible markers on the LUS transducer [12]. Our proposed augmented reality LUS system also uses visual tracking and eliminates the external base coordinate system. Furthermore, we address the problem that stereo laparoscopes have a narrow baseline (camera spacing of about 5 mm) which results in narrow triangulation and poor accuracy of stereo laparoscope augmented reality systems [18].

Our primary innovation is to separate ultrasound calibration and LUS transducer tracking. We use a 75 mm baseline stereo camera for ultrasound calibration and a stereo laparoscope for LUS tracking. For both ultrasound calibration and LUS tracking we use the same LUS optical fiducials and the same tracking method. This approach should reduce the ultrasound calibration error. We measure accuracy by using the tracked LUS to estimate the location of a pinhead of known location in the camera coordinate system. To our knowledge, Leven et al. [9] proposed, but did not report, results for direct visual tracking of a LUS with a stereo laparoscope, so this is the first such report. A second aspect of this project is to characterize the accuracy of an augmented reality LUS system as a function of a changing camera focal length. We do this to understand the consequences of a surgeon changing the focal length of the stereo laparoscope during surgery to optimize the view of the surgical field [16].

The objective and novelty of this paper is to show how the size of camera baseline during ultrasound calibration affects the error of an augmented reality LUS system.

2   Methods

This section describes the apparatus that was used, the calibration and tracking methods, and the experiments. We compared the combination of a wide baseline calibration and narrow baseline tracking (our proposal) to a combination of narrow baseline calibration and narrow baseline tracking (the standard approach of using the same sensor for calibration and tracking). Accuracy and precision of the two proposed augmented reality LUS systems are reported. Henceforth, the stereo laparoscope will be referred to as a narrow baseline camera.

2.1   Apparatus, Calibration and Tracking

We used a SonixTOUCH ultrasound machine (Ultrasonix Medical Corporation, Richmond, BC, Canada) with a 10MHz LUS transducer (28 mm linear array) [15]. The LUS transducer is designed to take advantage of the dexterity of the da Vinci tools. It can be picked up with the da Vinci Pro-Grasp tool and be moved in all 6 DOF. Furthermore, the surgeon at the da Vinci console controls the movement of the LUS transducer which allows the surgeon's natural hand-eye coordination to aid interpretation of the 3D anatomy from a set of 2D cross-sectional images. All ultrasound images were taken at an ultrasound image depth of 20 mm. All camera images (stereo camera calibration, ultrasound calibration and validation experiments) were taken simultaneously with the two camera systems allowing for a more controlled comparison of the accuracies of the respective camera combinations. The narrow baseline camera is a wide angle NTSC da Vinci stereo laparoscope from the da Vinci Surgical System (Standard). It has a narrow baseline of 5 mm and a resolution of 720×486 pixels. The wide baseline camera system has a baseline of 75 mm and consists of two Flea2 cameras (Point Grey Research, Richmond, Canada) with a resolution of 1280×960 pixels. It has previously been observed that a similar difference in camera resolution did not have a significant effect on camera calibration results [12], so the important difference is the baseline. The calculation of the intrinsic and extrinsic camera parameters and lens distortion coefficients was done with the Caltech Camera Calibration toolbox [2] using about 20 images of unique poses of a 8×10 checkerboard with 5 mm squares.

To define the LUS transducer marker coordinate system we used a similar approach to Pratt et al. [12] in which a small checkerboard is mounted onto the LUS. We placed a 6×2 and a 7×2 checkerboard with 3.175 mm squares on the two flat (9 mm $\times$ 27 mm) surfaces on each side of the LUS transducer [Figure 1]. Our checkerboard is made of surgical identification tape (KeySurgical Inc.,

Eden Prairie, MN, USA) which is approved for internal human use, repeated sterilization cycles and designed to be semi-permanently attached to surgical instruments. Using a camera to track an ultrasound transducer for construction of 3D ultrasound images has been done previously [1].

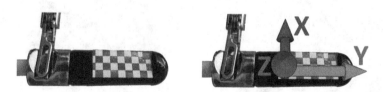

Fig. 1. Left: Picture showing the da Vinci Pro-Grasp tool holding the "pick-up" LUS transducer which has checkerboard markers on it. Right: Same picture as left with addition of 3D coordinate system overlay showing the axes of the LUS transducer marker coordinate system (T). The z axis and the normal of the ultrasound imaging plane are almost parallel.

We used the triple N-wire ultrasound calibration technique [10]. The triple N-wire phantom was precisely manufactured with the Objet30 desktop 3D printer (Objet Inc., Billerica, MA, USA) which has 28 micrometer precision. For defining the location of the N-wires in the coordinate system of the phantom we used an Optotrak Certus optical tracker (Northern Digital Inc, Waterloo, Ontario, Canada) to track four NDI markers on our phantom and an NDI tracked stylus that was used to select the 18 N-wire holes. An Optotrak is not strictly required for this step; we could have used the known geometry of our CAD model to calculate the same geometric relationships. The phantom bath was filled with distilled water and 9% by volume glycerol [11] to achieve a sound speed of 1540 m/s.

For ultrasound calibration and tracking experiments the LUS transducer was placed at a distance of 100 mm from the narrow baseline camera and 150 mm from the wide baseline camera. Figure 2 includes a picture of the experimental setup (left) and a diagram of the four coordinate systems. The coordinate systems are: #1) Ultrasound image coordinate system (I), #2) LUS transducer marker coordinate system (T), #3) Camera coordinate system (C) and #4) Phantom coordinate system (Ph). The camera coordinate system (C) represents either the coordinate system of the wide baseline or narrow baseline camera.

Equation (1) shows the transformation from the ultrasound image coordinate system (x,y with units of mm) to the camera coordinate system (a,b,c with units of mm). The ultrasound calibration matrix - the fixed 6DOF transformation from the ultrasound image to LUS transducer marker coordinate system $(^{T}T_{I})$ - is the part of that equation that is determined offline prior to LUS imaging during surgery. The transformation from the LUS transducer marker coordinate system to the camera coordinate system $(^{C}T_{T})$ is solved by using a corresponding point algorithm between the known location of the 21 saddle points on the transducer checkerboard in the transducer coordinate system and the camera coordinates of

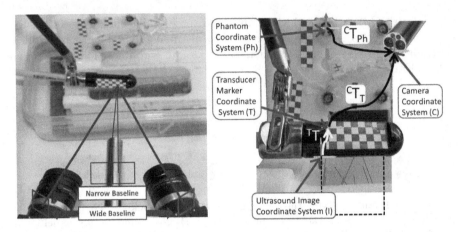

Fig. 2. Two pictures of the experimental setup. Left: The wide baseline and narrow baseline (stereo laparoscope) cameras are in the foreground and the pick-up LUS transducer and triple N-wire phantom are in the background. Right: The LUS transducer, held by the da Vinci Pro-Grasp tool, is directly above the N-wires. The phantom optical fiducials are in the background. The four experimental coordinate systems (I, T, C and Ph) and the transformations between them (^CT_T, ^TT_I, $^CT_{Ph}$) are shown.

those same saddle points as determined by a Harris corner detector and stereo-triangulation [5]. The transformation from the phantom to the camera ($^CT_{Ph}$) is solved in the same way except the points are the four centers of the NDI markers and their locations in the camera images are selected manually.

$$
\begin{bmatrix} a \\ b \\ c \\ 1 \end{bmatrix}^C = {}^CT_T\,{}^TT_I \begin{bmatrix} x \\ y \\ 0 \\ 1 \end{bmatrix}^I
\tag{1}
$$

For each LUS image of the N-wire phantom, the location in the phantom coordinate system where the wires intersect the ultrasound imaging plane (d,e,f) are calculated by segmenting the wire ultrasound points and using the distance between the points and the known geometry of the N-wire phantom. The ultrasound calibration matrix (^TT_I) is solved by using a corresponding point algorithm [5] between the N-wire points (d,e,f), projected from the phantom to LUS transducer marker coordinate system, (see equation (2)) and the same N-wire points (x,y) in the ultrasound image coordinate system. Ultrasound segmentation is done via a semi-automatic algorithm which finds the location of each wire by finding the centroid of the ultrasound image pixels associated with each wire.

$$
{}^TT_C\,{}^CT_{Ph} \begin{bmatrix} d \\ e \\ f \\ 1 \end{bmatrix}^{Ph} = {}^TT_I \begin{bmatrix} x \\ y \\ 0 \\ 1 \end{bmatrix}^I
\tag{2}
$$

In total, 30 LUS transducer poses were captured for calibration. The 30 poses were randomly assigned to ten groups of 10, ten groups of 15 and one group of 30 and the ultrasound calibration matrix for each group was calculated. During ultrasound calibration, the LUS transducer covered an approximately uniform range within a 5×5×20 mm cuboid and Euler angles of 23°, 11°, and 23° about the x, y and z axes of the LUS transducer marker coordinate system of the first LUS transducer pose [Figure 1].

In summary we built our experimental apparatus so we could compare the combination of a wide baseline camera for ultrasound calibration and a narrow baseline camera for tracking to the combination of a narrow baseline camera for both ultrasound calibration and tracking.

2.2   Experiments

2.2.1   Point Reconstruction Accuracy and Precision

To estimate the pinhead's location in the camera coordinate system, it is segmented from each ultrasound image and its location is transformed to the camera coordinate system as shown in equation (1). Its actual location is determined by stereo triangulation of the pinhead location after draining the fluid medium. Accuracy is the Euclidean distance from the average of the estimated pinheads location to the actual pinhead location. Precision is the average Euclidean distance from each estimated pinhead location point to the centroid of those points. These measures account for errors in calibration as well as alignment, segmentation, tracking and other errors [6]. However, we kept alignment, segmentation and tracking constant across experiments so the changes in accuracy and precision are primarily due to the different ultrasound calibration matrices. The same 22 LUS transducer poses were used for all point reconstruction experiments. The LUS transducer covered an approximately uniform range within a 6×8×10 mm cuboid and Euler angles ranged over 22°, 16°, and 28° about the x, y and z axes respectively of the LUS transducer marker coordinate system of the first LUS transducer pose. The pinhead is plastic and has a diameter of 2.5 mm.

2.2.2   Point Reconstruction Accuracy as a Function of Focal Length

In this experiment the change in accuracy and precision is calculated for a change of focal length from 100 mm to 160 mm. The focal length of the stereo laparoscope was changed to 160 mm, the LUS transducer was moved to a distance of about 160 mm from the stereo laparoscope and 16 new LUS transducer poses were captured. The location of the LUS transducer was calculated using the 100 mm focal length camera calibration parameters and separately with the 160 mm focal length camera calibration parameters. Both sets of camera calibration parameters were calculated with 20 images of an 8 × 10 checkerboard and the Caltech Camera Calibration toolbox [2]. The stereo laparoscope is set to a focal length of 100 mm or 160 mm by placing a checkerboard perpendicular to the viewing direction at those respective distances and adjusting the focus until the checkerboard is sharply in focus. This approach is necessary because the da Vinci application programming interface does not report the focal length.

3   Results

3.1   Point Reconstruction Accuracy and Precision

The wide baseline approach for calibration improved accuracy (reduced point target localization error) from 3.1 mm to 1.3 mm when 30 LUS transducer poses were used for calibration (Table 1). A similar trend was seen for 10 and 15 calibration poses. A greater number of poses appear to help repeatability of the calibration.

Table 1. Point reconstruction accuracy (mm) ± standard deviation for the combination of narrow baseline calibration and tracking and the combination of wide baseline calibration and narrow baseline tracking. 30 LUS transducer poses were captured for calibration and randomly assigned to ten groups of 10, ten groups of 15 and one group of all 30 poses.

Stereo camera type for ultrasound calibration	Stereo camera type for tracking LUS	# of calibration poses		
		10	15	30
Narrow baseline	Narrow baseline	3.3 ± 1.3	3.3 ± 0.9	3.1
Wide baseline	Narrow baseline	1.5 ± 0.4	1.4 ± 0.3	1.3

The wide baseline approach for calibration improved precision a small amount (Table 2).

Table 2. Point reconstruction precision (mm) ± standard deviation for the combination of narrow baseline calibration and tracking and the combination of wide baseline calibration and narrow baseline tracking. 30 LUS transducer poses were captured for calibration and randomly assigned to ten groups of 10, ten groups of 15 and one group of all 30 poses.

Stereo camera type for ultrasound calibration	Stereo camera type for tracking LUS	# of calibration poses		
		10	15	30
Narrow baseline	Narrow baseline	1.3 ± 0.2	1.4 ± 0.1	1.3
Wide baseline	Narrow baseline	1.2 ± 0.1	1.1 ± 0.1	1.2

3.2   Point Reconstruction Accuracy as a Function of Focal Length

Table 3 shows the accuracy and precision of the point reconstruction test after moving the LUS transducer from a distance of 100 mm to 160 mm and changing the focal length from a distance of 100 mm to 160 mm without updating the camera calibration parameters. The change of focal length without updating the camera calibration parameters decreases accuracy (increased point target localization error) to about 20 mm. When the stereo camera is calibrated at 160 mm

Table 3. Point reconstruction results (mm) ± std for the LUS transducer at a distance of 160 mm from the narrow baseline camera. The focal length (mm) is the focal length at which the stereo camera calibration parameters were calculated. 30 LUS transducer poses were captured for calibration and randomly assigned to ten groups of 15.

Stereo camera type for ultrasound calibration	Stereo camera type for tracking LUS	Focal Length (mm)	Accuracy (mm)	Precision (mm)
Narrow baseline	Narrow baseline	100	19.2 ± 0.7	1.8 ± 0.2
Wide baseline	Narrow baseline	100	20.2 ± 0.2	1.5 ± 0.1
Narrow baseline	Narrow baseline	160	2.6 ± 1.0	1.8 ± 0.2
Wide baseline	Narrow baseline	160	0.8 ± 0.4	1.5 ± 0.1

and those camera calibration parameters are used accuracy returns to 0.8 mm and 2.6 mm for wide baseline and low baseline camera tracking respectively. These results are similar to what was observed when the LUS transducer was at a distance of 100 mm.

4   Discussion and Conclusion

We have shown a millimeter level of accuracy for an augmented reality LUS system via direct visual tracking using a stereo laparoscope, suggesting it is a viable option for guidance in minimally invasive surgery. When we implement our proposed method of using a wide baseline (75 mm) stereo camera for ultrasound calibration and a narrow baseline (5 mm) stereo laparoscope for tracking the accuracy is 1.3 mm (Table 1). When the narrow baseline camera system is used for ultrasound calibration and tracking, accuracy of 3.1 mm is achieved. This reinforces the need for careful consideration of the ultrasound calibration step.

Most other research groups that developed augmented reality LUS systems used tracking systems that include an external base coordinate system such as optical tracking [9], electromagnetic tracking [3], and a combination of optical tracking and electromagnetic tracking [4]. These groups have reported point reconstruction errors in the approximate range of 1.5 mm and 3 mm. It should be noted that direct comparisons of accuracy results are difficult because of differences in apparatus, tests and definitions of accuracy. The novelty in our work is the use of a different stereo camera system for the ultrasound calibration and the direct visual tracking of the LUS transducer with a stereo laparoscope. The concept of using a different sensor for ultrasound calibration is broadly applicable. With the increasing adoption of the da Vinci, Viking and Olympus stereo laparoscopes, the need for understanding the challenges associated with direct visual tracking with a stereo laparoscope will continue to grow. Furthermore, direct visual tracking has an elegant simplicity that minimizes the extra equipment required to implement the system and electromagnetic field distortion is not a concern. One drawback is the need for a line of sight between the laparoscope and the LUS transducer, but this is naturally performed by the surgeon when placing the LUS transducer over a region of interest. A second drawback is that blood or other fluid may obscure part of the LUS checkerboard optical markers. However, as long as part of the checkerboard remains visible the LUS transducer can still be tracked, albeit with reduced accuracy.

To further understand the effect of camera baseline on accuracy we calculated the accuracy of the combination of wide baseline calibration and tracking and the accuracy of the combination of narrow baseline calibration with wide baseline tracking. The results were 0.6 mm and 2.45 mm respectively. For these experiments we used the same 30 LUS transducer poses that were captured for calibration and the same 22 LUS transducer poses that were captured to determine the accuracy and precision. Thus, the best case accuracy is 0.6 mm and we surmise that using a narrow baseline camera for tracking decreases accuracy (increases point target localization error) by about 0.7 mm to the overall accuracy of 1.3 mm (see Table 1).

The next steps for this project include real-time implementation, clinical validation and further accuracy improvements. The custom-built pick-up LUS [15] used in this experiment has a built-in EM sensor so visual tracking and EM sensor fusion is possible [4]. Further work will also address our finding that the change in stereo laparoscope camera focal length during the operation has a dramatic effect on the error of the point reconstruction accuracy. In future work we plan to match the camera calibration parameters to a range of pre-calibrated setting by using the checkerboard that is already mounted on the LUS transducer as a guide to the approximate camera calibration parameters. Several applications we may pursue for the stereo laparoscope augmented reality LUS system are guidance during MIS hepatic or renal tumour resections, pre-operative CT scan to intra-operative ultrasound registration and display of absolute elastography images [14]. Regardless, the stereo laparoscope augmented reality LUS system is broadly applicable across a large range of surgeries.

Acknowledgements. This work is supported by CIHR, NSERC and the Institute for Computing, Information and Cognitive Systems (ICICS) at UBC. The semi-automatic ultrasound segmentation and N-wire ultrasound calibration MATLAB code and GUI were written by Jeff Abeysekera at the University of British Columbia.

References

1. Ali, A., Logeswaran, R.: A visual probe localization and calibration system for cost-effective computer-aided 3d ultrasound. Computers in Biology and Medicine 37(8), 1141–1147 (2007)
2. Bouget, J.Y.: Camera calibration toolbox for matlab @ONLINE (2013), http://www.vision.caltech.edu/bouguetj/calib_doc/index.html
3. Cheung, C.L., Wedlake, C., Moore, J., Pautler, S.E., Peters, T.M.: Fused video and ultrasound images for minimally invasive partial nephrectomy: A phantom study. In: Jiang, T., Navab, N., Pluim, J.P.W., Viergever, M.A. (eds.) MICCAI 2010, Part III. LNCS, vol. 6363, pp. 408–415. Springer, Heidelberg (2010)

4. Feuerstein, M., Reichl, T., Vogel, J., Traub, J., Navab, N.: Magneto-optical tracking of flexible laparoscopic ultrasound: model-based online detection and correction of magnetic tracking errors. IEEE Transactions on Medical Imaging 28(6), 951–967 (2009)

5. Horn, B.K.: Closed-form solution of absolute orientation using unit quaternions. JOSA A 4(4), 629–642 (1987)

6. Hsu, P.W., Treece, G.M., Prager, R.W., Houghton, N.E., Gee, A.H.: Comparison of freehand 3-d ultrasound calibration techniques using a stylus. Ultrasound in Medicine & Biology 34(10), 1610–1621 (2008)

7. Hubens, G., Coveliers, H., Balliu, L., Ruppert, M., Vaneerdeweg, W.: A performance study comparing manual and robotically assisted laparoscopic surgery using the da Vinci system. Surgical Endoscopy 17(10), 1595–1599 (2003)

8. Langø, T., Vijayan, S., Rethy, A., Våpenstad, C., Solberg, O.V., Mårvik, R., Johnsen, G., Hernes, T.N.: Navigated laparoscopic ultrasound in abdominal soft tissue surgery: technological overview and perspectives. International Journal of Computer Assisted Radiology and Surgery 7(4), 585–599 (2012)

9. Leven, J., et al.: DaVinci canvas: A telerobotic surgical system with integrated, robot-assisted, laparoscopic ultrasound capability. In: Duncan, J.S., Gerig, G. (eds.) MICCAI 2005. LNCS, vol. 3749, pp. 811–818. Springer, Heidelberg (2005)

10. Mercier, L., Langø, T., Lindseth, F., Collins, D.L., et al.: A review of calibration techniques for freehand 3-d ultrasound systems. Ultrasound in Medicine and Biology 31(2), 143–166 (2005)

11. Oates, C.: Towards an ideal blood analogue for doppler ultrasound phantoms. Physics in Medicine and Biology 36(11), 1433 (1991)

12. Pratt, P., Di Marco, A., Payne, C., Darzi, A., Yang, G.-Z.: Intraoperative ultrasound guidance for transanal endoscopic microsurgery. In: Ayache, N., Delingette, H., Golland, P., Mori, K. (eds.) MICCAI 2012, Part I. LNCS, vol. 7510, pp. 463–470. Springer, Heidelberg (2012)

13. Schneider, C.M., Dachs II, G.W., Hasser, C.J., Choti, M.A., DiMaio, S.P., Taylor, R.H.: Robot-assisted laparoscopic ultrasound. In: Navab, N., Jannin, P. (eds.) IPCAI 2010. LNCS, vol. 6135, pp. 67–80. Springer, Heidelberg (2010)

14. Schneider, C., Baghani, A., Rohling, R., Salcudean, S.: Remote ultrasound palpation for robotic interventions using absolute elastography. In: Ayache, N., Delingette, H., Golland, P., Mori, K. (eds.) MICCAI 2012, Part I. LNCS, vol. 7510, pp. 42–49. Springer, Heidelberg (2012)

15. Schneider, C., Guerrero, J., Nguan, C., Rohling, R., Salcudean, S.: Intra-operative "Pick-up" ultrasound for robot assisted surgery with vessel extraction and registration: A feasibility study. In: Taylor, R.H., Yang, G.-Z. (eds.) IPCAI 2011. LNCS, vol. 6689, pp. 122–132. Springer, Heidelberg (2011)

16. Stoyanov, D., Darzi, A., Yang, G.Z.: Laparoscope self-calibration for robotic assisted minimally invasive surgery. In: Duncan, J.S., Gerig, G. (eds.) MICCAI 2005. LNCS, vol. 3750, pp. 114–121. Springer, Heidelberg (2005)

17. Våpenstad, C., Rethy, A., Langø, T., Selbekk, T., Ystgaard, B., Hernes, T.A.N., Mårvik, R.: Laparoscopic ultrasound: a survey of its current and future use, requirements, and integration with navigation technology. Surgical Endoscopy 24(12), 2944–2953 (2010)

18. Wang, D., Bello, F., Darzi, A.: Augmented reality provision in robotically assisted minimally invasive surgery. International Congress Series, vol. 1268, pp. 527–532. Elsevier (2004)

Evaluation of Multiple Voxel-Based Morphometry Approaches and Applications in the Analysis of White Matter Changes in Temporal Lobe Epilepsy

Wenjing Li[1], Huiguang He[1,*], Jingjing Lu[2], Bin Lv[1], Meng Li[1], and Zhengyu Jin[2]

[1] State Key Laboratory of Management and Control for Complex Systems,
Institute of Automation, Chinese Academy of Sciences, Beijing, 100190, China
[2] Department of Radiology, Peking Union Medical College Hospital, Beijing, 100730, China

Abstract. The purpose of this study was to compare multiple voxel-based morphometry (VBM) approaches and analyze the whole-brain white matter (WM) changes in the unilateral temporal lobe epilepsy (TLE) patients relative to controls. In our study, the performance of the VBM approaches, including standard VBM, optimized VBM and VBM-DARTEL, was evaluated via a simulation, and then these VBM approaches were applied to the real data obtained from the TLE patients and controls. The results from simulation show that VBM-DARTEL performs the best among these VBM approaches. For the real data, WM reductions were found in the ipsilateral temporal lobe, the contralateral frontal and occipital lobes, the bilateral parietal lobes, cingulated gyrus, parahippocampal gyrus and brainstem of the left-TLE patients by VBM-DARTEL, which is consistent with previous studies. Our study demonstrated that DARTEL was the most robust and reliable approach for VBM analysis.

1 Introduction

Voxel-based morphometry (VBM) is a computational quantitative magnetic resonance image (MRI) analysis technique which can detect the differences of the brain tissue composition between groups. Compared with the conventional region-of-interest (ROI) analysis, VBM is fully automated and unbiased, and is not restricted to the analysis of specific brain regions. VBM was first proposed by Ashburner and Friston [1], which allows a voxel-wise study of differences in tissue concentration throughout the whole brain between groups. An optimized VBM method was introduced by Good et al. [2], improving image registration and segmentation. More recently, the preprocessing steps of VBM have been improved with the Diffeomorphic Anatomical Registration Through Exponentiated Lie algebra (DARTEL) registration method [3]. DARTEL was proposed by Ashburner as an alternative to the traditional registration measures in statistical parametric mapping (SPM), which can achieve more accurate inter-subject registration of brain images.

---

* Corresponding author. Tel: +86 10 6265 0799; fax: +86 10 62650799. E-mail address: huiguang.he@ia.ac.cn (Huiguang He).

C.A. Linte et al. (Eds.): MIAR/AE-CAI 2013, LNCS 8090, pp. 268–276, 2013.

VBM has been applied to detecting the pathological changes in various diseases [4-6]. In particular, there have been lots of studies focusing on the application of VBM in temporal lobe epilepsy (TLE) [6-8]. TLE is one of the most frequent forms of partial epilepsy in adults, and is defined as a chronic neurological condition characterized by recurrent unprovoked seizures originating from temporal lobe. Many MRI studies have shown that structural abnormalities associated with TLE have been found in the hippocampus as well as other structures in extrahippocampal regions. Keller et al. [8] compared the standard and the optimized VBM for analysis of brain abnormalities in TLE, revealing that the optimized VBM might detect the subtle neuroanatomical changes that were not found in the standard VBM. According to previous studies, we found that most studies focused on finding gray matter (GM) atrophies in TLE patients, while a few studies on white matter (WM) abnormalities.

As DARTEL is a very recent technique used in VBM, only a few studies have applied this new method in VBM [9], and there has not been any studies detecting the structural changes in TLE with DARTEL. Yassa et al. [10] evaluated several registration approaches, concluding that DARTEL was a real improvement over the standard registration method. However, VBM-DARTEL was not compared with other VBM approaches in previous studies.

In our study, we first evaluated these VBM techniques (standard VBM, optimized VBM, and VBM-DARTEL) via simulated data to provide a ground truth. Then these VBM approaches were applied to the real data to detect the WM abnormalities between the unilateral TLE patients and controls. This is the first study to compare VBM-DARTEL with standard and optimized VBM and be applied to TLE, and the performance of these multiple VBM approaches was quantified in our study.

2   Materials and Methods

2.1   Simulation of Atrophy

Images with simulated atrophy can act as the gold standard for evaluating the relative merits of various VBM approaches. We employed 20 normal anatomical models from BrainWeb (http://www.bic.mni.mcgill.ca/brainweb/) and the algorithm developed by Karacali and Davatzikos, which automatically simulated anatomical deformations, was used to simulate the volumetric loss of 3D images [11]. To eliminate inter-individual differences, the 20 normal models were considered as the controls, and the corresponding images with simulated atrophies were the patients. We selected three regions (centered in the left hippocampus, the right frontal lobe and the right occipital lobe) to simulate atrophies (Fig. 1). The radius of the three regions was 5/5/2mm, and the atrophied degree was 25±1.62%, 10±1.75%, 25±1.62%, respectively. In addition, we add Gaussian noise to all the images (SNR=33).The acquisition parameters were as follows: TR/TE=22/9.2 ms, flip angle (FA) =30° and 1 mm isotropic voxel size.

2.2   Subject and Data Acquisition

The study group consisted of 20 left-TLE patients (age: 33.2±8.1 years; 9 males), 20 right-TLE patients (age: 34.1±7.2 years; 9 males) and 20 controls with no history of neurological or psychiatric symptoms (age: 32.2±6.2 years; 9 males). All of these groups were matched in age and gender. The laterality of the seizures origin was determined based on medical history, ictal EEG and hippocampal atrophy observed on MRI. Written informed consent was obtained from each subject before the study.

T1-weighted MRI scans were obtained using a 3 Tesla scanner with following parameters: TR/TE/TI = 7/3/400 ms, slice thickness = 1.6 mm, FA= 15°, matrix size = 256×256, field of view (FOV) = 24×24 cm^2, yielding axial slices with in-plane resolution of 1×1 mm^2.

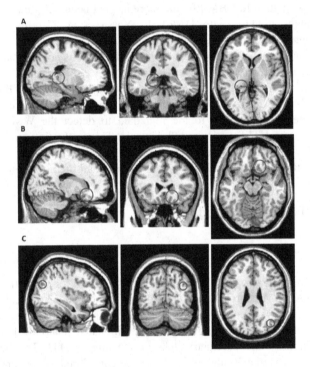

Fig. 1. Landmarks for simulated atrophies centered in (A) the left hippocampus, (B) the right frontal lobe and (C) the right occipital lobe

2.3   Image Preprocessing

All the 3D T1-weighted images were brain extracted to exclude the non-brain tissues and reoriented with the origin set close to the anterior commissure (AC). All these images were then preprocessed with multiple VBM approaches detailed as follows.

Preprocessing steps were performed by using Statistical Parametric Mapping (SPM8) (http://www.fil.ion.ucl.ac.uk/spm, Wellcome Department of Cognitive Neurology, London, UK, 2008) on a Matlab 7.6 platform (MathWorks, Natick, MA, USA).

The methodology of the standard VBM was proposed by Ashburner and Friston in 2000 [1], which was used to detect the differences in tissue density between groups. All the skull-stripped and reoriented images were spatially normalized to the Montreal Neurological Institute (MNI) space by minimizing the residual sum of squared differences between structural MRI and the ICBM 152 template image. The data were then resampled to $1.5\times1.5\times1.5$ mm^3. All these images were partitioned into GM, WM and CSF using the unified segmentation algorithm with bias correction incorporated in [12]. WM images were then smoothed with an 8-mm smoothing kernel.

The optimized VBM method customized a study-specific template obtained from all the subjects. Each reoriented image was normalized to MNI template and resliced to 1.5-mm isotropic voxels. Then, they were smoothed with an 8-mm Gaussian kernel. The whole-brain template was created by averaging all these images. The reoriented images were then normalized to the customized template and resliced to $1.5\times1.5\times1.5$ mm^3. After that, the unified segmentation algorithm [12] was performed. The segmented WM images were smoothed with 8-mm FWHM and the average image was the specific WM template. The reoriented images were segmented in native space. Each segmented WM image was normalized to the study-specific WM template with the normalization parameters applied to the reoriented images. Then, these normalized images were segmented again. Furthermore, modulation was alternative to correct for volume changes, creating the Jacobian scaled warped WM images. These images were then smoothed with an 8-mm Gaussian filter.

In VBM-DARTEL method, each reorientated image was first segmented into GM, WM and CSF in native space and then Procrustes aligned GM and WM images were generated by a rigid transformation. The resolution of the aligned images was specified as $1.5\times1.5\times1.5$ mm^3. The study-specific GM/WM templates were then created by the aligned images from all the patients and controls. The procedure began with the generation of an original template computing the average of all the aligned data, followed by the first iteration of the registration on each subject in turn. Thus, a new template was created and the second iteration began. After six iterations, the template was generated, which was the average of the DARTEL registered data. During iterations, all images were warped to the template yielding a series of flow fields that parameterized deformations, which were employed in the modulation step. Since the previous processing was in native space, it was a requirement to transform all the normalized, modulated data into MNI space. After the space transformation, all these images were smoothed with an 8-mm FWHM isotropic Gaussian kernel.

2.4   Statistical Analysis

Based on the general linear model, statistical parametric maps were created to identify brain regions with significant changes in patients relative to controls. As the simulated data, all the preprocessed WM images were analyzed with paired t test. An absolute threshold of 0.1 was used in the analysis. Since the images of controls and patients are from identical subjects, covariates (such as total intracranial volume (TIV), age and gender) were not considered in this model. The performance of the three VBM approaches was quantitatively evaluated by the ratio which was calculated by dividing the number of true positive voxels by the number of all the detected voxels with increasing t values. As the real data, the processed WM images were analyzed using two-sample t-test. The absolute threshold was set to 0.1. TIV, age and gender were incorporated in the design as nuisance covariates. The statistical parametric maps were thresholded at a p value of <0.05 by False Discovery Rate (FDR) to correct for multiple comparisons, and the extent threshold was set to 20.

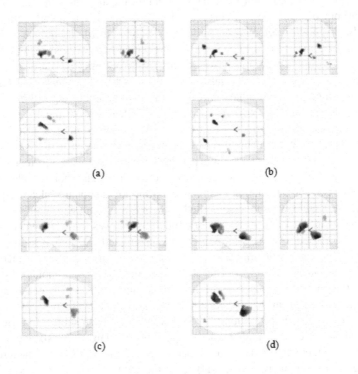

(a)   (b)

(c)   (d)

Fig. 2. Significant WM atrophies detected by (a) standard VBM, (b) optimized VBM (unmodulated), (c) optimized VBM (modulated), and (d) VBM-DARTEL using simulated data ($p < 0.05$, corrected for multiple comparisons using FDR, cluster size > 20 voxels)

3   Results

As the simulated data, significant WM atrophies detected by VBM approaches were shown in Fig. 2. We can see that all the VBM approaches have detected more or less degree of significant atrophies in the regions under the ground truth. With standard VBM (Fig. 2a), WM density changes were detected, but some false positive regions were also found. Using optimized VBM without modulation (Fig. 2b), less false positive regions were seen in the WM compared with standard VBM. For modulated data (Fig. 2c), the optimized VBM method examined more significant atrophies in WM, and fewer false positive regions were presented. With VBM-DARTEL (Fig. 2d), most true positive regions and least false positive regions displayed. The two regions with 5-mm radius were detected in each VBM method. However, the detected area of the region with 10% atrophy degree was smaller in each VBM approach except VBM-DARTEL. In addition, the atrophied region simulated with 2-mm radius and 25%-atrophy was only detected by VBM-DARTEL. Hence, a conclusion can be drawn that VBM-DARTEL is more robust and reliable than other VBM methods.

The ratio of the true positive voxels in the detected regions with increasing t values was calculated to quantitatively evaluate the performance of VBM approaches (Fig. 3). For the same t threshold, the higher the ratio is, the better the performance is. It is clear that with the t value increased, the ratio increased and reached 100% fastest with VBM-DARTEL method, indicating that VBM-DARTEL performed best. The order of the performance of these VBM approaches is: VBM-DARTEL > optimized VBM (modulated) > optimized VBM (unmodulated) > standard VBM.

As the real data, significantly reduced WM concentrations were detected by the standard VBM protocol in the left-TLE patients (Fig. 4 (a)) but not by the optimized VBM without modulation. For VBM-DARTEL and the optimized VBM with modulation, which contained a modulation step, WM volume reductions were found in the left-TLE patients (Fig. 4 (b), (c)). Fig. 4 shows that the locations of significant regions detected by standard VBM are more widely distributed. The distributions of significant atrophies detected by optimized VBM (modulation) and VBM-DARTEL were similar but obviously larger extents were found using VBM-DARTEL.

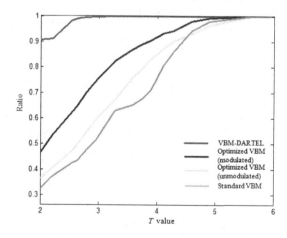

Fig. 3. The performance evaluated by the ratio of true positive voxels in the detected regions with increasing T values

Concluded from the simulation, VBM-DARTEL is more robust and reliable than other VBM approaches. Using VBM-DARTEL, the left-TLE patients showed WM volume decreases predominantly focused in the ipsilateral temporal lobe, the contralateral frontal and occipital lobes, the bilateral parietal lobes, cingulated gyrus, parahippocampal gyrus and brainstem (Table. 1). However, no significant WM concentration/volume reductions were examined in the right-TLE patients.

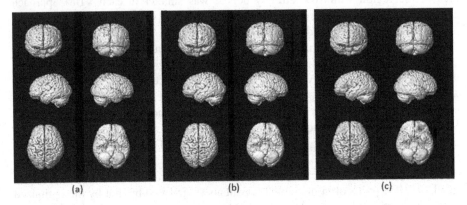

Fig. 4. Regions with significantly reduced white matter concentration/volume in the left-TLE patients ($p<0.05$, corrected for multiple comparisons using FDR) relative to controls by (a) standard VBM, (b) optimized VBM with modulation, and (c) VBM-DARTEL

Table 1. Significant reductions in white matter detected in the left-TLE patients versus controls by VBM-DARTEL ($p<0.05$, corrected for multiple comparisons using FDR, cluster size > 20)

Anatomical location	Side	Talairach coordinates			p(FDR-corr)	t	Cluster
		x(mm)	y(mm)	z(mm)			
Cingulate gyrus	L	0	-9	31	0.024	5.07	25173
		-12	-36	34	0.027	3.17	90
Superior temporal gyrus	L	-37	-1	-18	0.024	4.40	3911
ParaHippocampal gyrus	R	34	-8	-20	0.024	3.74	1482
Inferior frontal gyrus	R	45	17	13	0.025	3.38	113
Inferior parietal lobule	L	-49	-44	26	0.026	3.22	149
Middle occipital gyrus	R	34	-67	7	0.036	2.85	45
Precuneus	R	15	-47	49	0.037	2.83	32
Transverse temporal gyrus	L	-37	-33	14	0.038	2.80	28
Brainstem	R	10	-15	-3	0.039	2.79	54

4   Discussion and Conclusions

In the present study, the performance of various VBM approaches (standard VBM, optimized VBM and VBM-DARTEL) was first evaluated by simulation, concluding that VBM-DARTEL performed the best and the optimized VBM with modulation came second. In the left-TLE patients, WM reductions were found in the ipsilateral temporal lobe, the contralateral frontal and occipital lobes, the bilateral parietal lobes, cingulated gyrus, parahippocampal gyrus and brainstem by VBM-DARTEL. To the best of our knowledge, this is the first study to quantitatively evaluate VBM-DARTEL with standard and optimized VBM methods.

Previous studies [10] evaluated several registration approaches, concluding that DARTEL was a real improvement over the standard method. Keller et al. [8] revealed that the optimized VBM might detect more subtle neuroanatomical changes than standard VBM. In our study, VBM-DARTEL showed the best performance, next came the optimized VBM with modulation, which was a support to previous study.

There are many factors which may affect the results. First, voxels alignment is concernful in the preprocessing. Compared with other VBM methods, registration in DARTEL involves simultaneously minimizing the sum of squares difference between source and target images as well as the linear elastic energy of the deformations. While the normalization in SPM estimates nonlinear deformations by the linear combination of discrete cosine transformations, DARTEL provides high dimensional warping. Second, modulation is an important step in VBM. After nonlinear normalization, the volume of some regions may change. Modulation is the step to preserve the volume of a particular tissue within a voxel. With modulation, it is allowed to detect the volume changes. Third, template may also affect the results. In standard VBM, the template is ICBM 152 template. In optimized VBM, the template is generated by averaging the smoothed images from all subjects, which was matched with the study group. In DARTEL, the template is also created from all the subjects, but the procedure is iterative, which may improve the results. Many previous studies [8] have demonstrated the study-specific template might obtain more accurate results.

Some studies reported WM reductions of TLE patients in temporal lobe, frontal lobe and the corpus callosum [7]. Mueller et al. [8] found WM reductions in parietal lobe, parahippocampal gyrus and brainstem. Our results were consistent with these studies. Besides, our results from VBM-DARTEL showed more significant reductions in cingulated gyrus and occipital lobe, which was also detected in GM atrophy by Keller et al. [6]. Thus, our results have demonstrated the validity of VBM-DARTEL.

In our study, no significant WM atrophies were observed in the right-TLE patients. Coan et al. [13] reported that the atrophied progression was less intense in the right-TLE. Besides, less atrophies of hippocampus were observed in the right-TLE patients on MR images, suggesting that there might be less atrophy.

In the present study, some issues are still to be addressed. First, although VBM-DARTEL performed best among various VBM approaches, it has some disadvantages when compared with variable velocity models. The constant velocity vector field employed in DARTEL makes the model parameterization less suited to computational anatomy studies [3]. Second, the scanning parameters of simulated and real data were different, which might cause differences in the evaluation. However, the results from both simulated and real data revealed that VBM-DARTEL performs best, indicating VBM-DARTEL is appropriated to these two models.

The current study has some limitations. First, the images are resliced from $1\times1\times1$ mm^3 to $1.5\times1.5\times1.5$ mm^3 during the preprocessing step because of a memory problem in VBM-DARTEL. Thus, the atrophied size might be affected. Second, the TLE patient group was heterogeneous without subgroup stratification and no consideration of medication was included, which is to be considered in the future.

References

1. Ashburner, J., Friston, K.J.: Voxel-based morphometry-the methods. Neuroimage 11, 805–821 (2000)
2. Good, C.D., Johnsrude, I.S., et al.: A voxel-based morphometric study of ageing in 465 normal adult human brains. Neuroimage 14, 21–36 (2001)
3. Ashburner, J.: A fast diffeomorphic image registration algorithm. Neuroimage 38, 95–113 (2007)
4. Baron, J.C., Chetelat, G., et al.: In vivo mapping of gray matter loss with voxel-based morphometry in mild Alzheimer's disease. Neuroimage 14, 298–309 (2001)
5. Kubicki, M., Shenton, M.E., et al.: Voxel-based morphometric analysis of gray matter in first episode schizophrenia. Neuroimage 17, 1711–1719 (2002)
6. Keller, S.S., Mackay, C.E., et al.: Voxel-based morphometric comparison of hippocampal and extrahippocampal abnormalities in patients with left and right hippocampal atrophy. Neuroimage 16, 23–31 (2002)
7. Bernasconi, N., Duchesne, S., et al.: Whole-brain voxel-based statistical analysis of gray matter and white matter in temporal lobe epilepsy. Neuroimage 23, 717–723 (2004)
8. Keller, S.S., Wilke, M., et al.: Comparison of standard and optimized voxel-based morphometry for analysis of brain changes associated with temporal lobe epilepsy. Neuroimage 23, 860–868 (2004)
9. Bergouignan, L., Chupin, M., et al.: Can voxel based morphometry, manual segmentation and automated segmentation equally detect hippocampal volume differences in acute depression? Neuroimage 45, 29–37 (2009)
10. Yassa, M.A., Stark, C.E.L.: A quantitative evaluation of cross-participant registration techniques for MRI studies of the medial temporal lobe. Neuroimage 44, 319–327 (2009)
11. Karacali, B., Davatzikos, C.: Simulation of tissue atrophy using a topology preserving transformation model. IEEE Trans. Med. Imaging 25, 649–652 (2006)
12. Ashburner, J., Friston, K.J.: Unified segmentation. Neuroimage 26, 839–851 (2005)
13. Coan, A.C., Appenzeller, S., et al.: Seizure frequency and lateralization affect progression of atrophy in temporal lobe epilepsy. Neurology 73, 834–842 (2009)

Author Index